Register Now for Online Access to Your Book!

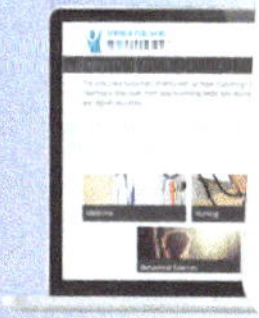

AF701009

Your print purchase of *Evidence-Based Physical Examination Handbook* **includes online access to the contents of your book**—increasing accessibility, portability, and searchability!

Access today at:

http://connect.springerpub.com/content/book/978-0-8261-6466-7

or scan the QR code at the right with your smartphone and enter the access code below.

76JH2GE0

Scan here for quick access.

If you are experiencing problems accessing the digital component of this product, please contact our customer service department at cs@springerpub.com

The online access with your print purchase is available at the publisher's discretion and may be removed at any time without notice.

Publisher's Note: New and used products purchased from third-party sellers are not guaranteed for quality, authenticity, or access to any included digital components.

Kate Sustersic Gawlik, DNP, APRN-CNP, FAANP, is an assistant professor of clinical nursing at The Ohio State University. She is certified by the American Nurses Credentialing Center as a family nurse practitioner. She has extensive background in primary care, with experience in family practice, college health, urgent care, and reproductive care. Her clinical interests are evidence-based practice, health professionals' education, population health, preventive care through lifestyle change, clinician well-being, wellness, and cardiovascular disease prevention. She currently serves as the director of Undergraduate Health and Wellness Academic Programming, codirector of the Health and Wellness in Healthcare program, and the project manager for the Million Hearts initiatives at Ohio State's College of Nursing. She has received multiple awards for her clinical practice and teaching including the 2018 American Association of Nurse Practitioner State Award for Excellence. She was inducted as a Fellow into the American Association of Nurse Practitioners in June 2018. She has taught undergraduate, RN-BSN, and graduate nursing students and has taught advanced health assessment for over 10 years.

Bernadette Mazurek Melnyk, PhD, APRN-CNP, EBP-C, FAANP, FNAP, FAAN, is the vice president for health promotion, university chief wellness officer, and professor and dean of the College of Nursing at The Ohio State University. She is also a professor of pediatrics and psychiatry at Ohio State's College of Medicine. In addition, she is the executive director of the Helene Fuld Health Trust National Institute for Evidence-Based Practice in Nursing and Healthcare. Dr. Melnyk is a nationally/internationally recognized expert in evidence-based practice, intervention research, child and adolescent mental health, health and wellness, and clinician well-being and is a frequent keynote speaker at national and international conferences. Dr. Melnyk has consulted with hundreds of healthcare systems and colleges throughout the nation and globe on how to improve quality of care and patient outcomes through implementing and sustaining evidence-based practice. Her record includes over $33 million of sponsored funding from federal agencies and foundations as principal investigator and over 430 publications along with seven books. Dr. Melnyk is an elected fellow of the National Academy of Medicine, the American Academy of Nursing, the National Academies of Practice, and the American Association of Nurse Practitioners. She currently serves as editor of *Worldviews on Evidence-Based Nursing* and is a member of the National Quality Forum's (NQF) Behavioral Health Standing Committee as well as the National Academy of Medicine's Action Collaborative on Clinician Well-Being and Resilience. In addition, she is the founder and current president of the National Consortium for Building Healthy Academic Communities and an elected board member of the National Forum for Heart Disease & Stroke Prevention.

Alice M. Teall, DNP, APRN-CNP, FAANP, is an assistant professor of clinical nursing at The Ohio State University. She was a founding member of the College of Nursing's team delivering distance education; while serving as director of the online Family Nurse Practitioner program, she was honored with the University Provost Award for Distinguished Teaching. She is currently director of Graduate Health and Wellness Academic Programming, and director of Telehealth Services. She has published and presented nationally about teaching telehealth competencies and wellness coaching. Dr. Teall has more than 35 years of experience in nursing, 25 years in nursing education, and 20 years in advanced nursing practice. An experienced educator, she has taught assessment online and on campus for students across nursing programs, including traditional undergraduate, RN-BSN completion, accelerated graduate entry, graduate, and doctoral programs. Dr. Teall has received leadership, alumni, and practice awards, and is a Fellow of the American Academy of Nurse Practitioners. As a certified nurse practitioner and an integrative nurse coach, her areas of clinical practice expertise include adolescent health, primary care of at-risk youth and families, college health, recovery from substance use disorder, and statewide quality improvement initiatives.

Evidence-Based Physical Examination HANDBOOK

Kate Sustersic Gawlik
DNP, APRN-CNP, FAANP

Bernadette Mazurek Melnyk
PhD, APRN-CNP, EBP-C, FAANP, FNAP, FAAN

Alice M. Teall
DNP, APRN-CNP, FAANP

Editors

SPRINGER PUBLISHING

Springer Publishing Company, LLC
11 West 42nd Street, New York, NY 10036
www.springerpub.com
connect.springerpub.com/

Acquisitions Editor: Adrianne Brigido
Compositor: S4Carlisle Publishing Services

ISBN: 978-0-8261-6465-0
ebook ISBN: 978-0-8261-6466-7
DOI: 10.1891/9780826164667

20 21 22 23 24 / 5 4 3 2 1

DISCLAIMER
The author and the publisher of this Work have made every effort to use sources believed to be reliable to provide information that is accurate and compatible with the standards generally accepted at the time of publication. Because medical science is continually advancing, our knowledge base continues to expand. Therefore, as new information becomes available, changes in procedures become necessary. We recommend that the reader always consult current research and specific institutional policies before performing any clinical procedure or delivering any medication. The author and publisher shall not be liable for any special, consequential, or exemplary damages resulting, in whole or in part, from the readers' use of, or reliance on, the information contained in this book. The publisher has no responsibility for the persistence or accuracy of URLs for external or third-party Internet websites referred to in this publication and does not guarantee that any content on such websites is, or will remain, accurate or appropriate.

Library of Congress Cataloging-in-Publication Data

Names: Gawlik, Kate, editor. | Melnyk, Bernadette Mazurek, editor. | Teall, Alice M., editor.
Title: Evidence-based physical examination handbook / Kate Sustersic Gawlik, Bernadette Mazurek Melnyk, Alice M. Teall.
Description: New York : Springer Publishing Company, [2022] | Includes bibliographical references and index.
Identifiers: LCCN 2020055312 (print) | LCCN 2020055313 (ebook) | ISBN 9780826164650 (cloth) | ISBN 9780826164667 (ebook)
Subjects: MESH: Physical Examination--methods | Evidence-Based Medicine | Handbook
Classification: LCC RC76 (print) | LCC RC76 (ebook) | NLM WB 39 | DDC 616.07/54--dc23
LC record available at https://lccn.loc.gov/2020055312
LC ebook record available at https://lccn.loc.gov/2020055313

Contact sales@springerpub.com to receive discount rates on bulk purchases.

***Publisher's Note*: New and used products purchased from third-party sellers are not guaranteed for quality, authenticity, or access to any included digital components.**

Printed in the United States of America.

To all of the health science students and practicing clinicians who need a little handbook to study, refresh, and renew their skills, thank you for demonstrating a willingness to learn and for your dedication to providing the best, evidence based, patient-centered care for individuals, families, communities, and populations. You make us proud.

Contents

Abbreviations Inside front and back covers
Contributors xi
Preface xix

1. Evidence-Based History-Taking Approach 1
2. Approach to General Survey and Developmental Assessment 13
3. Heart and Circulatory System 45
4. Evidence-Based Assessment of Lungs and Respiratory System 79
5. Evidence-Based Assessment of Skin, Hair, and Nails 101
6. Evidence-Based Assessment of the Lymphatic System 133
7. Evidence-Based Assessment of Head and Neck 147
8. Evidence-Based Assessment of the Eye 163
9. Evidence-Based Assessment of Ears, Nose, and Throat 189
10. Evidence-Based Assessment of Nervous System 217

11. Evidence-Based Assessment of the Musculoskeletal System 249

12. Evidence-Based Assessment of the Abdomen and Gastrointestinal and Urological Systems 287

13. Evidence-Based Assessment of Male Genitalia, Prostate, Rectum, and Anus 319

14. Evidence-Based Assessment of Breasts, Female Genitalia, and Reproductive System 343

15. Evidence-Based Obstetric Assessment 381

16. Evidence-Based Assessment of Mental Health and Substance Use 403

Index 435

Contributors

Melissa Baker, DNP, RN
Director for Prelicensure Programs
College of Nursing
The Ohio State University
Columbus, Ohio

Angela Blankenship, MS, RN, CPNP-AC/PC
APRN Clinical Leader
The Heart Center
Nationwide Children's Hospital College of Nursing
The Ohio State University
Columbus, Ohio

Sherry Bumpus, PhD, FNP-BC, CME
Associate Professor
College of Nursing
Michigan State University
East Lansing, Michigan

Amber Carriveau, DNP, FNP-BC
Assistant Professor
Family Nurse Practitioner Program Director
Michigan State University
East Lansing, Michigan

Kelly Casler, DNP, APRN, FNP-BC, EBP-C
Assistant Professor of Clinical Practice
College of Nursing
The Ohio State University
Columbus, Ohio

Maria Colandrea, DNP, NP-C, CORLN, CCRN, FAANP
Clinical Consulting Associate
Department of Otolaryngology
Duke School of Nursing
Durham VA Medical Center
Durham, North Carolina

Sandy Dudley, MS, BBA, PA-C
Instructor
Digestive Health Institute and Section of Pediatric Gastroenterology, Hepatology and Nutrition School of Medicine
University of Colorado
Aurora, Colorado

Kristie L. Flamm, DNP, FNP-BC, ACNP-BC, FAANP
Clinical Assistant Professor
College of Nursing
University of Arizona
Tucson, Arizona

Kate Sustersic Gawlik, DNP, APRN-CNP, FAANP
Assistant Professor of Clinical Nursing
College of Nursing
The Ohio State University
Columbus, Ohio

Retha D. Gentry, DNP, FNP-C
Assistant Professor
Graduate Programs College of Nursing
East Tennessee State University
Johnson City, Tennessee

Brenda M. Gilmore, DNP, CNM, FNP-BC, CNE, NCMP
Assistant Professor
College of Nursing
University of South Florida
Tampa, Florida

Matt Granger, APRN-CNP
Family Nurse Practitioner
Wexner Medical Center
Ross Heart Hospital
The Ohio State University
Columbus, Ohio

Emily Hill Guseman, PhD, ACSM-CEP
Assistant Professor
Diabetes Institute
Department of Family Medicine
Heritage College of Osteopathic Medicine
Ohio University
Athens, Ohio

Audra Hanners, DNP, RN, APRN-CNP, EBP-C
Instructor of Clinical Practice
College of Nursing
The Ohio State University
Columbus, Ohio

Brittany B. Hay, DNP, APRN, ANP-BC, FNP-BC
Assistant Professor
College of Nursing
University of South Florida
Tampa, Florida

Joyce Karl, DNP, RN, APRN-CNP
Assistant Professor of Clinical Nursing
College of Nursing
The Ohio State University
Columbus, Ohio

Jennifer Kosla, DNP, APRN-CNP, CPNP-PC, CNE
Assistant Professor of Clinical Practice
College of Nursing
The Ohio State University
Columbus, Ohio

Pamela Lusk, DNP, RN, FAANP, FNAP
Associate Professor of Clinical Practice
College of Nursing
The Ohio State University
Columbus, Ohio

Kady Martini, DNP, RN, NEA-BC
Assistant Professor of Clinical Practice
College of Nursing
The Ohio State University
Columbus, Ohio

Bernadette Mazurek Melnyk, PhD, APRN-CNP, EBP-C, FAANP, FNAP, FAAN
Dean and Professor
College of Nursing
The Ohio State University
Columbus, Ohio

Molly McAuley, DNP, CNL, RN
Assistant Professor of Clinical Practice
College of Nursing
The Ohio State University
Columbus, Ohio

Rosario Medina, PhD, FNP-BC, ACNP, CNS
Assistant Dean of Graduate Programs
College of Nursing
University of Colorado
Aurora, Colorado

John Melnyk, PhD, OD
Clinical Assistant Professor
Department of Ophthalmology
Wexner Medical Center
Dublin, Ohio

Mary Alice Momeyer, DNP, APRN, CNP, AGPCNP-BC
Assistant Professor of Clinical Nursing
College of Nursing
The Ohio State University
Columbus, Ohio

Hollie Moots, DNP, RN, CNE
Assistant Professor of Clinical Practice
College of Nursing
The Ohio State University
Columbus, Ohio

Emily Neiman, MS, ARPN-CNM, C-EFM
Certified Nurse Midwife
Wexner Medical Center
The Ohio State University
Columbus, Ohio

Lisa E. Ousley, DNP, FNP-C

Assistant Professor Graduate Programs
College of Nursing
East Tennessee State University
Johnson City, Tennessee

Vinciya Pandian, PhD, MBA, MSN, RN, ACNP-BC, FAAN, FAANP

Associate Professor
School of Nursing
Johns Hopkins University
Baltimore, Maryland

Oralea A. Pittman, DNP, APRN-CNP, FAANP

Assistant Professor of Clinical Nursing
College of Nursing
The Ohio State University
Columbus, Ohio

Linda Quinlin, DNP, RN, APRN-CNS, APRN-CNP, ACHPN

Assistant Professor of Clinical Nursing
College of Nursing
The Ohio State University
Columbus, Ohio

Eileen M. Raynor, MD, FACS, FAAP

Associate Professor Pediatric Otolaryngology
Duke Head and Neck Surgery & Communication Sciences
Duke University School of Medicine
Durham, North Carolina

Kerry Z. Reed, MS, RN, CPNP-PC

Senior Instructor
Digestive Health Institute and Section of Pediatric Gastroenterology, Hepatology and Nutrition
School of Medicine
University of Colorado Children's Hospital
Colorado Anschutz Medical Campus
Aurora, Colorado

Britta Shute, MSN, APRN, FNP-BC
Family Nurse Practitioner
UCONN Health
Farmington, Connecticut

Leslie E. Simons, DNP, ANP-BC
Certified Pain Management Nurse Assistant Professor Health Programs
College of Nursing
Michigan State University
East Lansing, Michigan

Leigh Small, PhD, RN, CPNP-PC, FNAP, FAANP, FAAN
Associate Dean of Academic Programs
College of Nursing
University of Colorado
Aurora, Colorado

Tammy Spencer, DNP, RN, CNE, ACNS-BC, CCNS
Assistant Dean of Academic Programs
College of Nursing
University of Colorado
Aurora, Colorado

Zach Stutzman, MS, PA-C, ATC
Physician Assistant
Total Joint Replacement
Sports & Orthopaedic Specialists
Minneapolis, Minnesota

Alice M. Teall, DNP, APRN-CNP, FAANP
Assistant Professor of Clinical Nursing
College of Nursing
The Ohio State University
Columbus, Ohio

Kathryn Tierney, MSN, APRN, FNP-BC
Family Nurse Practitioner
Middlesex Health
Middletown, Connecticut

Sinead Yarberry, MSN, RN, CNS
Instructor of Clinical Practice
College of Nursing
The Ohio State University
Columbus, Ohio

Rosie Zeno, DNP, APRN-CNP, CPNP-PC
Assistant Professor of Clinical Nursing
College of Nursing
The Ohio State University
Columbus, Ohio

Preface

I have no special talent. I am only passionately curious.

—Albert Einstein

Evidence-Based Physical Examination Handbook was developed as a guide to the strategies and best practices needed by clinicians to assess an individual's health and well-being. This handbook is intended to be used by a broad audience of health science students and clinicians across disciplines who strive to exemplify excellence in evidence-based assessment and practice.

The overall goal of the handbook is to provide a practical, scientific, and holistic approach to assessment, in a summarized format that provides ease of access to students and clinicians while in lab and clinical settings. Additional goals of this text include:

1. To promote evidence-based assessment to ensure that clinicians are using valid and reliable examination methods in which to base future decision-making.
2. To incorporate physical and mental dimensions of wellness, social determinants of health, prevention, and self-care needs into assessment in a manner that respects an individual's personal perspectives, family, and community.
3. To provide information on specific assessment skills that are often overlooked or misunderstood.
4. To summarize abnormal subjective (history) and objective (physical exam) findings for common disease states across the life span.
5. To ensure that clinicians are able to conduct a self-assessment of their own personal health and wellness.

Learning to effectively assess the health and well-being of an individual involves integrating skills of history taking, physical examination, and diagnostic decision-making within the context of patient-centered, culturally sensitive, evidence-based clinical practice.

Each chapter of *Evidence-Based Physical Examination Handbook* begins with priority clinical considerations. The first two chapters review evidence-based approaches to assessment—the importance of history taking and the approach to general survey. Chapters 3 to 11 review assessment priorities and common diagnoses relative to specific body systems. Chapters 12 to 15 focus on assessments related to sexual and reproductive health and obstetric assessment. Chapter 16 focuses on mental status and mental health. All chapters include life-span considerations pertinent to pediatric, adolescent, adult, and older adult populations.

Evidence-Based Physical Examination Handbook incorporates a broad understanding of wellness, presents evidence-based recommendations for history taking, reviews the physical examination components required to inform clinical decision-making, and lists the findings that are generally associated with differential diagnoses. Only with evidence-based assessment can a clinician ensure patient safety and high-quality, cost-effective care. The valid, reliable assessment techniques and approaches in this text are intended to prepare clinicians to deliver evidence-based, safe, quality clinical care.

Kate Sustersic Gawlik
Bernadette Mazurek Melnyk
Alice M. Teall

1

Evidence-Based History-Taking Approach

CLINICAL CONSIDERATIONS

- Individuals seek visits with clinicians primarily for three reasons: to address episodic concerns, for wellness exams, and to manage chronic illnesses. At all of these visits, clinicians assess a patient's history and obtain subjective information.
- A thorough patient history consists of the chief concern or reason for seeking care; history of present illness; past health history, including medication and allergy history, family history, social history, and review of systems.
- Although objective assessments can be made during history taking, data gathered is primarily subjective (i.e., information reported, experienced, or understood by the patient).
- Listening and responding empathetically to an individual's history serves to establish a therapeutic partnership, improves patient and clinician satisfaction, and results in improved health outcomes. Active listening requires the clinician to eliminate distractions and focus on an individual's verbal and nonverbal responses.

HISTORY TAKING FOR AN EPISODIC VISIT

- The episodic visit, scheduled for a recent, bothersome, or acute health problem, accounts for the majority of clinician visits.
- Episodic visits focus on a specific concern voiced by the patient. The patient can be either an established patient or a new patient.
- For an episodic visit, the extent of the history collected is variable and based on the clinician's judgment and the patient's presenting symptoms. For new patients, a comprehensive health history should be conducted. For established patients,

a more limited health history is collected, tailored to the chief concern.

- The following sections provide the general framework for the elements of history taking during an episodic visit. To begin the visit, the clinician introduces themselves and washes their hands.

CHIEF CONCERN OR REASON FOR SEEKING CARE

- History taking begins with clarifying the patient's main reason for the visit. Clarifying an individual's CC is a priority.
- The CC is the description of the symptom, problem, condition, diagnosis, or reason for seeking care. Often, documentation of the CC is in the patient's own words—for example, "my left elbow hurts."

HISTORY OF PRESENT ILLNESS

- The HPI provides key information required for developing differential diagnoses, determining a diagnosis, and guiding treatment. Often a diagnosis can be made from the history alone, so this step is crucial.
- In the HPI, the patient provides detailed reasons for the visit, and describes how the illness has progressed. Allow the patient to tell the story in their own words about their concerns, including their perception of the illness or health problem. The history of the present illness contains eight core elements to assess, summarized with the mnemonic OLDCARTS:
    - **Onset:** When did symptoms start? Are symptoms recent? How did symptoms begin?
    - **Location:** Specific location of symptoms?
    - **Duration:** Are symptoms persistent or transitory? Increasing or unchanged?
    - **Characteristics:** How would you describe the symptoms? Is there itching, burning, drainage, pain, swelling, bruising, or redness? How does the symptom feel (e.g., sharp, dull, stabbing, burning, crushing, throbbing, nauseating, shooting, twisting, or stretching)?
    - **Aggravating factors:** What actions or activities may have precipitated the symptoms, or caused the symptoms to worsen?
    - **Relieving factors:** What actions or activities decrease the symptoms? What medications has the individual taken to help with the symptoms? (Note that treatment may be listed as a distinct component of the HPI.)
    - **Temporal factors/timing:** How do symptoms respond to treatment, relieving factors, situations, or conditions? Are symptoms constant?

- **Severity:** How severe are the symptoms on a scale of 0 to 10? Do symptoms limit participation in activities at school/work/home?

PAST MEDICAL HISTORY

- Also referred to as *history of illness, health history,* or *past medical and surgical history,* the assessment of past medical history is important to obtain and review during all visits; even when established patients follow up with clinicians, their health history should be updated.
- Assessment includes asking the patient about experiences with illnesses both acute and chronic (may include pertinent childhood illnesses), hospitalizations, surgeries, sexual/reproductive health issues, and hereditary conditions that could place the patient at risk.
- When asking health history questions, review all current medications, prescribed, OTC, and/or herbal; when an individual shares history of allergies, ask specifics about their reaction to the allergens.
- Components of past medical history:
  - **History of physical or mental health conditions:** Ask whether ever diagnosed with specific conditions (e.g., heart disease, elevated blood pressure, cancer, diabetes, depression, arthritis, asthma); clarify whether conditions are current or past health problems.
  - **History of hospitalizations and surgeries:** Clarify reason and dates
  - Recent illness, accidents, injuries, or exposures
  - History of emergency department or urgent care visits
  - Immunization status, record of vaccines
  - **Gender identity and sexual orientation with age-appropriate considerations:** Women's health history (menstrual, gynecological, obstetric, sexual health), men's health history (sexual and reproductive health), pediatric health history (birth history, growth, development)
- **Medications:** Prescribed and OTC medications and supplements, including dose and frequency
- **Allergies:** To medications or seasonal, environmental, and/or food allergies, including reaction

FAMILY HISTORY

- Review of the immediate family members' history related to medical events, illnesses, and hereditary conditions that place the patient's current and future health at risk.

- Immediate family includes parents, grandparents, siblings, children, and grandchildren.
- As details are provided during the family history, inquire whether the relative is alive or deceased. If the person is deceased, ask about the age at death and the cause of death, especially for first-degree relatives.
- Assess family history for:
    - **Chronic diseases:** Hypertension, heart disease, obesity, diabetes, cancer, epilepsy, and asthma
    - **Acute or recent episodic illnesses:** Infectious diseases, allergies, environmental exposures
    - **Mental health disorders:** Anxiety, depression, bipolar disorder, or severe, persistent mental illness; substance use disorder, alcoholism, addiction
    - Intellectual disabilities, learning disorders, developmental delays
    - Genetic or hereditary conditions
- Family history provides valuable insight into health risks and supports recommendations for screening and/or referral for genetic counseling. Genetic conditions can be inherited in a variety of patterns, depending on the gene involved (e.g., autosomal dominant, autosomal recessive, X-linked dominant, X-linked recessive, Y-linked, codominant, mitochondrial, and polygenic). If any red flags are present (**Box 1.1**), referral to genetic counseling is necessary.

BOX 1.1 Red Flags in Subjective History That Indicate a Need for Genetic Counseling

- Significant family medical history—breast, ovarian, prostate, colon, melanoma, pancreatic, or other cancers
- Cancer occurs in every generation
- Early age of onset (<50 years)
- Condition in the less-often-affected gender (e.g., male breast cancer)
- Bilateral cancer, or multiple primary cancers in one individual
- Known family genetic mutation
- Ethnicity predisposition to certain genetic disorders (e.g., Ashkenazi Jewish ancestry)
- Consanguinity

SOCIAL HISTORY

- Provides information regarding one's health beliefs and behaviors, including support systems; it also allows a clinician to identify risk factors that may impact well-being. Note that the influence of culture on health beliefs, behaviors, practices, perceptions, and approaches is vast; this component of history requires a sensitive and humble approach that respects cultural, family, community, and personal values and norms. Components of social history:
    - Substance use history:
        - Tobacco use in any form (pipe, snuff, chewing tobacco, e-cigarettes, hookah, vaping, cigars, cigarettes)? If yes, assess smoking history, readiness to quit.
        - Alcohol use? If yes, screen for binge drinking, problematic use.
        - Other substances (e.g., medications not prescribed, illicit drugs)?
            - Ask whether has ever taken medications not specifically prescribed for them.
            - Ask whether has ever taken substance for how it would make them feel.
    - Relationships, including marital status; living arrangements:
        - Family dynamics
        - Friends and social support system
        - Strengths, including spiritual, religious, and ethnic/cultural support systems
        - History of trauma, victim of violence, and adverse childhood events
    - Safety of home, work, and/or school environments:
        - Exposure to hazards (e.g., fumes, radiation, chemicals, viruses)
        - Risk or current exposure to violence, trauma, stressors
        - Behaviors involving risk-taking, risk of falls
        - Safe participation in sports and physical activities
        - Screen for use of seat belts, bicycle/motorcycle helmets
        - Screen for smoke detectors in home
        - Screen for access to guns in home, neighborhood, and at work
        - Assess social determinants of health

Social Determinants of Health

Asking about the environments in which an individual resides, works, learns, plays, worships, and connects socially offers important insight into the determinants of their health. Key areas to consider related to the determinants that impact an individual's health:

- **Economic stability:** Access to employment and job training; access to resources to meet daily needs, including food
- **Physical environment:** Access to safe, affordable housing; public safety; exposure to violence, toxic substances, or physical hazards
- **Healthcare system:** Availability of evidence-based healthcare services; access to clinicians with linguistic and cultural competency; access to insurance coverage, and care meeting health literacy needs
- **Social context:** Availability of recreational and leisure-time activities; socioeconomic conditions; cohesion and social support; experiences of discrimination, isolation, bias
- **Education:** Access to quality education, including early childhood education; access to internet, smartphones, and emerging technologies

PREVENTIVE CARE CONSIDERATIONS

Assess an individual's participation in behaviors to prevent disease and illness:

- Healthy lifestyle behaviors, including diet/nutrition, physical activity/exercise, and sleep
- Management of stress, coping with stressors
- Recent/needed health screenings (e.g., blood pressure, anxiety, depression, mammogram, colonoscopy, cholesterol, lead, STIs, and vision/hearing)

REVIEW OF SYSTEMS

- Inventory of symptoms that is obtained by a series of questions that are organized by body systems.
- Offers essential information about current/potential disease processes or health problems that may otherwise go unnoticed.
- Includes pertinent positive and negative findings. Important: The ROS is subjective information provided by the patient, and not the clinician's observation or findings.
- Clinicians choose the depth of the ROS based on the acuity of the individual who is presenting to them, whether the patient is established or new, and according to the level of diagnostic decision-making that is required during a visit. The ROS can be focused, extended, or complete. Example ROS history questions:
    - **General or constitutional:** Recent illness? Weight gain or loss? Fatigue? Changes in sleep pattern? Night sweats? Fever? Frequent infections?

- **Integumentary:** Lesions or rashes? Changes in skin, hair, nails? Itching? Eczema?
- **Head, neck:** Headache? Neck pain? Dizziness? Pain related to head injury?
- **Lymphatic/hematologic:** Swollen or tender lymph nodes? Abnormal bleeding? Bruising?
- **EENT:** Eye drainage or redness? Vision changes? Itchy eyes/ears/nose? Ear pain? Hearing loss? Rhinorrhea or congestion? Sore throat? Trouble chewing or swallowing? Bleeding gums? Dental pain?
- **CV:** Chest pain? Palpitations? Exercise intolerance? Orthopnea? Edema?
- **Respiratory:** Cough? Dyspnea or shortness of breath? Wheezing? Hemoptysis?
- **Breast:** Tenderness? Palpable lumps or masses? Skin changes or discharge?
- **GI:** Pain? Change in bowel habits? Blood in the stool? Nausea? Vomiting? Heartburn? Change in appetite?
- **GU:** Urinary frequency? Pain with urination? Nocturia? Urgency? Hematuria? Unusual discharge or odor? Pelvic or groin pain? Dyspareunia?
- **MSK:** Back pain? Muscle aches? Joint swelling? Limitations of function?
- **Neurologic:** Numbness or tingling? Syncope? Memory loss? Restlessness? Changing level of consciousness? Loss of coordination? Tremors?
- **Endocrine:** Increased thirst? Heat or cold intolerance?
- **Psychiatric/mental health:** Worry? Sadness, helplessness, hopelessness? Insomnia? Change in mood? Irritability? Difficulty coping with stress? Trouble concentrating?

HISTORY TAKING FOR A WELLNESS EXAM

KEY CONSIDERATIONS

- Wellness exams can be an important health promotion and disease prevention strategy; goals include early identification of health risks, and/or detection of health problems at an early stage when treatment is most likely to be effective.
- Sports physicals, well-child exams, work physicals, and annual exams are examples of wellness exams; these clinician visits require age- and gender- appropriate history and physical exam.
- Because the patient history taking during wellness exams is not problem oriented, the history will not include a chief concern,

although the reason for the visit can be listed. In addition, there is not likely to be a need to collect HPI. Rather, a wellness exam should include a comprehensive history and physical examination appropriate to the patient's age and gender, counseling and anticipatory guidance, risk reduction interventions, the ordering or administration of vaccine-appropriate immunizations, and the ordering of appropriate laboratory and/or diagnostic testing.

- The wellness exam differs from the episodic visit and chronic care management visit because the components of the wellness exam are based on age and risk factors, not a presenting problem.

COMPONENTS OF WELLNESS EXAMS

- Comprehensive, culturally sensitive history and physical examination
- For infants and children, include assessment of growth and development
- Anticipatory guidance regarding risks to health and well-being
- Recommendations for immunizations, screenings, diagnostic testing
- Anticipatory guidance and support regarding reaching health and wellness goals

HISTORY TAKING AND CHRONIC CARE MANAGEMENT

KEY CONSIDERATIONS FOR CHRONIC CARE MANAGEMENT VISITS

- More than half of all adults in the United States have a chronic condition; chronic diseases are among the leading causes of death and disability.
- Common chronic diseases include heart disease, cancer, chronic lung disease, stroke, Alzheimer's disease, diabetes, chronic kidney disease.
- Health behaviors play an important role in the risk for chronic disease. Tobacco use and exposure to secondhand smoke, poor nutrition, lack of physical activity, and excessive alcohol use have been found to be key contributors to increasing a patient's risk of acquiring a chronic disease.
- Chronic conditions place patients at risk for adverse health events. Managing conditions effectively requires face-to-face visits along with non–face-to-face visits.
- The focus of chronic care management is the patient's relationship with the healthcare team (not just the clinician); establishing

and achieving individual health goals; coordination of community and social services; medical, functional, and psychosocial assessment; and preventive care.

- History taking during a chronic care management visit includes all of the components of an episodic visit, in addition to assessing and prioritizing the patient's ability to manage their chronic illness. Assessment priorities for chronic care management include:
    - Functional and psychosocial assessment, with disease-specific concerns
    - Assessment of wellness, dimensions of wellness, and healthy lifestyle behaviors
    - Individual health goals; motivation and readiness, confidence, and self-efficacy
    - Problem list, treatment goals, expected outcomes, and collaborative management
    - Self-management support; options for coaching, team-based care, and group visits

HISTORY CONSIDERATIONS FOR OLDER ADULTS WITH CHRONIC CONDITIONS

- Older adults have unique history considerations. Multiple comorbidities are often present, which require clinicians to assess and manage multiple medications and complex care needs.
- Age-appropriate screenings should be conducted to review a patient's functional ability and level of safety. The use of appropriate screening questions or standardized questionnaires to assess medication appropriateness, ADL, fall risk, hearing impairment, and home safety should be used for older adult populations.
- Evidence-based screening tools include:
    - American Geriatrics Society Beers Criteria® for Potentially Inappropriate Medication Use in Older Adults: https://qioprogram.org/sites/default/files/2019BeersCriteria_JAGS.pdf
    - Home Fall Prevention Checklist for Older Adults: www.cdc.gov/steadi/pdf/check_for_safety_brochure-a.pdf
    - Katz Index of Independence in Activities of Daily Living: www.alz.org/careplanning/downloads/katz-adl.pdf
- Changes in an older adult's functional assessment can be a first indicator of a mental/physical decline. Identifying functional decline early can trigger interventions that will maximize the person's independence and safety. Completing a functional screening will help the clinician establish a realistic and patient-focused treatment plan.

- Age-appropriate screenings to assess a patient's cognitive function should be conducted initially by direct observation, in addition to considering information reported by the patient, and concerns raised by family members, friends, caregivers, and others. If it is determined that additional screening is warranted, use validated structured cognitive assessment tools to further assess the patient's cognitive function. A thorough history includes assessment for depression in older adults. See Chapter 16 for evidence-based assessment of mental health.
- A discussion on advance directives should be conducted with age-appropriate patients. Advance directives assist individuals with end-of-life planning, include discussion about future care decisions that may be needed, and allow for identification of a healthcare decision-maker. Advance directives allow older adults to share their healthcare preferences in the event that they are unable to make their own healthcare decisions.

THERAPEUTIC COMMUNICATION

- Regardless of the type of patient visit, the goal during the history taking is to be attentive to the patient and receptive to the individual's needs.
- Conducting the patient history requires patient-centered interviewing skills, which includes skillful use of therapeutic communication. Therapeutic communication techniques include:
  - **Open-ended questions:** The use of open-ended questions allows the patient to express their concerns. Example: *You've reported you have shortness of breath; can you tell me more about that?*
  - **Active listening:** Providing an opportunity for an individual to share their history and concerns without interruption and with full engagement communicates nonverbally that what is being said is being heard. Example: The clinician nods their head and maintains eye contact while the patient is sharing the reason that they made the visit.
  - **Reflection:** The use of reflection demonstrates active listening and acknowledges the patient's response. Example: *I can see the news has been upsetting to you.*
  - **Empathy:** The patient's emotions are central to effective decision-making. Affirming the patient's emotions demonstrates that the clinician appreciates how the patient is feeling. Example: *You are experiencing lots of changes in your health; it's understandable that this would be difficult to accept right now.*

- **Seeking clarification:** Asking follow-up questions to history statements is helpful in obtaining an accurate history and with establishing trust with the patient. Example: *You said that you were unable to quit smoking; tell me more about that.*
- **Summary or restatement:** Summarizing patient statement to demonstrate an understanding of a patient's values and preferences allows the clinician to develop a partnership with the individual. Example: *I hear you say that you value your time with your family, and your preference is to receive treatment for your breast cancer.*

- In each chapter of this text, history questions specific to each system are listed; many are specific to the patient's CC. The questions are intended to be asked in a confidential, sensitive manner and will reveal the patient's perspectives about health, wellness, and illness. As each chapter is reviewed, remember to spend time in self-reflection and consider how to sensitively ask and respond to patient assessments. Implementing evidence-based, patient-centered assessment requires sensitivity and openness to the patient's responses as specific details of their history and perspectives are shared.

REFERENCES

References for this chapter draw from Chapter 2, "Evidence-Based History-Taking Approach for Wellness Exams, Episodic Visits, and Chronic Care Management," and Chapter 3, "Approach to Implementing and Documenting Patient-Centered, Culturally Sensitive Evidence-Based Assessment," of the textbook *Evidence-Based Physical Examination: Best Practices for Health and Well-Being Assessment*. The references may be accessed in the digital version of the handbook at connect.springerpub.com/content/book/https://connect.springerpub.com/content/book/978-0-8261-6466-7/chapter/ch01

2

Approach to General Survey and Developmental Assessment

CLINICAL CONSIDERATIONS

- Evidence-based assessment begins with observation. Skilled, systematic observation is essential for accurate clinical evaluation.
- Initial general survey includes assessing for problems, instability, or alterations in airway, breathing, circulation, and neurologic status, which involves exposing an individual as needed in order to complete the exam safely and effectively.
- Assessments of mental and physical status include an evaluation of pain and measurements of vital signs and body habitus.
- For some individuals, especially children, obtaining vital signs can precipitate anxiety. Be sure to take time to answer questions and alleviate concerns before beginning these assessments as anxiety can increase a patient's pulse rate, respiratory rate, and blood pressure.
- Surveillance of growth and development in children is key to recognizing those who may be at risk for developmental delays or mental health/behavioral disorders.

SUBJECTIVE HISTORY

COMMON REASONS FOR SEEKING CARE

- Routine wellness exam, including routine pediatric wellness and follow-up exams
- Urgent or emergent problems noted during general survey:
  - Syncope, loss of consciousness
  - Choking, wheezing, respiratory distress, hypoxia, tachypnea
  - Chest pain, dizziness, hypertension, hypotension, bradycardia, tachycardia
  - Pulselessness

- Diaphoresis, cyanosis
- Fever
- Pain: Acute, recurrent, episodic, or chronic
- Underweight, overweight, obesity, weight gain, weight loss, malnutrition
- Inattention, impulsivity, distraction, anxiety
- Confusion, disorientation, depressed mood

INITIAL STEPS TO DETERMINE PHYSIOLOGIC STABILITY

- The initial assessments of a general survey are completed to determine whether the individual being evaluated is in distress. Observing whether a patient is well or unwell is essential and can be completed quickly.
- Use the ABCDE mnemonic to determine whether an individual has physiologic stability—airway, breathing, circulation, disability, exposure. Note that each of these assessments is vital, with "C" being given the highest priority in adults.
- **Box 2.1** lists the red flags (signs and symptoms) of emergent or urgent medical problems.
- For the patient who is physiologically unstable, experiencing emergent distress, and is unconscious, unresponsive, or not breathing normally, the clinician should respond to the situation appropriately, which may require initiating CPR while continuing to assess.
- For the patient who is physiologically and functionally stable, the clinician's next steps include completing the history and physical exam.
- This chapter includes a significant review of vital signs, pain, body habitus, and developmental level (for children), which are key assessments in determining patient stability and function. Subsequent chapters will review additional priority assessments, including signs and symptoms of respiratory distress, hypoxia, heart failure, and neurologic disorders.
- Completing the initial general survey allows the clinician to determine an appropriate, subsequent history and physical exam.

History of Present Illness

- **Onset:** When did the symptoms start? Did they occur suddenly, or have they been developing gradually? When did the patient or the caregiver first notice this problem?
- **Location:** Does the individual have pain or discomfort? If so, where is the discomfort located? Multiple sites?

BOX 2.1 Red Flags in Initial General Survey That May Indicate Physiologic Instability (Emergent Distress)

- *Airway:* Paradoxical chest and abdominal movements with respirations, cyanosis, diminished breath sounds, noisy breath sounds, wheezing, and stridor
- *Breathing:* Wheezing, stridor, cyanosis, dyspnea, hypoxia, retractions, inability to speak in full sentences, apnea
- *Circulation:* Chest pain, dyspnea, bleeding, decreased perfusion, tachycardia, bradycardia, pulselessness
- *Disability:* Confusion, irritability, vomiting, seizure, loss of consciousness, non-responsiveness, sudden change in neurologic status
- *Exposure:* Trauma that may have caused functional instability; panic, feelings of impending doom, restlessness

- **Duration:** How long do the symptoms last? Are symptoms worsening? Persistent?
- **Characteristics:** Describe the symptoms being experienced.
- **Aggravating factors:** What actions, activities, exposures, or positions make the symptoms worse? Is the problem associated with a particular activity, food, or place? Additional temporal factors, such as recent illness, infection, travel?
- **Relieving factors:** What actions decrease symptoms? If relieved, how long does the relief last?
- **Treatment:** What medications have been taken to help with the symptoms? Clarify dosage and frequency of any medications.
- **Severity:** How severe are the symptoms on a scale of 0 to 10? Do the symptoms limit participation in activities, interrupt sleep, impact work or school attendance? Are there associated symptoms? Is the individual feeling anxious or fearful?

HEALTH HISTORY

Past Medical History

- Chronic illnesses (physical, mental/behavioral)
- Recent injury, trauma; emergency department or urgent care visits
- Hospitalizations, surgeries

- **Birth history, especially for children under 2 years of age**: Prenatal care, maternal health during pregnancy; labor and delivery complications, type of delivery; newborn hospital stay, including complications or support needed; newborn screening results, including hearing screen

MEDICATIONS

Prescribed and OTC medications or supplements, including dose and frequency

Allergies

Allergies to medications or seasonal, environmental, and/or food allergies. If "yes," clarify reaction.

Preventive Health Behaviors

- Physical activity and exercise
- Typical diet; access to fruits and vegetables; food handling and cooking
- Adequate sleep and rest
- Stress reduction/coping strategies
- Vaccine history

FAMILY HISTORY

- **Chronic illnesses**: Cardiac disease, hypertension, obesity, diabetes, cancer, epilepsy, asthma, bleeding disorders
- Intellectual disabilities, learning disorders, genetic disorders, developmental delays
- **Mental health disorders**: Anxiety, depression, bipolar disorder, ADHD, disorder, schizophrenia
- Trauma, physical or sexual abuse, neglect
- Infectious diseases or immune disorders

SOCIAL HISTORY

- Home situation and relationships:
  - Married/single/divorced/widowed/partnered?
  - Who lives in the home? Composition of family? Caregivers?
  - Substance use in the home?
  - Is housing /home/neighborhood safe?
  - Social support system? Close friends? Pets?

  - Sexual history (including risk factors for sexually transmitted illnesses)
- Substance use:
  - Smoking/vaping history/history of tobacco use/exposure to secondhand smoke?
  - Alcohol use?
  - Other substances (e.g., medications not prescribed, illicit drugs)?
- Safety (including work or school environment):
  - Trauma history, including adverse childhood events, bereavement, grief, isolation
  - Risk or current victim of violence?
  - Stress, anxiety, depression/suicidal risk, burnout related to workplace culture, school, or work expectations
  - Financial or career concerns

REVIEW OF SYSTEMS

- **General:** Fatigue, fever, weight changes, pain
- **Integumentary:** Dryness, itching, bruising, rashes, lesions, hair loss
- **HEENT:** Headache, congestion, eye or ear pain, sore throat
- **Lymphatic:** Bruising, bleeding, lymphadenopathy
- **CV:** Chest pain, shortness of breath, rapid pulse
- **Respiratory:** Dyspnea, wheezing, cough, breathlessness
- **GI/GU:** Appetite changes, dysphagia, nausea, vomiting, constipation, diarrhea, abdominal pain, dysuria, pelvic pain
- **Mental health:** Sadness/depression, helplessness, hopelessness, suicidal ideation, worry, insomnia, hypersomnia; changes in memory, concentration, or mood
- **Neurologic:** Weakness, numbness, fainting, falls, dizziness, confusion

NUTRITIONAL ASSESSMENT

- The primary determinants of nutritional status are food and nutrient intake, which can be assessed by estimating energy and protein intake of an individual. Estimates can be obtained through the history (e.g., verbal report, food diary, food tracking app) or, when feasible, by direct observation.
- There are many valid/reliable nutritional assessment tools for screening malnutrition in adults. The Malnutrition Screening Tool and the Mini Nutritional Assessment (www.mna-elderly.com/forms/mini/mna_mini_english.pdf) are two screening tools that should be considered if a patient presents

with recent weight loss, recent poor intake/appetite, and/or a low BMI. Both tools have a high sensitivity and specificity—Malnutrition Screening Tool, 93%/93%; Mini Nutritional Assessment, 97.9%/100%.

ASSESSMENT OF PAIN

- Verbalization of pain (subjective) is the most common way to assess pain. Although a patient may demonstrate nonverbal, objective signs that indicate pain (e.g., increases in heart rate, blood pressure, respiratory rate), assessing subjective experience is best practice.
- Noting symptom characteristics and responsiveness to treatment allows the clinician to appreciate whether pain is nociceptive or neuropathic, somatic, or visceral:
  - **Neuropathic pain**: Results from within the nervous system; described as sharp, shooting, tingling, burning; may respond poorly to traditional analgesic medications
  - **Nociceptive pain**: Usually responsive to medications; can be somatic or visceral:
    - *Somatic pain* originates from MSK tissue, sharp or dull, usually well localized
    - *Visceral pain* originates from internal organs, poorly localized, accompanied by symptoms of autonomic nervous system stimulation (nausea, vomiting, diaphoresis)
- Evidence-based tools are effective for assessing pain and monitoring response to treatment:
  - **Initial Pain Assessment Tool**: Eight questions regarding the onset, location, duration, quality, intensity, aggravating triggers, relieving factors, and effects of pain
  - **Numeric rating scales**: Patient chooses a number that best indicates current level of pain, with 0 being no pain and 10 being the worst pain that can be imagined
  - **Descriptor scales**: Key words that describe different levels of pain intensity (e.g., no pain, moderate pain, severe pain)
  - **Visual Analog Scale**: Combines a numeric scale and descriptor words; uses a red-yellow-green color scheme depending on the level of pain
  - **Wong–Baker FACES Scale**: A series of faces with different expressions to demonstrate varying levels of pain; used for children who can verbalize their pain level but may not be able to correlate it with a number
- Understanding is crucial before attempting to use any self-reporting pain scale or tool.
- For younger children and older adults who are not developmentally or cognitively able to describe pain, be aware that

interruptions in appetite, sleep, elimination, and/or activity may be indicators of pain intensity.

PHYSICAL EXAMINATION

- Assessment always begins with observation to determine whether the individual being evaluated is well or ill, and, if ill, whether they are experiencing distress.
- Review Box 2.1 for signs and symptoms that require emergent or urgent action.
- Once the clinician has determined that an individual is not experiencing acute distress, the next steps involve observation of the individual's appearance, behavior, and cognition. Much of these assessments are completed while the clinician assesses the patient's history; additional mental status assessments may also be considered part of the physical exam.

MENTAL STATUS ASSESSMENT

- An assessment of an individual's mental status provides the basis for identifying signs and/or symptoms related to their overall mental health functioning.
- Chapter 16, "Evidence-Based Assessment of Mental Health and Substance Use," contains information about completing a detailed and thorough mental status exam, including the interpretation of findings. Assessments of mental status can be remembered using the mnemonic "ABC":
  - **A—Appearance:** Affect (facial expression), posture, hygiene and grooming, body habitus
  - **B—Behavior:** Verbal and nonverbal expressions of pain, anxiety, illness, anger, fear, frustration, contentment, or sadness/depression; interactions; activity level; body movements and mobility
  - **C—Cognition:** Orientation to time, person, and place; attention and concentration; speech pattern, pace, and articulation; judgment, thought patterns, and content; sensory perceptions; impulse control; insight; memory; mood, including signs of anxiety, depression

MEASUREMENT OF VITAL SIGNS

Measurement of Temperature

- Multiple routes—Oral, rectal, axillary, temporal artery, tympanic membrane, infrared
- Consider advantages/disadvantages of each route when selecting the best method

- Temperature elevation that is considered "abnormal" can depend on the age, the site of measurement, and the clinical condition of the patient; in general, body temperature elevated above 100.4 °F (38 °C) rectally is considered a fever

Oral Temperature

- Generally considered a reliable means of measuring body temperature.
- The thermometer probe is positioned in either the right or the left posterior sublingual pocket, which has a rich blood supply and offers an indirect reflection of core temperature.
- Ask the individual to close their mouth around the probe during measurement. Most electronic thermometers will alert with an audible tone once the body temperature is registered.
- Disposable sheaths or probe covers offer protection from transmission of infection between patients.

Rectal Temperature

- Considered the best reflection of core temperature; however, it is used less frequently in practice because it is more invasive.
- Do not use oral thermometers rectally as these can cause injury. Rectal thermometers have a security bulb designed specifically for safely taking rectal temperatures.
- Place the patient in the Sims position. Lubricate the tip of the thermometer's probe cover. While wearing gloves, insert the thermometer probe 1 to 1½ inches into the adult rectum (½ inch for babies); hold it in place until the temperature is registered. Care should be given to ensure patient privacy throughout the procedure.

Axillary Temperature

- Most commonly conducted using an electronic thermometer.
- Probe is placed in the middle of the axilla, and the corresponding arm is held against the body to keep it in place until the audible tone is heard and the temperature is recorded.
- The axilla provides greater surface vasculature in newborns and infants than in adults, making it a better reflection of core temperature and a more appropriate site for temperature assessment.
- Axillary temperatures are about 1° lower than oral temperature readings; however, as axillary temperatures can vary widely, no standard conversion to core temperature exists.

Temporal Artery Temperature

- Measured using an infrared scanning thermometer. Accuracy is dependent on user technique.
- Place the thermometer probe flat on the center of the patient's forehead. Press and hold the scan button. Keeping the sensor flat

against the skin, slide the thermometer across the forehead to the hairline.

- If perspiration is present on the forehead, continue to depress the scan button, lift the probe from the forehead, and touch the probe to the neck behind the earlobe. This will account for the potential cooling effect of perspiration. Release the scan button to display the reading.

Tympanic Temperature

- Tympanic thermometers use infrared scanning to measure the temperature at the tympanic membrane in the ear.
- Gently pull the ear back to help straighten the canal (pull up and back for adults; pull down and back for children under 3). Insert thermometer probe into the ear to seal the canal. Press and hold the scan button until an audible tone is noted (1–3 seconds). Remove from the ear canal; thermometer will display the patient's temperature.
- Disposable probe covers should be used to prevent cross-contamination between patients.

Noncontact Infrared Temperature

- Infrared "no-touch" thermometers use the same type of technologies as tympanic thermometers.
- Advantage is the reduction of cross-contamination risk; strict adherence to manufacturer guidelines and instructions are required for accuracy.
- Ensure environment is appropriate; use a draft-free space, away from direct sunlight and radiant heat sources. The test area of the forehead should be uncovered, clean, and dry. Hold the sensing area perpendicular to the forehead, instruct patient to remain stationary, and press the scan button.
- Normal temperature readings should be below 99.0 °F (37.2 °C).

Assessment of Pulse Rate

- Clinician should note the pulse rate (number of beats/minute), rhythm (pattern or regularity of the beats), and the amplitude (strength of the pulse).
- To determine the rate, the clinician should count the number of beats for a full 60 seconds, or for 30 seconds and multiply times 2. Normal pulse rate for an adult is 60 to 100 beats/minute or bpm. If the rhythm of the pulse is irregular, default to using the full 60 seconds to calculate a rate.
- Peripheral pulses can be assessed at multiple locations, including over the carotid, brachial, radial, femoral, popliteal, dorsalis pedis,

and posterior tibial arteries. See Chapter 3, "Evidence-Based Assessment of the Heart and Circulatory System," for a review of the locations for palpating peripheral pulses. The most common site for determining the pulse rate in adults is over the radial artery. Gently compress the radial artery with the fingertips of the middle and index fingers; this allows for easy assessment of the pulse rate.

- Apical pulse is located over the apex of the heart at the fifth intercostal space left of the midclavicular line. Place the bell of the stethoscope over this area and listen, noting the rhythm and amplitude of the heartbeats, as well as the heart rate. Chapter 3, "Evidence-Based Assessment of the Heart and Circulatory System," delineates placement locations on the chest wall for additional, more thorough evaluation of heart sounds.

Assessment of Respiratory Rate

- Observe the rise and fall of the chest; count the number of breaths that occur in 1 minute. In practice, clinicians do not always count respirations for a full minute, but instead count for 30 seconds and multiply by two. This practice should be avoided as it decreases the accuracy of the respiratory assessment, especially in younger populations.
- The normal rate of respirations depends on age, recent physical activity, and level of alertness (i.e., waking/sleeping states). Respiration rates may increase with fever, illness, or medical conditions.
- The normal respiratory rate for an adult is 12 to 20 breaths/minute. Clinicians should assess for tachypnea, an elevated respiratory rate, and bradypnea, an abnormally slow breathing rate. If either condition exists, further assessment is needed. Chapter 4, "Evidence-Based Assessment of Lungs and Respiratory System," includes review of abnormal respiratory findings.

Blood Pressure Measurement

- BP measurement/monitoring can be completed using home, ambulatory, or office-based methods.
- In the United States, office-based BP monitoring is the standard of care for screening, diagnosis, and management of elevated BP (hypertension).
- The correct measurement of an office-based BP requires attention to the time of day, type of device, cuff size, cuff placement, technique of measurement, and recent use of nicotine or caffeine. Considerations for accurate measurement:
    - **Select equipment:** Length of the BP cuff bladder should be 80% of the circumference of the upper arm; width should be

at least 40% of the circumference of the upper arm. A too-small cuff will result in artificially high BP readings; a too-large cuff will result in artificially low readings. Measurement also requires an available, functioning manometer.

- **Assess circumstances:** Patient should have had no caffeine in the hour preceding the BP reading, no smoking in the 30 minutes prior, and no recent decongestant use. The environment should be quiet and warm.
- **Posture and positioning**: Proper patient positioning is essential for accuracy. Patient should be seated with their back supported, legs uncrossed, and arm supported at the level of the heart (**Figure 2.1**). Patient should be allowed to sit quietly for 5 minutes before BP is measured. Factors that can influence the measurement include bladder distention, background noise, and talking. Patient's arm should be free of clothing; do not roll the sleeve up, as this can create a tourniquet effect and alter the reading. Place the midline of the cuff bladder over the palpated brachial artery pulsation. The lower end of the cuff should be 2 to 3 cm above the antecubital fossa to minimize artifact noise from the stethoscope rubbing the cuff. The cuff should fit snugly on the patient's arm. Once the cuff is placed, the arm should remain supported at the level of the heart; neither the patient nor the clinician should talk.
- **Technique:** The estimated SBP should be palpated initially to avoid misinterpretation of the BP, which is more likely if the patient has an auscultatory gap. An auscultatory gap is a period of diminished or absent Korotkoff sounds during BP measurement, which can be missed if the cuff is inflated without first palpating the SBP. To palpate the SBP, place the fingers of one hand over the brachial or radial artery, and feel for the pulsation. Rapidly inflate the cuff with the hand bulb 30 mmHg above the point at which the pulse was not palpable. Slowly deflate the cuff at a rate of 2 to 3 mmHg/second until the pulse is palpated again, which is the estimated SBP, then quickly deflate the cuff completely. Once

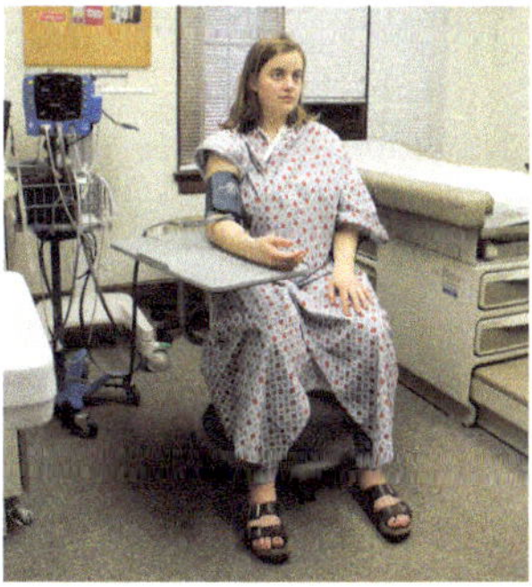

FIGURE 2.1 In-office blood pressure measurement.

the palpable SBP has been determined, place the bell of the stethoscope lightly over the brachial artery, and inflate the cuff quickly to 30 mmHg above the palpable SBP. Slowly release the cuff at a rate of 2 to 3 mmHg/second; listen for the first audible pulse (Korotkoff sound), which is the SBP. Continue to deflate the cuff slowly below the SBP and listen for the beginning of muffled sounds; approximately 8 to 10 mmHg below the muffled sounds, there is a disappearance of sound, which is the DBP. Once the DBP has been noted, rapidly deflate the cuff completely.

- **Number of readings:** Evidence-based recommendation for accurate measurement is to take at least two readings (1–2 minutes apart), while the individual is seated, one from each arm. If there is a substantial (>10 mmHg) and consistent SBP difference between the arms, the arm with the higher values should be used for future measurements.
- **Optional assessment using leg cuff:** If the arm pressure is elevated, take the pressure in one leg, particularly in patients under 30 years of age. Principles to obtain a leg BP reading are the same as in the arm. The SBP in the leg is expected to be 10% to 20% higher than when using the brachial artery.
- **Optional assessment of postural changes:** Check for postural changes by taking readings after the individual has been supine for 5 minutes, then immediately and 2 minutes after standing. This is particularly important for older adults, individuals with diabetes, or patients taking antihypertensive medication.

Considerations for Measurement of Vital Signs in Children

- Vital signs for infants and children can vary greatly in comparison with the normal range for adults. Normal vital signs by age are listed in **Table 2.1**.
- Technique for temperature measurement is age dependent. Rectal temperature is preferred for infants and young children; oral temperature can be obtained when the child is developmentally able to hold/maintain the thermometer under the tongue. In general, fever is defined by a temperature ≥100.4 °F. Newborns and some children with neurologic conditions may demonstrate a lower than normal temperature, even in the presence of serious infection.
- Heart rate can be assessed in a manner similar to adults, by auscultation of the apical pulse or palpation of the radial, for older children and adolescents; for infants, assess brachial or femoral pulse. In infants, each femoral pulse should be palpated simultaneously with a brachial or radial pulse. A delayed or diminished femoral pulse in comparison with the brachial or radial pulse is suggestive of coarctation of the aorta.

TABLE 2.1 Pediatric Vital Signs

Age	Heart Rate (Beats/Minute)	Blood Pressure (mmHg)	Respiratory Rate (Breaths/ Minute)
Premature	110–170	SBP 55–75 DBP 35–45	40–70
0–3 months	110–160	SBP 65–85 DBP 45–55	35–55
3–6 months	110–160	SBP 70–90 DBP 50–65	30–45
6–12 months	90–160	SBP 80–100 DBP 55–65	22–38
1–3 years	80–150	SBP 90–105 DBP 55–70	22–30
3–6 years	70–120	SBP 95–110 DBP 60–75	20–24
6–12 years	60–110	SBP 100–120 DBP 60–75	16–22
>12 years	60–100	SBP 110–135 DBP 65–85	12–20

DBP, diastolic blood pressure; SBP, systolic blood pressure.

- Respiratory rate varies not only with age but also with activity or distress. It is most accurately assessed for a full minute while the infant or young child is calm or sleeping.
- BP measurement in children not only varies with age but is also evaluated against a standard reference population of sex and height percentile. Annual, routine BP monitoring begins at 3 years of age. At any age, BP is taken in response to other findings suspicious of underlying cardiac or renal disease. It is imperative to use an appropriately sized BP cuff to obtain an accurate measurement for children. Cuff should cover approximately two-thirds of the upper arm.
- Many young children are fearful of the measurement of vital signs. To facilitate measurement and alleviate fear, the clinician can allow the child to touch and examine the equipment first and should be mindful of the language used for children who are concrete thinkers.

PHYSICAL EXAMINATION OF BODY HABITUS

Height

- *Height (stature)* is defined as the distance from the plantar surface of the foot to the crown of the head. It is measured in the standing position once an individual reaches 2 years of age and is able to stand independently. Measurement is completed using a *stadiometer*, which consists of a vertical ruler and a sliding horizontal piece with a flat bottom.
- To measure height with a stadiometer, make sure the patient's shoes, any hat, and excess or bulky clothing are removed prior to measurement; ask the patient to keep their eyes looking straight ahead, stand straight with feet together, and place heels and back against the vertical measuring surface (**Figure 2.2**).

Weight

- Weight represents total body mass. Body weight alone is a poor predictor of health because it is strongly correlated with height and not reflective of body composition. To evaluate health risks that may be related to an individual's weight, it must be considered in relation to height.
- Scales must be placed on a solid, flat surface and should be balanced appropriately (consult the operating manual for the

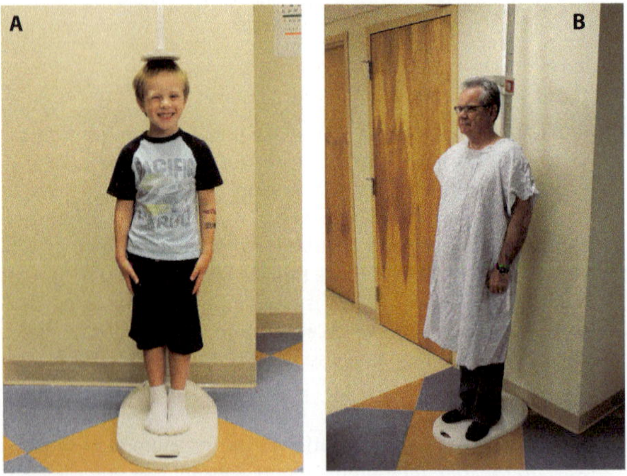

FIGURE 2.2 Correct measurement of height using a stadiometer. (**A**) Child. (**B**) Adult.

device). Weight should be measured to the nearest 0.1 kg (or nearest 0.1 lb.). Ensure patient's shoes and any excess or heavy clothing are removed. Ask patient to remove any belongings from their pockets, including wallets, keys, and phones. Have the patient place both feet in the center of the scale and avoid movement during measurement.

Body Mass Index Calculation

- Weight may be evaluated relative to height by calculating BMI. Divide weight in kilograms by height in meters squared (expressed as kg/m^2; if measuring in inches and pounds, it may be calculated as $[lb/in^2] \times 703$. Online BMI calculators can be accessed for ease of calculation: https://www.nhlbi.nih.gov/health/educational/lose_wt/BMI/bmi-m.htm
- BMI status may be classified according to standard cut points outlined by the National Heart, Lung, and Blood Institute (**Table 2.2**).
- Despite widespread use in clinical practice, the BMI metric has limitations. It does not capture information on distribution of body fat, and in general:
  - At the same BMI, women tend to have more body fat than men.
  - At the same BMI, Blacks have less body fat than Whites.
  - At the same BMI, older adults tend to have more body fat than younger adults.
  - At the same BMI, athletes have less body fat than non-athletes.

TABLE 2.2 Classification of BMI in Adults and Children

Classification	Adults	Children (2–20 years)
Underweight	<18.5 kg/m^2	<5th percentile
Normal	18.5–24.9 kg/m^2	5th–84.9th percentile
Overweight	25.0–29.9 kg/m^2	85th–94.9th percentile
Obesity	≥30.0 kg/m^2	≥95th percentile

Adult obesity may be further classified in increments of 5 kg/m^2: Class I, 30.0 to 34.9 kg/m^2; Class II, 35.0 to 39.9 kg/m^2; Class III, >40.0 kg/m^2.

Sources: From Centers for Disease Control and Prevention. (n.d.). *About child & teen BMI*. https://www.cdc.gov/healthyweight/assessing/bmi/childrens_bmi/about_childrens_bmi.html#percentile; National Heart, Lung, and Blood Institute. (n.d.). *Classification of overweight and obesity by BMI, waist circumference, and associated disease risks*. https://www.nhlbi.nih.gov/health/educational/lose_wt/BMI/bmi_dis.htm

Waist and Other Circumferences

- Presence of elevated waist circumference and/or elevated waist:hip ratio is an indicator of proportionally more adipose tissue distribution around the abdomen compared with the hip and thigh. Distribution of adiposity around the abdomen is referred to as an *android (or apple) distribution*, as opposed to a *gynoid (or pear) distribution*. Android pattern of adiposity is associated with increased risk of adverse health outcomes, including CV diseases and diabetes, and remains so even after statistically accounting for BMI.
- To measure waist circumference, have the patient remove any constricting clothing from their waistline. Tell the patient to breathe normally and avoid "sucking it in." The clinician should use their hands to walk up both sides of the patient's hips. Place the tape measure at the top of the iliac crest (**Figure 2.3**). Use a flexible tape measure that measures in inches or centimeters. Make sure that the tape measure is snug but does not compress the skin and that the tape measure lies parallel to the floor. Have the patient relax and exhale.
- It is not necessary to do a waist circumference on any patient with a BMI of 35 or greater or any individual with a height under 5 feet because of inaccuracies. Monitoring changes in waist circumference over time may be helpful, in addition to measuring BMI, since it can provide an estimate of increased abdominal adipose tissue even in the absence of a change in BMI. In obese patients with metabolic complications, changes in waist circumference are useful predictors of changes in CV risk factors.
- It may be necessary to measure the circumference of other body areas. These objective circumference measures to assess nutritional status are typically completed by nutritional specialists to ensure accuracy and consistency for long-term comparisons:
  - The mid-upper arm circumference is an independent anthropometric assessment tool used to determine undernutrition.
  - Calf circumference is used to assess nutritional status in adults and has been shown to have good diagnostic capacity.

Percentage of Body Fat

- Assessment of body composition accounts not only for an individual's body weight, but also the proportion of weight that is made up of fat and lean tissue. The most widely utilized term to reflect fat content of the body is *percentage of body fat*, calculated by dividing fat body weight by total body weight. Body weight is not a perfect reflection of body composition because

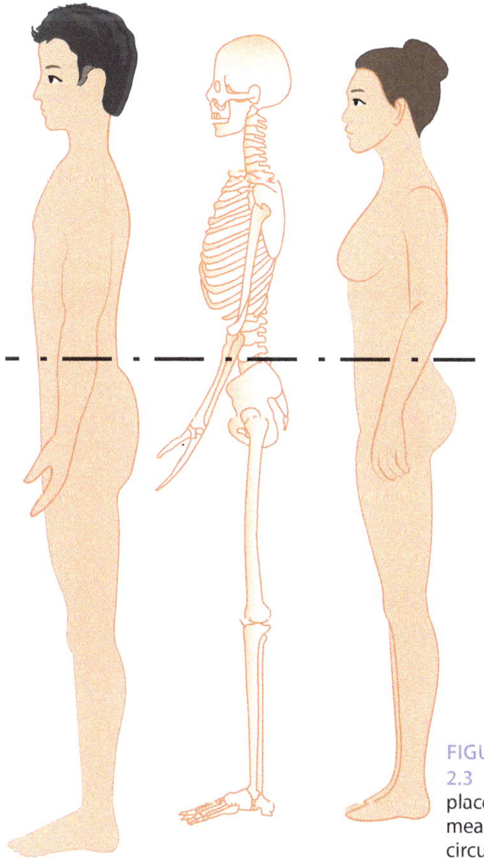

FIGURE 2.3 Correct placement for measuring waist circumference.

the densities of lean and fat tissues vary. Lean tissue is composed primarily of skeletal muscle, which is more dense than fat. Therefore, two individuals of the same body weight can vary greatly in body composition.

- Techniques used to estimate % BF may include assessment of skinfold thickness—measurement of the thickness of a fold of skin and the underlying subcutaneous adipose tissue at multiple body sites. Several methods and body density equations exist, including methods that assess as few as three body sites to as many as seven. The clinician locates the site to be measured, lifts the skin firmly by grasping between the thumb and forefinger, and uses specialized calipers to measure the thickness of the fold in millimeters. The clinician should rotate through all of the measurement sites until two consistent measurements are obtained at each site. The sum of skinfolds is used to calculate body density and % BF using sex-, age-, and ethnicity-specific equations.

PEDIATRIC GROWTH AND DEVELOPMENT

Measurements of Growth

- Infants and children undergo anthropometric assessment at each well child visit beause growth is the primary outcome measure of wellness in children. Deviations in growth trajectories may be indicative of neglect, chronic illness, malnutrition, hormonal conditions, or congenital syndromes. The CDC recommends using the WHO international growth charts for children aged 0 to 23 months and the CDC growth charts for children and adolescents aged 2 to 18 years.
- Regular assessment should include height/length, weight, head circumference, BMI (beginning at age 2), and associated percentiles. Because children are continuously growing, growth measurements are interpreted differently than for adults. Trends are compared with a reference population of children of the same age and sex and reported as a percentile. These measures should be assessed and documented to allow the clinician to monitor changes over time.
- Infants and young children under age 2 should be measured lying supine with a recumbent infant length board (**Figure 2.4**), and should be weighed nude or in a clean, dry disposable diaper on an accurately calibrated scale (**Figure 2.5**).

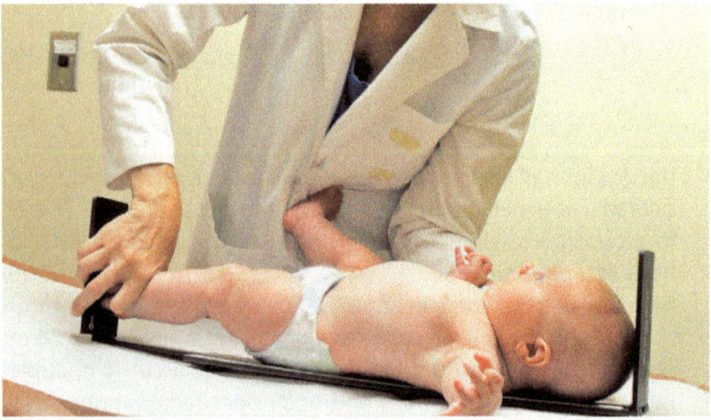

FIGURE 2.4 Obtaining length measurement in an infant.

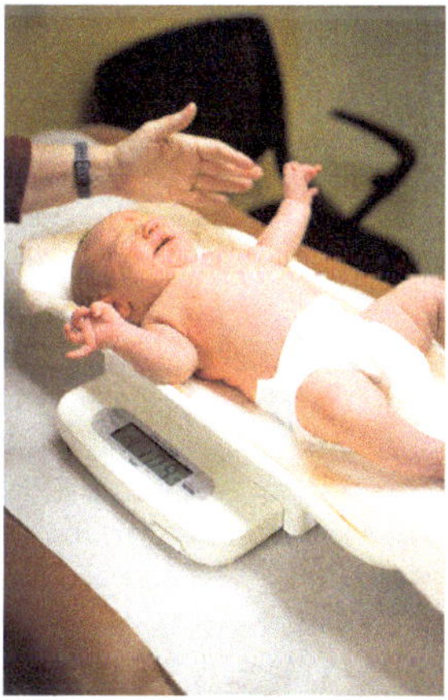

FIGURE 2.5 Infant weighed on calibrated scale.

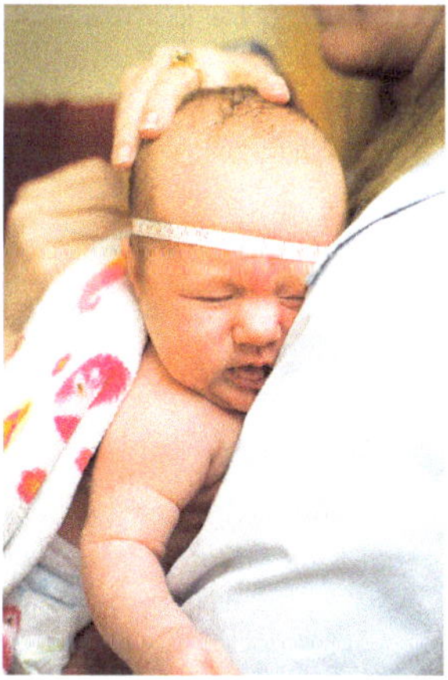

FIGURE 2.6 Measurement of occipito–frontal circumference.

- Head circumference should be measured for all children up to age 3 with a flexible, nonelastic measuring tape placed just above the brow line anteriorly and over the occipital prominence posteriorly (**Figure 2.6**). It is advisable to measure the head circumference three times in one encounter to ensure the accuracy of the recording.
- Length, weight, length-for-weight percentile, and head circumference measurements should be plotted according to age on the WHO growth chart designated for the infant's natal sex.
- Newborns are expected to lose up to 10% of their birth weight in the first few days of life; >10% weight loss should be urgently investigated.
- Normal weight gain for the newborn is 15 to 30 g/day (0.5–1 oz/day). It is normal for breastfed newborns to gain weight on the lower end of the normal range. The newborn should recover birth weight by at least 2 weeks of age. The average infant will double their birth weight by 6 months of age and triple it by 12 months.
- The average newborn length is 20 to 21 inches (51 cm). Linear growth velocity averages 2.5 cm/month from birth to 6 months, 1.3 cm/month from 7 to 12 months, and about 7.6 cm/year between 12 months and 10 years of age on average.
- Infants with poor weight gain or growth measurements that trend downward or fall below the third percentile may have a failure to thrive, and the cause should be investigated. If

neglect, organic disease, or severe malnutrition is suspected, the child should be hospitalized for evaluation.

- An upward-trending head circumference may indicate hydrocephalus or other intracranial pathology. A head circumference that stalls in growth may indicate a premature fusion of sutures/fontanels or a congenital syndrome associated with microcephaly.
- For adolescents and children older than age 2, height, weight, and BMI should be plotted on the CDC growth chart relative to the child's natal sex. Young children and adolescents who can stand steadily without assistance should be weighed with a calibrated electronic scale or beam balance scale. Height should be measured with a portable or wall-mount stadiometer, with the child standing erect, looking forward, with heels and occiput against the wall. Height and weight should be obtained without shoes. Prior to the accelerated growth period in adolescence, school-aged children typically grow an average of 2.5 inches and gain an average of 5 to 7 pounds/year.
- Although calculated using the same formula, BMI is interpreted differently for children and teens. Interpretation of BMI in children and adolescents requires the consideration of age and gender, as body fat percentages differ as children develop. The CDC BMI-for-age growth charts reflect these differences and visually show BMI as a percentile ranking.
- Obesity in children is indicated by a BMI greater than or equal to the 95th percentile on the CDC standardized growth chart. A BMI between the 85th and the 95th percentiles is considered overweight. A BMI between the 5th and the 85th percentiles is considered normal weight.

Developmental Assessment

- Evidence-based guidelines recommend that clinicians perform developmental surveillance at every routine health encounter and a standardized developmental screening at ages 9, 18, and 24 or 30 months.
- *Developmental surveillance* refers to the process of recognizing children who may be at risk for developmental delays. The clinician performs surveillance through physical observation of the child's development and by asking the caregiver whether the child has met age-appropriate developmental milestones.

- *Developmental screening* refers to the use of standardized tools to identify children at risk for delays in the developmental domains of motor (gross and fine), language, cognitive, emotional, and psychosocial.
- All clinicians working with children should be familiar with the early childhood developmental milestones that follow (CDC, 2019).
  - **Age: 2 months**
    - Social/emotional: Smiles, makes eye contact with caregiver, self-soothes briefly
    - Language/communication: Coos, makes gurgling sounds, turns head toward sounds
    - Cognitive: Pays attention to faces and follows with eyes
    - Motor: Develops head control and smoother movement in arms and legs
  - **Age: 4 months**
    - Social/emotional: Smiles spontaneously at people, copies some facial expressions
    - Language/communication: Begins to babble; copies sounds; cries in different ways when hungry, tired, or in pain
    - Cognitive: Responds to affection, reaches for things; follows movement
    - Motor: Holds head steady, rolls front to back
  - **Age: 6 months**
    - Social/emotional: Knows familiar faces, recognizes strangers, responds to others' emotions, likes to look at self in mirror
    - Language/communication: Responds to sounds by making sounds, responds to own name
    - Cognitive: Brings things to mouth, shows curiosity about things out of reach, passes things from one hand to another
    - Motor: Rolls back to front; begins to sit without support; when standing, supports weight on legs
  - **Age: 9 months**
    - Social/emotional: May have stranger anxiety, has favorite toys
    - Language/communication: Understands "no," copies sounds and gestures, uses finger to point
    - Cognitive: Plays peek-a-boo, develops object permanence (looks for things out of sight)

  - Motor: Stands, holding on; sits without support; pulls to standing; crawls
- **Age: 1 year**
  - Social/emotional: Cries when caregiver leaves, has favorite things and people, plays games such as pat-a-cake
  - Language/communication: Responds to simple requests; waves bye-bye; shakes head "no"; says words like *mama, dada, uh oh*!
  - Cognitive: Copies gestures; puts things in a container and takes things out of it; explores things by shaking, banging, throwing
  - Motor: Pulls up to standing, cruises (walks while holding on), may stand alone, may take a few steps
- **Age: 18 months**
  - Social/emotional: Plays simple pretend, like feeding a doll; may have temper tantrums; shows affection to familiar people
  - Language/communication: Says several single words; points to show someone what they want, points to pictures in a book
  - Cognitive: Knows what ordinary things are, like brush, spoon, phone; points to one body part; scribbles; follows command like "sit down"
  - Motor: Walks alone, drinks from a cup, eats with a spoon, pulls toys or carries toys while walking, may walk up stairs
- **Age: 2 years**
  - Social/emotional: Imitates others, gets excited when with other children and begins to involve them in games and play, shows more independence and defiance
  - Language/communication: Says sentences of two to four words, points to things in a book, follows simple commands, knows names of familiar people and body parts
  - Cognitive: Begins to sort shapes and colors, plays simple make-believe games, builds a tower of four cubes, finds things when hidden
  - Motor: Stands on tiptoe, kicks a ball, begins to run, climbs onto and down from furniture without help, walks up and down stairs while holding on
- **Age: 3 years**
  - Social/emotional: Copies adults and friends; shares, cooperates, shows concern and affection without prompting; dresses and undresses self

    - Language/communication: Follows instructions with two or three steps, understands prepositions (on, in, under), words are 75% understandable to strangers
    - Cognitive: Can button, complete puzzles with three or four pieces, copy a circle; turns book pages one at a time; builds towers of more than six blocks
    - Motor: Climbs well, runs easily; jumps forward; pedals a tricycle; walks up and down stairs, one foot on each step
  - **Age: 4 years**
    - Social/emotional: Enjoys doing new things, remembers parts of stories; uses scissors; starts to understand time; brushes teeth
    - Language/communication: Can say first and last names, uses pronouns correctly; can sing a song or recite a nursery rhyme from memory
    - Cognitive: Names some colors, numbers, draws a person with two to four body parts; plays board games, card games; can print some letters
    - Motor: Hops, stands on one leg for 2 seconds; catches a bounced ball most of the time; climbs stairs, alternating feet
  - **Age: 5 years**
    - Social/emotional: Likes to sing, dance, act, participate in imaginative play; knows the difference between real and make-believe
    - Language/communication: Speaks clearly, tells a simple story with complete sentences, uses future tense, says name and address
    - Cognitive: Prints letters and numbers, copies a triangle and shapes, knows about everyday things (e.g., food, money), draws a person with at least six body parts
    - Motor: Stands on one foot for 10 seconds or longer; may be able to skip, somersault; uses toilet on own; swings, climbs
- When a child is not developing skills in one or more domains according to the expected time frame, they are exhibiting signs of *developmental delay*.
- Identification of a developmental problem or delay should prompt further diagnostic evaluation and referral for early intervention services (**Box 2.2**).
- *Early intervention* is a collective term describing programs or services (e.g., speech therapy, physical therapy, occupational therapy) that support development for children aged 0 to 3 years with developmental delays or disabilities. Children aged 0 to 3 years

have greater neuroplasticity and therefore higher capacity for improved outcomes the earlier services are established.

BOX 2.2 Red Flags Indicating Need for Referral and Possible Early Intervention in Children With Developmental Delay

- Any child who fails to move ahead developmentally
- Any child who begins to deteriorate developmentally
- Failure to achieve developmental milestones, including:
    - Inconsistent or lack of response to auditory stimuli
    - Not sitting with support by 6 months
    - Unable to sit alone by 9 months
    - Unable to transfer objects hand to hand by 1 year
    - Abnormal pincer grasp at 15 months
    - Unable to walk alone by 18 months
    - No understandable speech by 18 months
    - Failure to speak recognizable words by 2 years
    - Speech predominately unintelligible at 3 years old

EVIDENCE-BASED RESOURCES

- **American Academy of Family Physicians (JNC-8 Guidelines):** www.aafp.org
- **American Academy of Pediatrics:** www.aap.org
- **American Heart Association:** www.heart.org
- **Centers for Disease Control and Prevention:** www.cdc.gov/growthcharts/data/set2clinical/cj41c070.pdf
  www.cdc.gov/mmwr/pdf/rr/rr5909.pdf
  www.cdc.gov/vaccines/hcp/acip-recs/index.html
- **Choosing Wisely Campaign:** www.choosingwisely.org
- **National Heart, Lung, and Blood Institute:** www.nhlbi.nih.gov
- **U.S. Food and Drug Administration:** www.accessdata.fda.gov/scripts/interactivenutritionfactslabel/assets/InteractiveNFL_Vitamins&MineralsChart_March2020.pdf
- **U.S. Preventive Services Task Force:** www.uspreventiveservicestaskforce.org

ABNORMAL FINDINGS

FEVER

An elevation in body temperature above 100.4 °F (38 °C) in response to internal and/or external factors.

Hyperthermia

History

- Prolonged exposure to hot, humid weather
- Flushing, excess sweating
- Chills or shivering, body aches
- Loss of appetite, nausea, vomiting
- Weakness, fatigue

Physical Examination

- Fever above 104.0 °F (40.0 °C)
- Tachycardia, tachypnea
- Delirium

Consideration

- Older age, certain illnesses, and certain medications increase risk

Hypothermia

History

- Prolonged exposure to cold air or water
- Drowsiness, confusion, loss of coordination

Physical Examination

- Body temperature <95.0 °F (35.0 °C)
- Respiratory distress
- Bradycardia, slow weak pulse

Considerations

- Assessment of temperature in newborns is a priority. Cold stress in a newborn can lead to hypoglycemia, hypoxia, and hypothermia
- Fever can be induced to manage certain medical conditions

HYPERTENSION: ELEVATED BLOOD PRESSURE

History

- May be asymptomatic
- Severe hypertension may result in headaches, blurred vision, chest pain

- Modifiable risk factors: smoking, obesity, poor diet, including excessive alcohol and sodium intake, or physical inactivity
- Nonmodifiable risk factors: older age, family history, race/ethnicity

Physical Examination

- Elevated blood pressure (may be the only sign)
- Obesity
- Retinal changes including papilledema, arteriovenous (AV) nicking, exudates
- Carotid and/or abdominal bruits; adventitious heart sounds
- Peripheral edema

Considerations

- Secondary hypertension is caused by a specific medication or disease state.
- Medications that can elevate BP include oral contraceptives, NSAIDs, decongestants, stimulants.
- Medical conditions that cause hypertension include obstructive sleep apnea, primary renal disease, pheochromocytoma, Cushing's syndrome, hyperthyroidism, and coarctation of the aorta (**Table 2.3**).

SHOCK

A life-threatening condition due to lack of blood flow that leads to hypotension and hypoxia. Identifying the cause is essential.

- **Septic shock**: Response to overwhelming infection
- **Systemic inflammatory response syndrome**: Results from noninfectious conditions like burns, amniotic fluid embolism, air embolism, and crush injuries

TABLE 2.3 Definitions of Hypertension for Adults

<table>
<tr><th>Blood Pressure</th><th>ACC/AHA 2017</th><th>JNC8</th></tr>
<tr><td><120/<80</td><td>Normal</td><td>Normal</td></tr>
<tr><td>120–129/80</td><td rowspan="2">"Prehypertension"</td><td>"Elevated"</td></tr>
<tr><td>130–139/80–89</td><td>Stage 1 HTN</td></tr>
<tr><td>140–159/90–100</td><td>Stage 1 HTN</td><td rowspan="2">Stage 2 HTN</td></tr>
<tr><td>≥169/≥100</td><td>Stage 2 HTN</td></tr>
</table>

ACC/AHA, The American College of Cardiology/American Heart Association; HTN, hypertension; JNC8, Eighth Joint National Committee.

- **Neurogenic shock**: Result of severe traumatic brain or spinal cord injury
- **Anaphylactic shock**: Results from severe allergic reactions
- **Cardiogenic shock**: Result of myocardial infarction
- **Hypovolemic shock**: Occurs from hemorrhagic or non-hemorrhagic fluid loss
- **Endocrine shock**: Associated with adrenal failure
- **Drug- and toxin-induced shock**: Associated with drug overdoses, snakebites, transfusion reactions, and poisonings

MALNUTRITION

Defined as imbalances, deficiencies, or excesses in intake of energy and/or nutrients

Undernutrition

Lack of adequate nutrition, caused by not having enough food or by not eating enough foods that contain the nutrients needed for proper growth and development

History

- Loss of appetite, or weight loss with normal appetite
- Dental pain or problems
- Unbalanced diet, lack of specific nutrients
- Pagophagia, compulsive craving, chewing, or consumption of ice, iced drinks
- Diarrhea, steatorrhea, change in stooling pattern
- Fatigue, weakness, dizziness, paresthesia
- Elderly adult, resident of a nursing home or rehabilitation facility
- May have functional decline, dementia, or Alzheimer's disease
- May have history of a malabsorption syndrome(s) and/or cancer(s)

Physical Examination

- Anemia, glossitis, cheilosis, or angular stomatitis
- Pallor
- Weight loss, wasting, muscle atrophy
- Growth delay
- Dermatitis or dermatoses
- Low bone density, pathologic fractures

Consideration

- Very young and very old are more at risk

Overweight/Obesity

A multifactorial disease, defined by BMI, which increases risks for chronic conditions, including CV disease, diabetes, cancer, stroke, sleep apnea, and mental illnesses.

History

- Imbalance in caloric intake and caloric expenditure
- Reported diet high in sugar, trans fats, saturated fats
- Sedentary lifestyle; little to no exercise
- Menstrual cycle changes
- Fatigue, sluggishness
- May have associated changes in body image, mental health, metabolism
- May have modifiable risk factors related to diet choices, dietary patterns, excessive alcohol intake, physical inactivity, stress
- May have nonmodifiable risk factors, including older age, genetics, chronic conditions

Physical Examination

- **Adults**: BMI of 25 or greater (overweight) or 30 or greater (obese)
- **Children**: BMI from 85th to 94th percentile (overweight) and at or above the 95th percentile (obese); note that percentiles are determined by age and gender

Consideration

- It is possible to be both overweight and micronutrient deficient.

Weight Gain

Similar to obesity, weight gain may arise from one of many causes. Consider secondary causes if weight gain cannot be attributed to alterations in diet or activity, or is associated with dyspnea, edema, headache, substance use, or changes in mental health.

Weight Loss

Results from energy expenditure that is in excess of energy intake. May result from a change in dietary habits and/or physical activity, or more complex causes, including medications, endocrine factors, psychosocial factors, and other illnesses.

History

- Imbalance in caloric intake and caloric expenditure
- Reported reduction in energy intake; diet low in fats, protein, calories
- Reported increase in physical activity

- Medications
- Diarrhea, abdominal pain
- Decreased appetite (anorexia), nausea, dyspepsia, dysphagia

Physical Examination
- Poor dentition
- Generalized muscle wasting
- Decreased hand/grip strength

Consideration
- Can result from decreased intake, decreased absorption, increased metabolic requirements, and/or increased loss of nutrients

Cachexia

A multiorgan syndrome that is characterized by anorexia, a dramatic loss of skeletal muscle mass and adipose tissue, substantial weight loss, and inflammation.

History
- Anorexia, dramatic weight loss
- Fatigue, weakness
- Often associated with advanced cancers, AIDS, certain autoimmune diseases, and other chronic conditions like heart failure and chronic kidney disease

Physical Examination
- Weight loss in adult or growth failure in children
- Insulin resistance
- Increased muscle protein breakdown; decreased muscle strength
- Low FFMI
- Increased inflammatory markers
- Significant anemia; low serum albumin

Consideration
- Cancer data strongly suggests that cachexia hinders treatment responses and patients' ability to tolerate treatment. Inflammatory cytokines, in particular, have been closely associated with cachexia and mortality in cancer patients.

Sarcopenia

A complex and multifaceted process that involves the degenerative (involuntary) loss of skeletal muscle mass, quality, and strength; most often the result of healthy aging.

History

- Loss of muscle mass, strength, and function
- Difficulty performing ADL
- Most commonly seen in inactive people but can also affect those who remain physically active throughout their lives

Physical Examination

- Loss of balance, slowed gait
- May require assistive devices

Consideration

- One of the most important causes of functional decline and loss of independence in older adults; adequate nutrition and targeting exercise remain gold standard for prevention and treatment.

PHYSICAL EXAMINATION DOCUMENTATION

Documentation of physical exam includes appraisal of illness and wellness, vital signs, body habitus; growth and developmental assessment in children

EXAMPLE DOCUMENTATION OF GENERAL SURVEY: ADULT

Height 5′5,″Weight 185 lbs, BMI 30.8
Temp 98.6 °F orally
Pulse rate 72/minute, Respiratory rate 12/minute
BP 144/88 right arm, 140/82 left arm; both after 5 minutes seated
Repeat BP right arm, 138/84

70-year-old White female. Affect pleasant. Oriented to time, person, and place. Nontoxic appearance. Respirations easy without distress. Pulse regular in rate and rhythm. Mucosa pink. Thoughts coherent; able to articulate health history with clarity. Steady gait; ambulates without assistive devices or abnormal movements. Transfers to table easily. Seated upright.

EXAMPLE DOCUMENTATION OF GENERAL SURVEY: CHILD

Temp 37.5 °C by temporal scan
Pulse 92/minute with normal rhythm
Respiratory rate 24/minute, easy with no retractions
See growth charts for length (75th percentile), weight (50th percentile), head circumference (75th percentile); consistent growth along the curve since birth

Well-nourished 1-year-old Black male. Awake and alert, responsive to caregiver (dad with child today). Nontoxic, no distress. Mucosa pink. Respirations easy. Recent developmental milestones: Can crawl on hands and knees, pulls self to standing, cruises around furniture, walks with one hand held; says "dada" and three other words, waves good-bye, points to objects; feeds self, is eating table foods, finger foods, drinks from cup; enjoys peekaboo and board books (no parental concern regarding development).

REFERENCES

References for this chapter draw from Chapter 4, "Evidence-Based Assessment of Children and Adolescents," Chapter 5, "Approach to the Physical Examination: General Survey and Assessment of Vital Signs," and Chapter 8, "Approach to Evidence-Based Assessment of Body Habitus (Height, Weight, Body Mass Index, Nutrition)," of the textbook *Evidence-Based Physical Examination: Best Practices for Health and Well-Being Assessment*. The references may be accessed in the digital version of the handbook at connect.springerpub.com/content/book/https://connect.springerpub.com/content/book/978-0-8261-6466-7/chapter/ch02

Centers for Disease Control and Prevention. (2019). *Milestone checklist*. https://www.cdc.gov/ncbddd/actearly/pdf/checklists/Checklists-with-Tips_Reader-2019_508.pdf

3

Heart and Circulatory System

CLINICAL CONSIDERATIONS

- Understanding the structure and function of the CV and PV systems provides the foundation for evidence-based assessment.
- Completing a comprehensive, evidence-based history and physical examination when an individual presents with concerns, symptoms, and/or risks related to the CV and PV systems provides a clinician with the opportunity to identify and distinguish between normal and abnormal findings.
- Early recognition of acute coronary syndrome, acute MI, arrhythmias, heart defects, heart failure, and heart disease can reduce costs and improve and save lives.
- Auscultation is a sensitive, specific, and effective method of detecting how the cardiac system is functioning. S1 indicates the beginning of systole and coincides with the apical pulse. S2 indicates diastole, closure of the aortic and pulmonic valves, and is heard best at the base.

SUBJECTIVE HISTORY

COMMON REASONS FOR SEEKING CARE

Chest pain, palpitations, lower extremity edema

HISTORY OF PRESENT ILLNESS

- **Onset:** When did the symptoms start? What was the individual doing when they became symptomatic? Did this occur suddenly, or has it been developing gradually?

- **Location:** Does the symptom have associated pain or discomfort? If so, where is the discomfort located? Does the pain radiate? Is there pain in the left jaw, neck, or arm? Is the edema in one or both legs?
- **Duration:** How long do symptom(s) last? Do the symptoms come and go? Over what period of time have the cardiac symptoms developed?
- **Characteristics:** Would you describe the pain/discomfort as an ache, burn, sharp, shooting, squeezing, crushing, tight, or dull?
- **Associated symptoms:** Presence or absence of numbness, tingling, weakness, nausea, vomiting, fever, heaviness in the arms or chest, neck pain; heartburn/GERD, hemoptysis, shortness of breath, unusual fatigue, feeling clammy or sweaty?
- **Aggravating factors:** What actions, activities, or body positions make the symptoms worse? If exertion worsens symptoms, clarify level of exertion that causes exacerbation. Are the symptoms worse at night or in the early morning?
- **Relieving factors:** Does rest decrease the symptoms? If relieved, how long does the relief last? Does elevating the legs or wearing TED hose relieve the edema?
- **Treatment:** What medications has the individual taken to help with the symptoms? Did the patient use nitroglycerin? Do antacids provide relief? Clarify dosage and frequency of any medications.
- **Severity:** How severe are the symptoms on a scale of 0 to 10? Do the symptoms limit participation in activities? Are the symptoms worsening? Is the individual feeling anxious or fearful about them?

HEALTH HISTORY

Past Medical History

- History of CVD throughout life span:
    - Premature birth history or fetal heart defect diagnosed during the prenatal, infancy, or childhood periods (including treatments and correctional surgeries)
    - HTN or history of elevated blood pressure readings
    - HLD
    - Stroke or TIAs
    - Blood clots (including pulmonary embolism)
    - ACS
    - Acute MI
    - PVD
    - CHF

  - History of stress tests, echocardiograms, EKGs, Holter monitors (including results)
- Comorbidities or risk factors related to CV/PVD:
  - Diabetes (insulin or noninsulin dependent)
  - Obstructive sleep apnea (including use of CPAP)
  - COVID-19
  - Kidney disease
  - Erectile dysfunction
  - Depression
  - Anxiety
  - Stress (acute or chronic)
  - History of pregnancy-associated conditions that increase later CVD risk (e.g., preeclampsia, eclampsia, gestational hypertension)
  - History of premature menopause
  - Previous surgeries, emergency room visits
  - Adverse childhood experiences

Medications

- Prescribed medications with dose, frequency, side effects, consistency of taking medications, and barriers to medication adherence (including anti-hypertensive medications, statins, nitroglycerin, anti-arrhythmic medications, and anticoagulants including warfarin)
- OTC medications or supplements, including aspirin, fish oil, coenzyme Q10, garlic, niacin
- Use of nitroglycerin; frequency and timing of use
- Chemotherapy (past or present)

Allergies

- Allergies to medications or seasonal, environmental, and/or food allergies; if "yes" to being allergic to any substance or environmental trigger, clarify reaction

Pediatric Considerations

- Birth history:
  - Any respiratory distress after birth? Any apneic episodes? Did the child require oxygen, pulse oximetry monitoring, or support for breathing as an infant? Apgar scores at birth?
  - Mother's health during pregnancy? Exposures during pregnancy? Maternal illnesses, illicit drug use, and medication use when pregnant?
  - Fetal abnormalities identified during the prenatal stage?

- Growth and development history:
  - Meeting developmental milestones?
  - Suboptimal growth or poor weight gain (based on pediatric growth charts)?
- Eating and nutritional history:
  - Is the child exhibiting intolerance of feeding? Note vomiting, diarrhea, decreased intake, little interest in feeding, easily fatigued or perspiring during feeding, and/or any color changes including cyanoses during feeding.

FAMILY HISTORY

- Acute MI (especially if occurred at a young age), congenital heart disease, CAD, CHF, long QT syndrome, sudden cardiac death
- Stroke
- Depression
- Diabetes
- Down syndrome
- HLD
- HTN
- Inherited hypercoagulable conditions, including Factor V Leiden, prothrombin gene mutation, and/or deficiencies of natural proteins that prevent clotting (such as antithrombin, protein C, and protein S)

SOCIAL HISTORY

- Tobacco use (type, pack years)
- Alcohol intake (type, amount, daily intake)
- Recreational drug use (specifically cocaine, heroin use, and whether drug use was in the past or present)
- Stress level (acute vs. chronic)
- Sleep (patterns, duration)
- Diet (specifically sodium intake, trans fats, red meat consumption)
- Exercise (frequency, duration, type)
- Home monitoring of blood pressure and/or daily weight

REVIEW OF SYSTEMS

- **General**: Fever, fatigue, dizziness, weight changes, recent travel (long car or plane ride)
- **HEENT**: Visual disturbances/visual difficulty, periodontal disease, recent strep infections, or history of untreated/undertreated strep infections

- **Respiratory**: Shortness of breath, orthopnea, snoring with or without witness apneas
- **CV**: Chest pain (with activity, at rest, or both); left arm, jaw, or neck pain; use of nitroglycerin; palpitations; skipping beats; racing heart rate; lower extremity edema; pain in lower extremities during activity; hair loss on the lower legs; history of stress test or EKG with results
- **GI**: Abdominal pulsations, abdominal pain, GERD
- **GU**: Use of oral contraceptives
- **Neurologic**: Weakness, numbness and tingling, syncope, headache, falls, dizziness
- **MSK**: Weakness, recent activity, or overuse
- **Mental health**: Depression, anxiety; changes in mentation, memory, or mood; current stress level and coping mechanisms

RED FLAGS IN SUBJECTIVE HISTORY

- Family history of premature atherosclerotic CVD, sudden death, bleeding disorders
- Chest pain
- Unstable angina
- Calf pain or unilateral lower extremity edema suggestive of DVT
- Sudden severe headache
- Dyspnea
- Hemoptysis
- Trauma to the chest, abdomen, or extremities

PHYSICAL EXAMINATION

- A systematic approach to the CV and PV exams should be taken to ensure that all components of the exam are completed.
- CV exam is completed with the patient in the seated, supine, or left lateral positions, and in some cases the standing/squatting position.
- The CV and PV exams follow the order of most system exams: inspection, palpation, auscultation. Some techniques are not completed in all positions or for all portions of the exams.
- Keep in mind the location of the heart valves and chambers—the second right (aortic valve) and left (pulmonic valve), ICSs, the left LSB (mitral valve and right ventricular area), and the fifth ICS MCL (mitral valve and left ventricular area). See **Figure 3.1** for depiction of these sites.

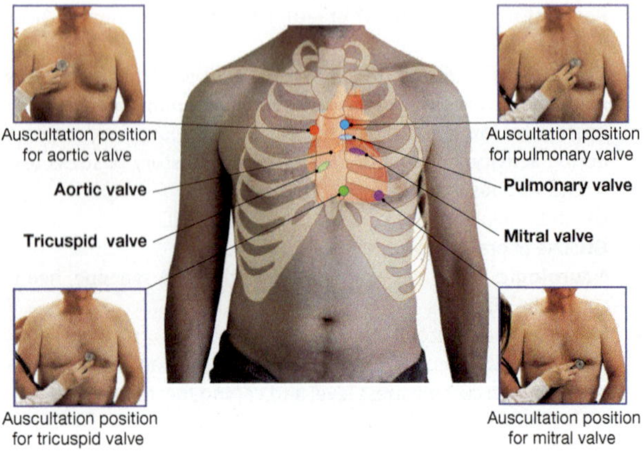

FIGURE 3.1 Auscultatory sites for heart sounds. Positioning for the aortic valve, pulmonary valve, tricuspid valve, and mitral valve.

GENERAL SURVEY

- Important general observations:
  - Does the patient appear comfortable? Those presenting with chest pain or shortness of breath should especially be observed for an urgent or emergent situation.
  - Observe skin color, respiratory effort, and mental status. Abnormalities in these parameters may indicate CV compromise.
  - Discoloration or ulceration of the skin of exposed extremities may indicate peripheral PVD.
- Refer to Box 2.1 (in Chapter 2, "Approach to General Survey and Developmental Assessment") for a reminder of the assessment to determine physiological stability. If the patient's status is unstable, immediate intervention is warranted.

CARDIOVASCULAR EXAMINATION OF THE PATIENT: SEATED POSITION

Blood Pressure and Vital Sign Assessment

- BP, pulse and respiratory rates, temperature, and pulse oximetry are all indices of the CV and PV systems. An increase in an individual's weight over a relatively short period of time may be due to vascular congestion and volume retention due to conditions such as CHF.

- An accurate blood pressure reading in both arms is imperative to both the CV and PV assessments. See Chapter 2, "Approach to General Survey and Developmental Assessment," for more information on vital signs and taking an accurate BP.

Inspection

- Inspect the chest surface. Note the skin color, scars (which may be evidence of prior surgery or an implanted cardiac pacemaker or defibrillator), apparent heaves, lifts, or abnormal pulsations. Heaves and lifts are abnormal outward thrusting or focal movement of the chest wall during the cardiac cycle that may indicate enlarged chambers, aneurysm, or an underlying valvular disorder.
- The apical impulse is visualized at the same anatomic location where the PMI is palpated. This normal pulsation is observed, in normal-size hearts, in the left fifth ICS at or just medial to the MCL. Reference any abnormalities to the known cardiac anatomical landmarks so that consideration is given to the area during palpation of the chest wall.

Palpation

Typically done during the supine portion of the exam; will be discussed in the text that follows.

Auscultation

- Auscultate the apical pulse, noting the heart rate and rhythm. The rhythm should be regular, and the rate should be between 60 and 100 impulses/minute. For any irregular rhythm, note whether there is a regular or irregular pattern. Assess the radial pulse in conjunction with auscultation of the apical pulse. Any difference between the apical rate and the radial pulse rate is noted as a pulse deficit and may indicate an abnormal cardiac rhythm.
- Identify S1 and S2. These heart sounds will allow the clinician to identify systole and diastole and assist in identifying the timing of abnormal heart sounds. S1 indicates the beginning of systole and is heard as a "lub." S1 also coincides with the carotid artery pulse.
- Auscultate the apical pulse while gently palpating the carotid artery (refer to "Carotid Pulse Palpation" later in this chapter for correct carotid palpation technique) to ensure the sound is S1. S1 is heard with each pulsation of the carotid artery. S2 indicates diastole, follows S1, and is heard as "dub." S1, representative of the closure of the mitral and tricuspid valves (AV valves), is heard best at the apex and is louder than S2 at this location. S2, indicating

the closure of the aortic and pulmonic (semilunar) valves, is heard best at the base and is louder than S1 here.

- Listen to the two sounds individually, denoting systole from diastole. A split in the S1 sound (heard best along the LSB) and a physiological S2 split (heard best at the left second and third ICS) are normal. Persistent S2 splitting may indicate underlying conduction or valvular disorder. A fixed S2 split with no variation with respiration may indicate an ASD or a VSD.
- The auscultatory exam may start at the apex or the base of the heart. Regardless of the approach used, follow a "Z" pattern inching along the path, listening throughout systole and diastole at each site. Starting at the base of the heart, from the second right ICS move the stethoscope in turn to the second left ICS, the right sternal border (RSB), and the apex in the fifth ICS near the MCL. The order is reversed if starting at the apex. Listen with the bell first, then repeat the pattern listening with the diaphragm.
- Before completing the seated portion of the exam, the patient is asked to lean forward and hold the breath after full exhalation while the clinician uses the diaphragm to listen along the left LSB. This position brings the left ventricular outflow tract closer to the chest wall and enhances the high-pitched sounds of the semilunar valves.
- At each precordial site, listen first for systole and then diastole relative to S1 and S2. Once these are identified, listen carefully for abnormal or extra heart sounds, such as the third (S3) and fourth (S4) heart sounds or murmurs. S3 and S4 may be auscultated in diastole and can be normal or abnormal. A pathological S3 is also referred to as a ventricular gallop and indicates decreased compliance of the ventricle and volume overload, as might occur in HF or high CO states. Although not often detected in the outpatient setting, evidence strongly supports the utility of an S3 in the diagnosis of HF. S4, occurring immediately before S1, is a soft sound with low pitch. It is heard best with the bell of the stethoscope when the patient is in the left lateral position. A pathological S4, or atrial gallop, may occur as a result of decreased compliance of the ventricle and increased afterload.
- A variety of abnormal heart sounds may be auscultated over the precordium. These can include a variety of murmurs and pericardial friction rubs. Murmurs may be heard as a whooshing, clicking, snapping, vibrating, rumbling, or blowing sound. Murmurs can be benign (physiological) or pathological, related to congenital or acquired abnormalities, such as valvular disease and CHD. Murmurs are described according to eight characteristics: timing, loudness, pitch, pattern, quality, location, radiation, and posture (**Table 3.1**).

TABLE 3.1 Characteristics of Heart Murmurs

Type of Murmur	Precordial Location	Timing in Cardiac Cycle	Radiation	Pitch	Sound Quality	Special Maneuvers
Aortic stenosis	Right second and third intercostal spaces	Mid-systolic	Toward carotid arteries	Crescendo–decrescendo; medium	Harsh	Best heard with patient sitting and leaning forward
Mitral stenosis	Apex	Diastole	None	Decrescendo; low	Rumbling	Use bell of stethoscope at PMI; best heard with patient in left lateral decubitus position
Aortic regurgitation	Left second to fourth intercostal spaces	Diastole	Toward apex	High	Blowing	Best heard with patient sitting and leaning forward with breath held following exhalation
Mitral regurgitation	Apex	Holosystolic	Toward left axilla	Medium/high	Harsh	Murmur should not vary with respiration
Tricuspid regurgitation	Lower left sternal border	Holosystolic	Toward xiphoid process	Medium	Blowing	Murmur will increase with inspiration
Pulmonic stenosis	Left second and third intercostal spaces	Mid-systolic	May radiate to left shoulder	Crescendo–decrescendo; medium	Harsh	None

PMI, point of maximal impulse.

CARDIOVASCULAR EXAMINATION OF THE PATIENT: SUPINE POSITION

Inspection

- The precordial exam is also completed with the patient supine. Lower the HOB so that the patient's head and chest are at a 30° to 45° angle. Young patients and healthy patients with no known or suspected cardiopulmonary disease may be examined lying flat.
- Visual inspection of the chest with the patient in the supine position replicates the inspection completed while in the seated position.

Palpation

- Palpating with the palm of the hand and then the pad(s) of the finger(s), locate the apical pulse (**Figure 3.2A**). It is <2.5 cm in diameter, approximately the size of a quarter. Note the location, size, amplitude (upstroke), intensity (strength/force), and duration of the pulse. The apical impulse represents the brief contraction of the LV and, as such, is located at the apex of the heart, approximately fifth ICS MCL. The apical impulse is the PMI in patients with normal-sized hearts and surrounding anatomy. PMI locates the left border of the heart and is typically in the fifth ICS, 7 to 9 cm lateral to the MSL. Palpation of the apical impulse and PMI provides information about the size of the heart. Displacement of the apical impulse suggests increased LVEDV and left ventricular mass. The apical impulse is palpated with the patient in the supine position but can also be performed in the left lateral position if there is difficulty identifying it while the patient is supine.
- Palpate over the heart region to determine any thrills, lifts, or heaves (**Figure 3.2B**). A *thrill* is a palpable murmur, and any grade 4/6 murmur or louder will have an accompanying palpable thrill. Evidence demonstrates a systolic thrill to be strongly suggestive of significant valvular disease.

Auscultation

- Auscultation of the heart with the patient in the supine position is identical to the exam completed in the seated position, listening over all auscultatory sites with both the bell and the diaphragm. In addition, the patient is asked to turn to the left lateral position and the clinician auscultates over the apex of the heart, left fifth ICS MCL, with the bell. In this position, the LV is closer to the chest wall accentuating S3, S4, and mitral murmurs, specifically mitral valve stenosis.

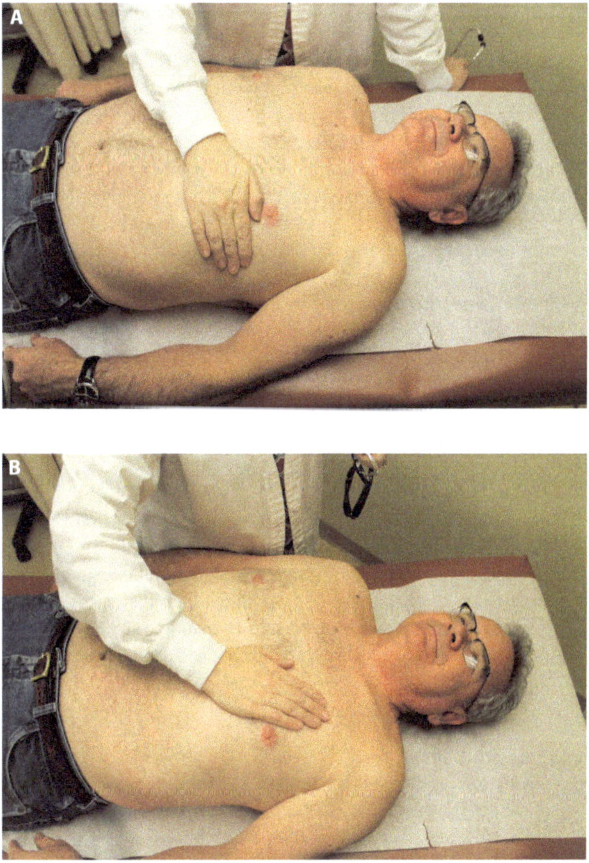

FIGURE 3.2 Palpation of the chest. (**A**) Palpation with palm of hand to locate the apical pulse. (**B**) Palpation over the heart region to determine thrills, lifts, or heaves.

- Patients in whom a systolic murmur has been identified should be examined in additional positions in an attempt to further delineate the origin of the murmur. Examining a patient in the squatting and standing positions can help to distinguish between the systolic murmurs of AS and HCM. AS is best heard in the second right ICS while the murmur of HCM is best heard in the third to fourth left ICS. With the patient in the standing position, and preferably using the exam table for balance, the clinician stands next to the patient and places the stethoscope on the chest. The clinician asks the patient to squat and then stand while auscultating the heart. The patient is asked to momentarily pause while in the squatting position, then rise. The murmur of AS intensifies while the murmur of HCM deceases in intensity during the squatting phase as a result of increased arterial blood pressure, stroke volume, and left ventricular volume. The standing phase decreases arterial blood pressure, stroke volume, and left ventricular volume, thus decreasing the intensity of the AS murmur and intensifying the murmur of HCM. Patients may also be asked to perform the Valsalva maneuver (bear down as when having a bowel movement) while supine. The murmur of HCM intensifies during the Valsalva.

PERIPHERAL VASCULAR EXAMINATION OF THE PATIENT: SUPINE POSITION

- This portion of the exam includes evaluation of the carotid artery, JVP, and vascular aspects of the abdomen and extremities.
- As noted previously, the PV exam of the extremities may be performed with the patient seated. For individuals in whom vascular disease is suspected, it is important to examine the legs supine and seated as color changes can indicate certain disorders.

Inspection

Jugular Venous Pressure

- Identify the jugular vein to be used for measurement of JVP. The internal jugular vein lies deep in the sternomastoid muscle and can be difficult to see. Its pulsation is best visualized in the sternal notch. The top of the external jugular vein is visualized where it overlies the sternomastoid muscle.
- Raise the HOB 30° to 45° for visualization of the jugular vein and measurement of JVP. The angle may be more or less depending on at what elevation or height the jugular column (venous meniscus) is visualized. For patients suspected of hypovolemia, the HOB may need to be lowered for visualization of the jugular pulsation. For those suspected of fluid overload, the HOB may need to be raised higher.
- Use a folded pillow or blanket behind the patient's head to elevate the head off the mattress while maintaining the shoulders on the mattress. Turn the patient's head away and elevate the jaw

slightly. Shine a tangential light across the neck to help visualize the venous motion.

- Place a ruler vertically on the sternal angle (the bony prominence on the sternum below the sternal notch). Use another straight edge as the horizontal reference line. Place the straight edge perpendicular to the ruler across the highest point of the internal jugular pulsation or the point just above where the external jugular appears to collapse (**Figure 3.3**).
- Round the identified measurement to the nearest centimeter. If a jugular pulsation is not noted, it may lie below the level of the sternum and, as such, the venous pressure is not elevated. A measurement of 3 cm above the sternal angle indicates an elevated JVP. An elevated JVP, and thus elevated right heart pressure, is a sign of HF. Traditionally, the right internal jugular vein has been used for this measurement; however, it can be difficult to locate. Studies affirm that using either the right or left internal jugular or right or left external jugular vein provides accurate results.
- If venous pulsations are not visualized in the neck, JVP is likely normal. Lower the HOB until a pulsation is visualized to ensure that the pressure is not so high that it cannot be visualized.
- If JVP is elevated, perform the HJR, also known as the *abdomino-jugular reflux*. With the patient supine, the clinician places their right hand over the mid-abdomen below the right costal margin and pushes firmly for 10 to 15 seconds, observing the right

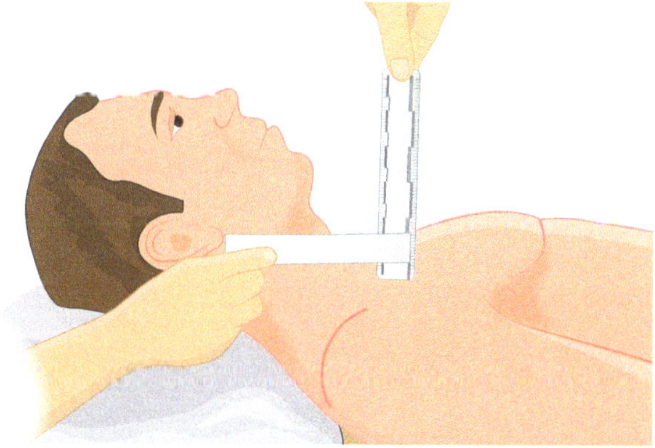

FIGURE 3.3 Assessment for jugular venous distention or pressure measurement.

jugular. If the jugular rises for a few seconds and then returns to baseline, the CVP is considered normal. Sustained elevation of the jugular is consistent with elevated CVP. In conjunction with an elevated JVP, positive HJR increases the likelihood (LR+ 8.0) of elevated venous pressure.

Palpation

- Palpate the right and left carotid arteries, located just medial to the sternomastoid muscle. The patient should be in the supine position with the HOB elevated to 30° to 45°. Do not apply firm pressure or palpate both carotids at the same time; this can compromise blood flow to the brain, causing syncope. Using several fingers, palpate the artery at the level of the cricoid cartilage. Use the right fingers to palpate the left carotid pulse and vice versa. Avoid palpating near the top of the thyroid cartilage, the location of the carotid sinus, as pressure on this may cause slowing of the heart rate. Note the symmetry, rhythm, rate, amplitude (or upstroke), and intensity (or strength, force) of the pulse. It should be smooth and symmetric with a brisk upstroke.
- Palpation of the carotid artery may be done in conjunction with cardiac auscultation during identification of S1 and S2. Palpation of the carotid and femoral arterial pulses simultaneously is done for suspected coarctation of the aorta. With this condition, there is delayed transmission and amplitude of the femoral pulse as compared with the carotid.

Auscultation

- Carotid artery auscultation is completed after palpation, when there is an indication of neurologic signs or symptoms consistent with decreased cerebral blood flow, as occurs with carotid artery stenosis, or when a palpable bruit is identified.
- Place the bell of the stethoscope over the identified carotid artery (**Figure 3.4**). Ask the patient to take a breath, exhale, and hold the breath. Holding the breath helps to avoid interpreting tracheal sounds as turbulent blood flow. This technique also avoids contraction of the levator scapulae muscle in the neck from dampening the sound. As when listening for other turbulent blood flow, note a blowing or swishing sound, a carotid bruit. Cardiac murmurs may be transmitted from the heart to the carotids. To avoid interpreting a heart murmur for a bruit, perform a complete precordial exam.

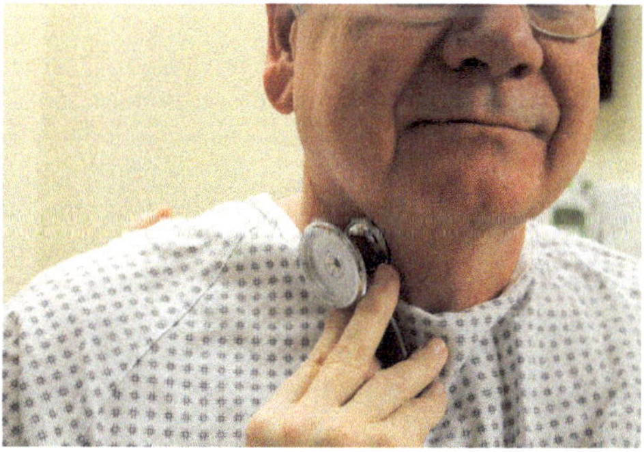

FIGURE 3.4 Auscultation of carotid artery.

ABDOMEN

Refer to Chapter 12, "Evidence-Based Assessment of the Abdomen and Gastrointestinal and Urologic Systems," for information on completing the PV exam for the abdomen, including inspection, auscultation, and palpation of the aortic, renal, and femoral arteries.

EXTREMITIES

Inspection

- Inspect the extremities. Note the skin color (keeping in mind the patient's ethnicity). Assess the color of the nails, noting any cyanosis. Check for capillary refill (see Chapter 4, "Evidence-Based Assessment of Lungs and Respiratory System").
- Examine the lower extremities for skin color, hair distribution, lesions, and edema. Arms and legs should be symmetric in size. Decreased hair distribution, cool skin, skin ulcerations, pale legs on elevation, and dusky red skin in the dependent position may be signs of PAD. Brown pigmentation or petechiae of the skin, cyanosis with leg dependency, stasis dermatitis (dry, scaling, hyperpigmented skin), and ulcerations may indicate venous insufficiency. Note any varicosities (engorged veins) of the legs. Note edema of the lower extremities as this may indicate poor venous return (as in venous insufficiency) or fluid retention, as occurs in HF.

Palpation

- Palpate the arms and legs for skin temperature, texture, turgor, and edema. Lower-extremity edema is identified as either pitting or nonpitting, with pitting edema graded 1 to 4. Press firmly and gently with the thumb over the dorsum of the foot and pretibial area of the lower leg (shin). Hold the pressure for 5 seconds. Pitting is present if an indentation remains in the tissue after the thumb is removed (**Figure 3.5**). Grade the pitting and note the extent to which the edema ascends the extremity. See **Box 3.1** for information on grading and documenting edema.

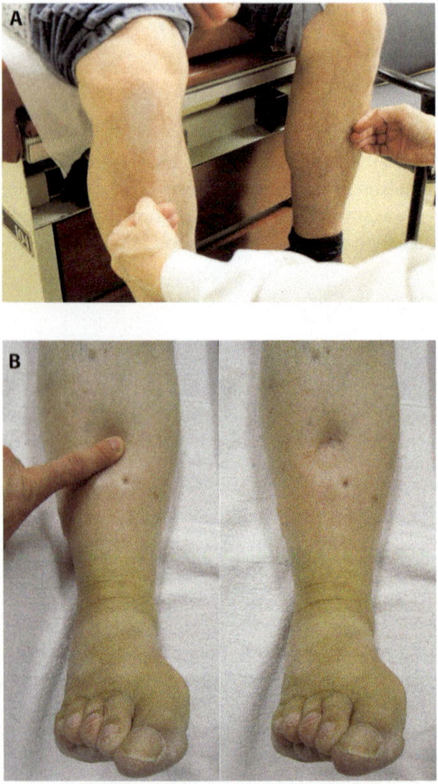

FIGURE 3.5 (**A**) Palpation of the legs. (**B**) Pitting edema.

Source: Part B image courtesy of James Heilman, MD.

BOX 3.1
DOCUMENTING EDEMA

The following scale is used to grade pitting edema:

- 1+: Mild pitting with only slight indentation and no appreciable extremity edema
- 2+: Moderate pitting; thumb indentation resolves rapidly
- 3+: Deep pitting; indentation remains for brief period of time and appreciable extremity edema present
- 4+: Severe pitting; indentation remains for a long time and the extremity is obviously swollen

Nonpitting edema is graded according to severity:

- Mild
- Moderate
- Severe

Documentation also includes the extent to which the edema ascends the extremity (e.g., moderate nonpitting edema of the feet, ankles, and halfway up the calf).

BOX 3.2
GRADING SCALE FOR PULSES

Pulses are graded on a 3-point scale according to the strength or force of the pulse:

- 3+: Bounding
- 2+: Normal
- 1+: Weak
- 0: Absent

- If unilateral edema is present, use a tape measure to document the difference between the two extremities. Measure at the smallest and largest difference of the calf and the circumference of the mid-thigh (if edema is present here). While there is a slight difference in the measurement of extremities, a difference of more than 1 to 2 cm is considered abnormal. Unilateral edema may be due to an injury, a venous thrombosis, lymphatic obstruction, or impaired venous return from a proximal obstruction.
- Note the symmetry, rate, rhythm, amplitude (or upstroke), and intensity (strength or force) of the peripheral pulses (**Box 3.2**). The

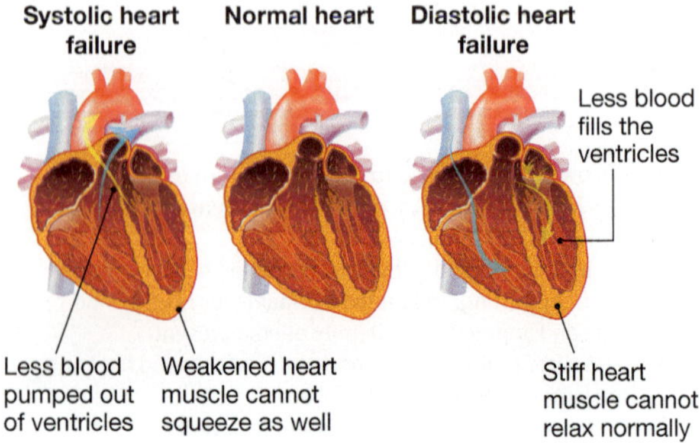

FIGURE 3.6 Heart failure.

peripheral pulses include the radial, brachial, femoral, popliteal, posterior tibial (PT), and dorsalis pedis (DP). Light pressure on the pulse is important as firm pressure may obliterate the pulsation. In some adults, this pulse may be absent bilaterally (**Figure 3.6**).

PEDIATRIC CONSIDERATIONS

- Many aspects of the physical exam in infants and children are the same as adults.
- Auscultation of heart sounds may indicate different disease processes in the pediatric population; however, they occur at the same landmarks and are described and classified in the same fashion.
- General appearance of the infant or child (happy or cranky), as well as nutritional and respiratory status, are very important in infants and children. Subtle changes in these systems can signal warning signs for CHD.
- Palpation of pulses is another very important exam technique in infants and children as differentials in pulses between extremities can be indicative of a coarctation of the aorta while bounding pulses may be indicative of a shunt lesion.
- BP evaluation in children is just as important as it is in adults and can help screen for heart diseases. Clinicians should be familiar with appropriate techniques for obtaining BP as well as normative blood pressure ranges for infants and children by age. See Chapter 2, "Approach to General Survey and Developmental Assessment," Table 2.1, for normal BPs by age.

CONSIDERATIONS FOR THE OLDER ADULT

History questions and the physical exam for older adults presenting with cardiac symptoms are not different from those used for the adult. However, age itself is an independent risk factor for CV disease so the likelihood of CV disease being present is much higher in the older adult.

RED FLAGS IN OBJECTIVE EXAM

- Diaphoresis with reported chest pain, nausea/vomiting
- Bleeding
- Tachycardia or bradycardia
- Pulselessness
- Sudden confusion; change in mental status
- Unilateral weakness; facial drooping
- Slurred speech
- Sudden trouble walking or seeing
- Cold with color changes to extremity

EVIDENCE-BASED RESOURCES

- **American College of Cardiology Guidelines:** www.acc.org/guidelines#tab1
- **American Heart Association Guidelines:** www.professional.heart.org/professional/GuidelinesStatements/UCM_316885_Guidelines-Statements.jsp
- **American Society of Echocardiography Guidelines:** www.asecho.org/guidelines/guidelines-standards
- **Choosing Wisely Guidelines:** www.choosingwisely.org
- **Heart Rhythm Society Clinical Resources:** www.hrsonline.org/guidance/clinical-resources
- **Society for CV Magnetic Resonance Guidelines:** www.asecho.org/guidelines/guidelines-standards
- **Society for Vascular Medicine Guidelines:** vascular.org/research-quality/guidelines-and-reporting-standards/clinical-practice-guidelines
- **United States Preventive Services Task Force Guidelines:** www.uspreventiveservicestaskforce.org/uspstf/recommendation-topics/uspstf-and-b-recommendations

ABNORMAL FINDINGS

The abnormal findings and differential diagnoses listed in this section are in alphabetical order, rather than order of prevalence. The list not exhaustive.

ABDOMINAL AORTIC ANEURYSM

A ballooning or weakening of the aortic wall that is predisposed to rupturing.

History

- History of atherosclerosis and/or hypertension; family history of aneurysms
- Older age
- History of smoking
- Caucasian males are more affected
- Asymptomatic in the majority of patients; if symptomatic but not ruptured, pain is typically near the position of the aneurysm (epigastric region of the abdomen, back, flank, or pelvic region)
- Has an indolent onset
- Pain does not change with position or movement
- History of syncope or feeling faint

Physical Examination

- Pulsatile abdominal mass
- Bounding pulse
- Ruptured AAA triad: severe acute pain, a pulsatile abdominal mass, and hypotension occurs in approximately 50% of patients

Consideration

- Most often this condition is diagnosed with an ultrasound.

ACUTE CORONARY SYNDROME

A constellation of symptoms caused by a prolonged period of decreased myocardial oxygenation, due to decreased blood flow in the coronary arteries.

History

- Older age
- Smoking
- History of HTN, atherosclerosis, PAD, diabetes, HLD
- Lack of exercise; unhealthy diet
- Recent cocaine use
- Overweight/obese

- Family history of heart disease
- History of an abnormal stress test
- Chest pain that is described as aching, pressure, squeezing, tightness, or burning; occurs at rest and with activity; does not change with respiration or position; change in pain pattern over the past 24 hours and pain is unrelieved with nitroglycerin; pain radiating to both arms, left arm, jaw, or neck
- Nausea/vomiting
- Shortness of breath
- Fatigue
- Dizziness, lightheadedness, syncope
- Feeling of impending doom

Physical Examination

- Diaphoresis
- General appearance of distress and unrest
- Changes in blood pressure (hypotension, hypertension, or can be normotensive)
- Changes in pulse (tachycardia or bradycardia)
- EKG abnormalities (ST depression)
- Elevated cardiac serum markers (troponin)
- HEART Score (Than et al., 2014) range 7 to 10
- TIMI risk score (Antman et al., 2000) of 5 or higher

Considerations

- Patients with a history of ACS experience a decrease in ability to perform ordinary activities, and experience other comorbidities and mental health issues that affect their quality of life.
- About 10% of patients who present with acute chest pain are diagnosed with ACS.

ATHEROSCLEROSIS AND CORONARY ARTERY DISEASE

Atherosclerosis is a condition that causes thickening and loss of elasticity of the arterial wall due to plaques. Atherosclerosis causes CAD. See **Box 3.3** for the American Heart Association and American College of Cardiology Risk Calculator for Estimating 10-Year Risk for Atherosclerotic CV Disease.

History

- HLD, HTN, metabolic syndrome, intermittent claudication, TIAs, heart attacks, angina, and/or stroke
- Smoking
- Diabetes
- Asymptomatic in mild disease

BOX 3.3

RISK CALCULATOR FOR ESTIMATING 10-YEAR RISK FOR ATHEROSCLEROTIC CARDIOVASCULAR DISEASE*

Calculation Information:

- Age, gender, race
- Systolic and diastolic blood pressure
- Total cholesterol, HDL, and LDL
- History of diabetes, smoking (current, former, never)
- Current (yes/no) medications for HTN, statin, or on aspirin therapy

Factors Increasing ASCVD Risk Included in Clinician-Patient Risk Discussion:

- Family history of premature ASCVD
- Primary hypercholesterolemia
- Metabolic syndrome
- Chronic kidney disease
- Chronic inflammatory conditions
- History of premature menopause
- History of pregnancy-associated conditions that increase later ASCVD risk (e.g., preeclampsia)
- High-risk race/ethnicity (e.g., South Asian ancestry)
- Lipids/biomarkers associated with increased ASCVD risk

10-year risk for ASCVD:

- Low-risk (<5%)
- Borderline risk (5%–7.4%)
- Intermediate risk (7.5%–19.9%)
- High risk (≥20%)

*Calculations are for those without ASCVD only. Calculator can be found online at http://tools.acc.org/ASCVD-Risk-Estimator-Plus/#!/calculate/estimate

ASCVD, atherosclerotic cardiovascular disease; HDL, high-density lipoprotein; HTN, hypertension; LDL, low-density lipoprotein.

- Chest pain in the middle or left side (can extend into left arm, jaw, or neck pain); pain worsens with activity or emotional stress
- Shortness of breath

Physical Examination

- High BP
- Abdominal obesity
- Weak pulses
- Bruits

- Decreased blood pressure in limbs
- Elevated inflammatory biomarkers (C-reactive protein)
- Coronary artery calcium score >100 (moderate disease), >300 (severe disease)
- Ankle–brachial index <0.9 or >1.4

Considerations

- Signs and symptoms of transient ischemia (e.g., stable angina, TIAs) may appear when lesions decrease blood flow by narrowing the arterial lumen by 70% or more and/or by rupturing and acutely occluding a major artery.
- Atherosclerosis and CAD can also lead to aneurysms, arterial dissection, or sudden death without any prior symptoms of angina.

ATRIAL SEPTAL DEFECT

An opening between the RA and the LA, or the upper two chambers of the heart. ASD is common in combination with other heart defects and is often critical to blood flow and oxygenation in some congenital heart diseases.

History

- Family history of ASD
- Genetic syndromes: Holt–Oram syndrome, trisomy 21, Noonan's syndrome
- Young infants and children are often asymptomatic
- Occasionally an infant with isolated ASD may present as symptomatic with signs of CHF
- Older children may present with mild fatigue or dyspnea
- Adults with an unrecognized or untreated ASD may develop right-sided HF, pulmonary HTN, or Eisenmenger's syndrome

Physical Examination

- Wide fixed split S2: hallmark finding
- Systolic ejection murmur at the left parasternal area (midway between sternal border and midclavicular line); murmurs may be very soft in early childhood
- Those with long-standing left to right shunting: Left precordial bulge, and prominent RV impulse
- Abnormalities on chest x-ray, transesophageal echocardiogram, and occasionally on EKG (NSR) but may have prolonged QRS

Considerations

- ASD is common in combination with other heart defects and is often critical to blood flow and oxygenation in some CHD.
- As an isolated heart defect, ASD accounts for approximately 8% to 10% of congenital heart defects in children.

CHRONIC VENOUS INSUFFICIENCY

A condition caused by stasis and reflux of venous blood flow.

History

- History of prolonged sitting or standing throughout the day
- Obesity, physical inactivity
- Older age
- Female gender
- Prior injury to the extremity
- Pregnancy
- Can be asymptomatic, especially early in disease
- Aching in lower legs is the most commonly reported symptom
- Heaviness and itching in lower legs

Physical Examination

- Pitting edema in lower legs (cardinal sign)
- Varicose veins
- Will often see combined edema and hyperpigmented skin, sometimes called *brawny edema*
- Reduced ankle motion
- Hyperpigmentation and lipodermatosclerosis (inflamed and thickened skin) signal more advanced disease
- Lower-extremity ulcerations
- Normal sensory and motor exams (helps exclude diabetic neuropathy)
- Abdominal exam should be normal and helps exclude abdominal mass as cause for venous insufficiency.

Considerations

- CVI exists along a continuum that progresses from small telangiectasic "spider" veins to varicose veins, and, in severe cases, venous ulcers.
- CVI can occur at various anatomical levels, including superficial, deep, and perforating veins. Location of venous ulcers can be a clue to the location of the disease.

COARCTATION OF THE AORTA

A defect of the aortic arch involving a narrowing of the arch often occurring at the insertion site of the ductus arteriosus.

History

- Family history of coarctation
- Genetic syndromes: Turner's syndrome, 22q11.2 (DiGeorge's) syndrome
- Many infants will present with symptoms within the first week of life as the ductus arteriosus closes, hence limiting blood flow past the obstruction

- Infants with a critical obstruction to blood flow will present with acute symptoms of shock, metabolic acidosis, renal failure, and necrotizing enterocolitis

Physical Examination

- Murmur: Systolic ejection murmur along the left sternal border
- Gallop rhythm common
- Older children or adults may present with systemic HTN and a murmur
- Signs of CHF
  - Pulse abnormalities: Weak or absent femoral pulses; a delay between upper and lower extremity pulses
  - Tachypnea and tachycardia
  - Skin mottling, delayed capillary refill, and peripheral cyanosis
  - Chest x-ray abnormalities
- EKG abnormalities
  - Infants: Normal right ventricular dominance with right axis deviation
  - Older child or adult: LVH
- Echocardiogram: Shows location and degree of coarctation as well as velocity measurements to determine severity.

Considerations

- Coarctation can present in varying degrees depending on the amount of narrowing.
- Critical coarctation in the infant is a life-threatening condition if not quickly recognized and treated. Coarctation can be repaired with surgery or by stenting the narrowed segment.
- Children or adults with repaired coarctation require lifelong cardiology follow-up, as they can have re-coarctation or complications arising from the initial surgical repair.

CONGESTIVE HEART FAILURE

A complex syndrome caused by ventricular dysfunction and results in the inability of the heart to sufficiently meet the body's metabolic needs required to sustain life (see Figure 3.6).

History

- Fatigue, anorexia, nausea, weakness
- Medical history of AMI, LVH, diabetes, obesity, and/or hypertension
- Smoking, sedentary lifestyle
- Nocturia
- Chest pain, heaviness, or tightness (if caused by an AMI)
- Dyspnea at rest or with exertion
- Difficulty completing ADL

Physical Examination

- Arrhythmia or tachycardia
- Abdominal fluid accumulation (ascites)
- JVD
- Cough with white or pink blood-tinged exudate
- Edema, swelling
- Displacement of PMI
- Weight gain (can be rapid from fluid retention)
- Elevated ANP, BNP; elevated Gal-3 and sST2 proteins

Considerations

- HF has a significant impact on HRQoL, including higher rates of depression, higher BMI, low perceived control, and uncertainty about prognosis.
- The term *heart failure* is not the same as *cardiomyopathy* or *LV dysfunction* because the latter two terms describe structural or functional abnormalities that cause HF.
- There are two main classifications of HF based on EF of LV; HFpEF and HFrEF (Yancy et al., 2013). HFrEF is defined as HF with LVEF ≤40%, and HFpEF is HF with LVEF ≥50% EF. More recently, patients with an LVEF between 40% and 50% have been classified as HFmrEF (Yancy et al., 2013).
- HF classification is important because it helps describe severity and development of disease progression. It can also guide therapy choices. There are several different classification systems. The New York Heart Association functional classification system and the ACC/AHA classification are two of the most widely used.

DEEP VEIN THROMBOSIS

Occurs when clots develop in the deep venous systems of the extremities.

History

- Active cancer
- History of recent immobilization, bed rest, or surgery
- Recent travel
- Mostly occurs in the lower extremities but can occur in the upper extremities
- History of prior DVT or coagulation disorders
- Estrogen use (including birth control pills)
- Pregnancy

Physical Examination

- Unilateral leg edema
- Visible collateral superficial veins

TABLE 3.2 Wells' Clinical Prediction Tool

Criteria	Point
Active cancer	1
Immobilization or paralysis of lower extremity	1
Recent bed restrictions	1
Tenderness along the deep venous system	1
Leg swelling (ankle to thigh)	1
Symptomatic leg swollen >3 cm compared with asymptomatic leg	1
Pitting edema of symptomatic leg > asymptomatic leg	1
Prior DVT	1
Visible collateral superficial veins other than varicose veins	1
Other diagnosis than DVT more or as likely	–2
Low pretest probability of DVT = score of 1 or less high pretest probability = score of 2 or higher	

DVT, deep vein thrombosis.
Source: From Wells, P. S., Anderson, D. R., Bormanis, J., Guy, F., Mitchell, M., Gray, L., Clement, C., Robinson, K. S., & Lewandowski, B. (1997). Value of assessment of pretest probability of deep-vein thrombosis in clinical management. *The Lancet*, *350*(9094), 1795–1798. doi:10.1016/S0140-6736(97)08140-3

- Pitting edema in the leg
- Leg size greater than opposite leg
- In the outpatient, a score of one or less on the Wells' criteria (**Table 3.2**) combined with a negative D-dimer test reduces the probability of DVT to <2%

Considerations

- There is risk for serious sequelae, like pulmonary embolus, especially if the diagnosis is missed.
- The Well's Clinical Prediction Tool, which can be used to determine the need for further imaging, can be found in Table 3.2.

HYPERTENSION

See Chapter 2, "Approach to General Survey and Developmental Assessment," for information on hypertension.

INFECTIVE ENDOCARDITIS

An infection of the endocardial surface of the heart, which may include one or more heart valves, the mural endocardium, or a septal defect that causes severe valvular insufficiency, which may lead to intractable CHF and myocardial abscesses.

History

- Fever, chills, malaise
- Dyspnea, cough
- Arthralgias
- History of dental disease
- History of IV drug use

Physical Examination

- Petechiae: Common, but nonspecific, finding
- Subungual (splinter) hemorrhages: Dark-red, linear lesions in the nail beds
- Osler's nodes: Tender subcutaneous nodules usually found on the distal pads of the digits
- Janeway lesions: Nontender maculae on the palms and soles
- Focal neurologic deficits, including paralysis, hemiparesis, aphasia
- Delirium
- Gallops
- Rales
- Cardiac arrhythmias
- Pericardial or pleural friction rub

Consideration

- Many organisms have been identified as causative agents; however, *Staphylococcus aureus* has become the primary pathogen of endocarditis. Untreated, it is often fatal.

MITRAL VALVE PROLAPSE

Displacement or prolapse of the mitral valve leaflets into the LA during systole.

History

- Family history of MVP
- History of Graves' disease, sickle cell, or RHD
- Can be asymptomatic
- Chest pain
- Fatigue

- Dyspnea on exertion
- Anxiety
- Heart palpitations or arrhythmias

Physical Examination

- Midsystolic click on auscultation of heart
- Mitral valve leaflet thickness ≥5 mm by echocardiography

Considerations

- There is evidence that suggests a good prognosis exists with MVP; however, there are instances of serious complications such as sudden cardiac death, endocarditis, or severe MVP.
- The degree of leaflet thickness can help ascertain the severity of disease as it is associated with a 14-fold higher risk of complications, including sudden death.

PERICARDITIS

An inflammation of the pericardium, which is the fibroelastic membrane that surrounds the heart.

History

- History of acute trauma or infection
- Autoimmune disease
- Can be acute or chronic
- Chills or weakness
- Chest pain that worsens with breathing and lying down
- Chest pain that improves with sitting upright or leaning forward

Physical Examination

- Tachypnea and nonproductive cough
- Fever >100.4 °F
- Pericardial friction rub
- If cardiac tamponade (pressure on heart secondary to accumulation of fluid in the pericardial sac) occurs, additional signs (rare) are cool extremities, cyanosis, hypotension, and decreased systolic BP >10 mmHg during inspiration

Considerations

- Pericarditis may be secondary to a systemic disease process or a primary process unrelated to another systemic disease.
- The disease can cause cardiac tamponade, which is the presence of fluid in the pericardial sac.

PERIPHERAL ARTERY DISEASE

An atherosclerotic disease that affects the arteries of the lower extremities (**Figure 3.7**).

History

- Past or present smoking history
- African American race
- History of HTN, HLD, chronic kidney disease, diabetes, or metabolic syndrome
- Older age (>65)
- Pain in the calves or other parts of the lower extremity (iliac, femoral, popliteal, peroneal, and/or tibial arteries); exacerbated by exercise
- Can be bilateral or unilateral
- 20% can be asymptomatic

Physical Examination

- Femoral and iliac bruits (present in advanced and/or proximal disease)
- Weak or no posterior tibialis and/or DP pulses
- Asymmetric temperature to feet
- Hairless lower extremities and atrophic skin
- Lower-extremity ulcers/wounds usually found on the toes and feet and have a well-demarcated border
- Ulcers are painful and lack edema

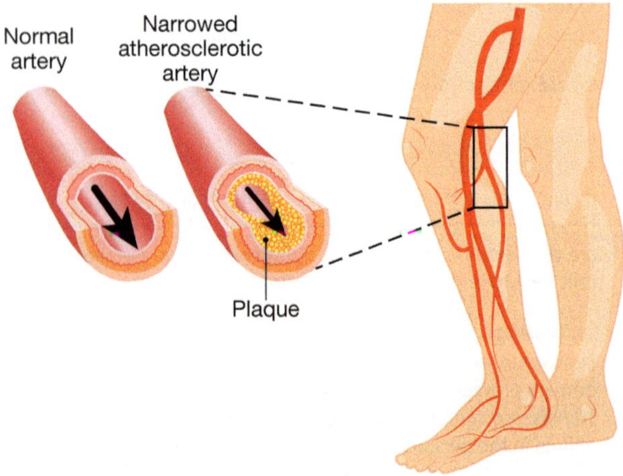

FIGURE 3.7 Peripheral artery disease.

RAYNAUD'S PHENOMENON

Occurs from vasomotor dysfunction that affects the distal arterial circulation of the fingers, toes, earlobes, face, nipples, or nose.

History

- Females are more affected than males
- Family history of Raynaud's
- History of co-occurring vascular diseases like PAD and CVI
- Vasospasms last a few minutes to a few hours
- Most often, the fingers (index, middle, and ring fingers) are affected, followed by the toes
- Can affect a single digit or only part of a digit
- Triggered by cold or stress
- As the recovery of pallor ensues, the affected extremities can become hyperemic and patients may experience pain, numbness, and tingling

Physical Examination

- Thinner patients
- Color change of digits, "tricolor" phase of symptoms (from white to blue to red)
- Sclerodactyly, or thickening and tightness of the skin of the affected areas, is highly associated with Raynaud's phenomenon

Consideration

- Primarily diagnosed through history and physical exam; however, diagnostic tests can be used.

RHEUMATIC HEART DISEASE

Sequelae of RF characterized by permanent damage to the heart valves. RF is an inflammatory response in the body that is a result of untreated strep throat and/or scarlet fever.

History

- History of suspected RF or untreated or undertreated strep throat
- Living in poverty or a lower socioeconomic status
- Little access to healthcare
- Joint pain and/or arthritis symptoms
- Children may not have any initial symptoms

Physical Examination

- Pathological heart murmur (mitral or aortic valve stenosis or regurgitation)
- Chest pain or swelling due to myocarditis or pericarditis
- Flat or slightly raised, painless rash with a ragged edge
- Small, painless bumps beneath the skin

Considerations

- Symptoms of RHD show up 10 to 20 years after the original illness.
- Most often, the mitral valve is damaged but the aortic valve can also be affected.
- Usually, RHD can be prevented by preventing strep infections or treating them with antibiotics when they do occur.

TETRALOGY OF FALLOT

A cyanotic congenital heart defect that comprises four different defects: VSD, overriding aorta, PS, and RV hypertrophy.

History

- Family history of CHD
- 70% are diagnosed prenatally with a 90% accuracy on ultrasound
- Genetic syndromes: 22q11.2 deletion (DiGeorge's syndrome); trisomy 21, 18, 13; Holt–Oram syndrome; Alagille's syndrome
- Reports irritability and/or prolonged crying
- Reports tiring easily during play or exercise
- Episodes of loss of consciousness and "tet spells"

Physical Examination

- "Tet spells" (an acute decrease in blood across the right ventricular outflow tract, causing the infant to suddenly develop deep blue skin, nails, and lips after crying or feeding)
- Poor weight gain
- Murmur: Systolic ejection murmur at left lower sternal border with a single S2
- Clubbing
- Cyanosis: Varying degrees
- Abnormalities on chest x-ray, EKG, and echocardiogram

Consideration

- Most infants with TOF do well with surgical intervention and survive into adulthood.

VENTRICULAR SEPTAL DEFECT

An opening between the RV and the LV. A VSD often occurs in combination with other heart defects as well as in isolation.

History

- Family history of VSD
- Genetic syndromes: Trisomy 13, 18, and 21; Holt–Oram syndrome

- Maternal use of marijuana, cocaine, and paint stripping
- Poor eating
- Failure to thrive
- Easy tiring, fatigue, and weakness

Physical Examination

- Tachypnea
- Murmur; dependent on the size of defect:
  - Large defect: May not have a significant murmur or may have a short systolic ejection murmur
  - Small defect: Loud holosystolic murmur often recognized in early infancy
- Abnormalities on chest x-ray, EKG, and echocardiogram

Considerations

- Small VSDs are pressure restrictive, and infants do not develop volume overload or CHF symptoms. Smaller defects may spontaneously close over time.
- Large VSDs, that are left untreated, can result in development of CHF, pulmonary vascular disease, and Eisenmenger's syndrome.

PHYSICAL EXAMINATION DOCUMENTATION

CV SYSTEM

Documentation should include results of inspection, palpation, and auscultation.

Example of Normal Findings

Skin on chest and back without lesions, rashes, or erythema. No visible heaves, or lifts over precordium; apical impulse visualized at 5th ICS of left chest at MCL. No palpable heaves, lifts or thrills over precordial area, apical impulse palpable at 5th ICS of left MCL. Auscultation: S1 and S2 crisp. S1 more prominent at heart's apex, S2 more prominent at base; rate and rhythm regular without extra heart sounds, murmurs, gallops, clicks, or friction rubs audible.

PERIPHERAL VASCULAR SYSTEM

Documentation should include results of inspection, palpation, and auscultation.

Example of Normal Findings

Skin on extremities are without lesions, rashes, varicosities, or stasis changes. JVP is 3 cm above sternal angle with head of bed at 30 degrees. No visible pulsations on the chest or abdomen. Carotid arteries are symmetric, brisk, and without bruits bilateral. Extremities are warm, non-edematous, and non-tender to palpation. Radial, brachial, femoral, popliteal, DP, and posterior tibialis 2+ bilateral. No abdominal or femoral bruits noted.

REFERENCES

References from this chapter draw from Chapter 6, "Evidence-Based Assessment of the Heart and Circulatory System," of the textbook *Evidence-Based Physical Examination: Best Practices for Health and Well-Being Assessment*. The references may be accessed in the digital version of the handbook at connect.springerpub.com/content/book/ https://connect.springerpub.com/content/book/978-0-8261-6466-7/ chapter/ch03

Antman, E. M., Cohen, M., Bernink, P. J. L. M., McCabe, C. H., Horacek, T., Papuchis, G., Mautner, B., Corbalan, R., Radley, D., & Braunwald, E. (2000). The TIMI risk score for unstable angina/non–ST elevation MI: A method for prognostication and therapeutic decision making. *Journal of the American Medical Association, 284*(7), 835–842. https://doi.org/10.1001/jama.284.7.835

Than, M., Aldous, S., Lord, S. J., Goodacre, S., Frampton, C. M. A., Troughton, R., George, P., Florkowski, C. M., Ardagh, M., Smyth, D., Jardine, D. L., Peacock, W. F., Young, J., Hamilton, G., Deely, J. M., Cullen, L., & Mark Richards, A. (2014). A 2-hour diagnostic protocol for possible cardiac chest pain in the emergency department: A randomized clinical trial. *JAMA Internal Medicine, 174*(1), 51–58. https://doi.org/10.1001/jamainternmed.2013.11362

Yancy, C. W., Jessup, M., Bozkurt, B., Butler, J., Casey, D. E., Jr, Drazner, M. H., Fonarow, G. C., Geraci, S. A., Horwich, T., Januzzi, J. L., Johnson, M. R., Kasper, E. K., Levy, W. C., Masoudi, F. A., McBride, P. E., McMurray, J. J. V., Mitchell, J. E., Peterson, P. N., Riegel, B., Sam, F., Stevenson, L. W., Wilson Tang, W. H., Tsai, E. J., & Wilkoff, B. L. (2013). 2013 ACCF/AHA guideline for the management of heart failure. *Circulation, 128*(16), e240–e327. https://doi.org/10.1161/CIR.0b013e31829e8776

4

Evidence-Based Assessment of Lungs and Respiratory System

CLINICAL CONSIDERATIONS

- Assessing respiratory status is a key factor in determining the extent or severity of illness.
- Best practice for the examination of the respiratory system is not to assess over clothing.
- Clean the entire surface of a stethoscope after use, including the ear tips.
- Pertinent health history includes assessment for recent travel and illness exposures.
- Ask about smoking status and exposure to secondhand smoke. Advise individuals that it is never too late to quit smoking.

SUBJECTIVE HISTORY

COMMON REASONS FOR SEEKING CARE

Shortness of breath or dyspnea, cough, chest congestion

HISTORY OF PRESENT ILLNESS

- **Onset:** When did the symptoms start? What was the individual doing when they became symptomatic? Did this occur suddenly or has it been developing gradually?
- **Location:** Does the symptom have associated pain or discomfort? If so, where is the discomfort located?
- **Duration:** How long do symptom(s) last? Over what period of time has the respiratory symptom developed?
- **Characteristics:** Is the patient winded, unable to take air in, feeling short of breath, wheezing, or coughing? If coughing, is the

cough deep, barking, whooping, spasmodic, or productive? If productive, is sputum frothy, foul-smelling, thick, large volume, blood-streaked, or with frank bleeding? Is the patient experiencing or noticing any color changes of lips, mucosa, or nails associated with the symptom(s)?

- **Aggravating factors:** What actions, activities, or body positions make the symptoms worse? If exertion worsens symptoms, clarify level of exertion that causes exacerbation. If lying flat worsens symptoms, clarify number of pillows needed to rest easy. Has exposure to smells, dust, pollen, smoking, or activities caused an increase in symptoms?
- **Relieving factors:** What actions, activities, or body positions decrease the symptoms? If relieved, how long does the relief last?
- **Treatment:** What medications has the individual taken to help with the symptoms? Did the patient use any breathing treatments or inhaled respiratory medications? Clarify dosage and frequency of any medications.
- **Severity:** How severe are the symptoms on a scale of 0 to 10? Do the symptoms limit participation in activities? Are there associated symptoms? Are the symptoms worsening? Is the individual feeling anxious or fearful?

HEALTH HISTORY

Past Medical History

- History of respiratory illnesses throughout their life span:
  - Premature birth history or lung disease diagnosed during childhood
  - Previous diagnoses of asthma, bronchiolitis, bronchitis, pneumonia, emphysema
  - Previous emergency room visits or hospital stays for respiratory problems
  - History of need for intubation, mechanical ventilation, or respiratory resuscitation
  - Previous thoracic procedure or surgery
  - Recurrent respiratory illnesses that caused shortness of breath, wheezing, or cough
  - History of eczema or allergic rhinitis
  - Similar symptoms (note circumstances)
- Comorbidities or risk factors related to pulmonary disease:
  - Recent travel (note mode of transportation, location, & length of stay)
  - Recent exposure to individual with flu, flu-like symptoms, or COVID-19

   - Known or suspected pulmonary, cardiac, or renal disease
   - History of malignancy
   - Recent surgery, hospitalization, or immobility
   - Pregnancy status, note likelihood of pregnancy or if currently or recently pregnant

Medications

- Prescribed and OTC medications or supplements, including dose and frequency
- Use of inhalers, nebulizers, and/or spacers, and how they are being used
- Recent antibiotic and/or oral steroid use
- Recent start of ACE inhibitors

Allergies

- Allergies to medications or seasonal, environmental, and/or food allergies
- If yes to being allergic to any substance or environmental trigger, clarify reaction:
   - Nausea, intestinal upset? Vomiting?
   - Skin rashes, itching? Hives?
   - Swelling of tongue, lips, face?
   - Dyspnea, wheezing, dizziness?

Immunizations

Risks for vaccine-preventable illnesses: Vaccine status; date of last influenza, pertussis, and pneumococcal vaccinations; risks for tuberculosis, flu, pertussis, pneumonia

Pediatric Considerations Related to Health History

- Additional assessments for children under 3 years of age and/or presenting with respiratory symptoms:
   - Birth history:
      - Delivery eventful or uneventful, vaginal or C-section, prolonged or abrupt?
      - Any respiratory distress after birth? Any apneic episodes? Did the child require oxygen, pulse oximetry monitoring, or support for breathing as an infant? Apgar scores at birth?
      - Mother's health during pregnancy? Exposures during pregnancy?
      - Fetal abnormalities identified during the prenatal stage?

- Growth and development history:
  - Meeting developmental milestones?
  - Suboptimal growth or poor weight gain (based on pediatric growth charts)?
- Eating and nutritional history:
  - How has the child been eating? Specifically for the infant: Is the infant breast or bottle fed? Has the child's eating patterns changed?
  - Is the child exhibiting intolerance of feeding (which can be associated with COVID-19 and other illnesses)? Note vomiting, diarrhea, decreased intake, little interest in feeding, easily fatigued or perspiring during feeding, and/or any color changes including cyanoses during feeding.

FAMILY HISTORY

- Asthma, reactive airway, allergies, or breathing problems
- Chronic bronchitis, lung cancer, asbestosis, or lung problems
- Cystic fibrosis, congenital anomalies, or respiratory illnesses related to genetics
- Influenza, COVID-19, tuberculosis, or contagious illnesses caused by viruses or bacteria

SOCIAL HISTORY

Environmental Exposures

- Exposure to pollutants and/or irritants in the work environment
- Low-level chronic exposure to hazardous substances at work or at home
- Safety/protective measures; handwashing practices, masks worn at work, at home, or in public
- Air quality and exposures where the individual lives
- Exposure to secondhand or thirdhand smoke

Lifestyle Behaviors (Including Substance Use)

- Typical use of alcohol, episodes of binge drinking, alcohol misuse
- Use of prescription medications or illicit substances for nonmedical purposes
- Use of OTC drugs for reasons other than health, especially inhalants
- Use of tobacco, including cigarettes, smokeless tobacco, e-cigarettes or vaping, cigars; note amount of use and length of time to determine *pack years*; use the 5 A's as steps to intervene in response to positive tobacco use history for every individual (**Box 4.1**).

BOX 4.1

THE 5 A'S: STEPS TO INTERVENTION IN TOBACCO USE DISORDER

1. **Ask:** Identify and document tobacco use status for every patient at every visit.
2. **Advise:** Support the self-efficacy of every person who uses tobacco to quit.
3. **Assess:** Determine each individual's willingness and readiness to quit.
4. **Assist:** Individuals willing to make a quit attempt should be offered options, including counseling and pharmacotherapy, as appropriate.
5. **Arrange:** Schedule follow-up, in person or by phone, within the first week of a quit date.

REVIEW OF SYSTEMS

- **General:** Fever, fatigue, chills, night sweats, weight changes, appetite changes
- **Skin, hair, nails:** Rashes, lesions, changes in mucosa, changes in skin, hair
- **Lymphatic:** Generalized or localized lymph node swelling and/or tenderness
- **HEENT**: Headache, throat pain, ear pain, eye drainage or redness, congestion
- **Respiratory (additional review):** Orthopnea, snoring, hemoptysis, postural dyspnea
- **CV:** Chest pain, palpitations, edema; if positive for chest pain, note whether pleuritic (i.e., sudden, intense, stabbing, sharp, or burning pain exacerbated by deep breathing, coughing, or sneezing)
- **GI:** Nausea, heartburn, abdominal pain, epigastric discomfort, vomiting
- **Neurologic:** Weakness, numbness and tingling, tremors, dizziness, syncope
- **MSK:** Weakness, chest wall tenderness or pain, myalgias, leg pain or swelling
- **Mental health:** Sadness; insomnia; uncontrolled worry; changes in mentation, memory, or mood; current stress level and coping mechanisms; history of panic attacks

BOX 4.2 Red Flags in Subjective History That Indicate Risk for Pulmonary Embolus

- Sudden onset of pleuritic chest pain
- Breathlessness
- Dizziness or syncope
- Recent long-distance travel
- Prolonged immobility
- History of trauma to lower extremities or pelvis surgery in the last 3 months
- Previous deep vein thrombosis, emboli, malignancy
- Comorbid heart failure or chronic lung disease
- Pregnancy
- Use of hormonal contraception
- History of smoking and/or vaping

RED FLAGS IN SUBJECTIVE HISTORY

- Shortness of breath, difficulty breathing, breathlessness, wheezing, confusion, "coughing up blood," drooling, and/or any swelling of the lips or throat indicate the need for immediate physical exam and intervention.
- Key symptoms in individuals with pulmonary disease include pleuritic chest pain, dyspnea, and cough. Clarify characteristics of these symptoms and review the individual's history of chronic lung disease and smoking.
- See **Box 4.2** for red flags that indicate risk for pulmonary embolus.

PHYSICAL EXAMINATION

GENERAL SURVEY

- **Vital signs**: Temperature, pulse rate, respiratory rate, blood pressure
- Rate, rhythm, depth, and effort of breathing
- Posture and position
- Ability of the patient to speak in full sentences
- Wheezing or audible breath sounds
- Tracheal deviation, nasal flaring, or retractions (suprasternal, substernal, or intercostal)

INSPECTION

Peripheral Assessment

- Observe the lips, oral mucosa, and conjunctiva for cyanosis or pallor.
- Assess for purse-lipped breathing (i.e., exhaling through tightly pressed lips).
- Evaluate nailbeds for color and capillary refill; assess for clubbing (**Figure 4.1**). Normally, the angle between the skin and nailbed is 160 degrees, which creates a diamond-shaped window (Schamroth's window) when opposing fingers are held back-to-back.

Inspection of the Thoracic Cage and Chest Movement

- Observe the rate, rhythm, and depth of respirations for a full minute:
  - Rate of respiratios depends on several factors, including age, recent physical activity, and level of alertness. Adult respiratory rate is normally 12 to 20 breaths/minute.
  - Rhythm of breathing at rest should be even, with occasional sighs.
  - Depth and ease of breathing, which should be unlabored, quiet, without use of accessory muscles. Nasal flaring; tracheal

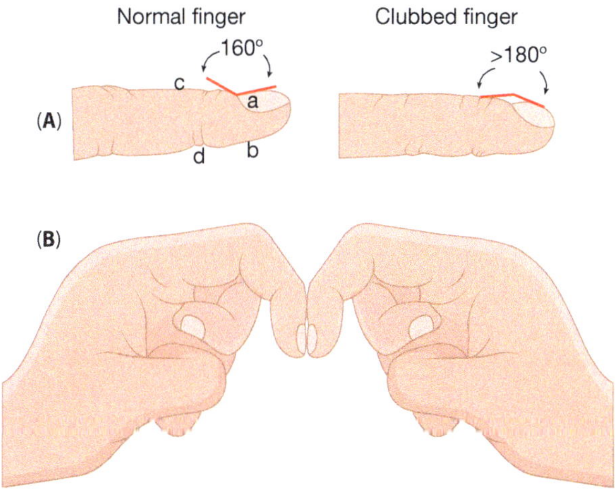

FIGURE 4.1 Assessment for clubbing. (**A**) Assessment of nail bed angle. (**B**) Schamroth's window.

deviation; suprasternal, substernal, or intercostal retractions are associated with respiratory distress and/or disorders.

- Inspect anterior and posterior chest wall:
  - Presence of any skin lesions, masses, or discolorations
  - Shape and symmetry, noting presence of chest or spine deformities. The AP diameter of the chest is ordinarily half of the lateral diameter, or 1:2. The thoracic cage is described as being a barrel chest when the AP diameter is equal to or greater than the lateral (transverse) diameter, or 1:1.

PALPATION

- Palpate the entire chest wall using the palmar surface of the hands to assess for tenderness, depressions, masses, deformities, or crepitus.
- Palpate the spine to identify any tenderness.
- Palpate the posterior thorax for symmetric chest expansion (**Figure 4.2**). Ask the patient to take a deep breath in, and then exhale. During inspiration, thumbs should separate, and each hand should rotate away from the midline equally. Asymmetric chest wall expansion is suggestive of unilateral lung pathology, and limited movement is associated with poor diaphragmatic excursion and hyperinflation, changes that occur with COPD.

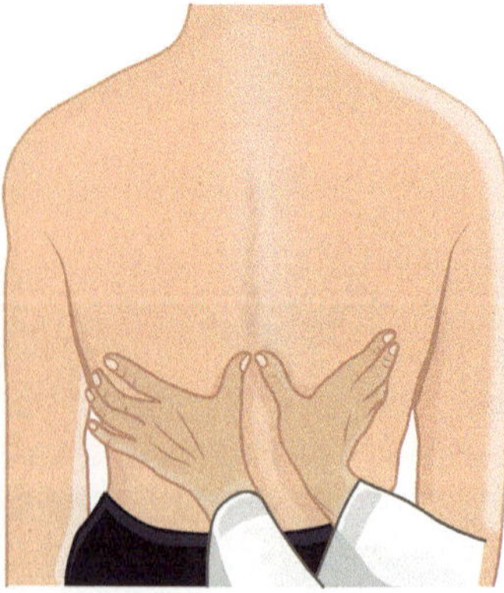

FIGURE 4.2 Palpation for symmetric chest expansion.

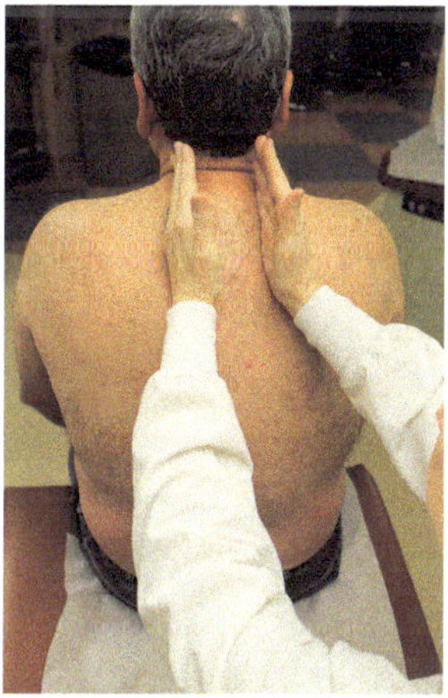

FIGURE 4.3 Palpation for tactile fremitus using the ulnar aspect of both hands.

- *Tactile fremitus* refers to the palpable vibratory sensation transmitted to the surface of the chest during speech. Palpate the posterior and anterior chest wall for fremitus (**Figure 4.3**). Ask the patient to say "99" and to repeat this while palpating the entire chest wall. Increased or decreased tactile fremitus is a finding that is understood to be a component of a constellation of signs and symptoms indicating respiratory disorders and is not solely diagnostic of pathology. The degree of fremitus found will vary. Tactile fremitus is usually stronger in the anterior versus posterior thorax, stronger at the apex than at the bases, and notable in the right upper back because that area is closer to the bronchial bifurcation.

PERCUSSION

- Percuss the posterior, lateral, and anterior chest wall, comparing each area bilaterally.
- Place the nonstriking finger of the nondominant hand on the chest wall firmly, while the remaining fingers are lifted slightly off the chest wall. Then use a quick, sharp wrist motion to strike the pressed finger at the midpoint between the proximal and distal interphalangeal joints with a plexor finger of the dominant hand to produce a sound. Strike the finger at least twice, lightly, sharply, and consistently, to produce a clear percussive sound (**Figure 4.4**).

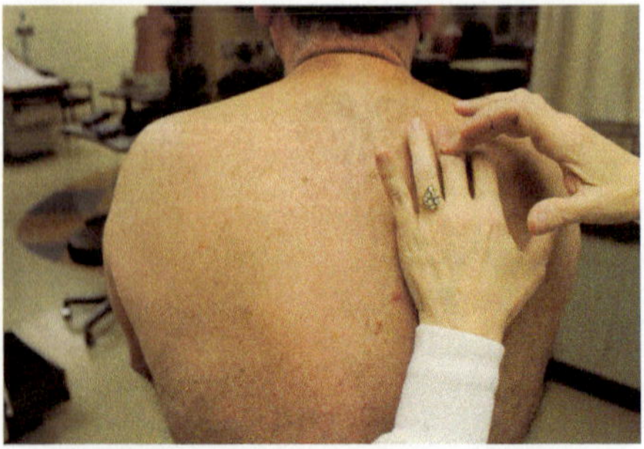

FIGURE 4.4 Percussion technique.

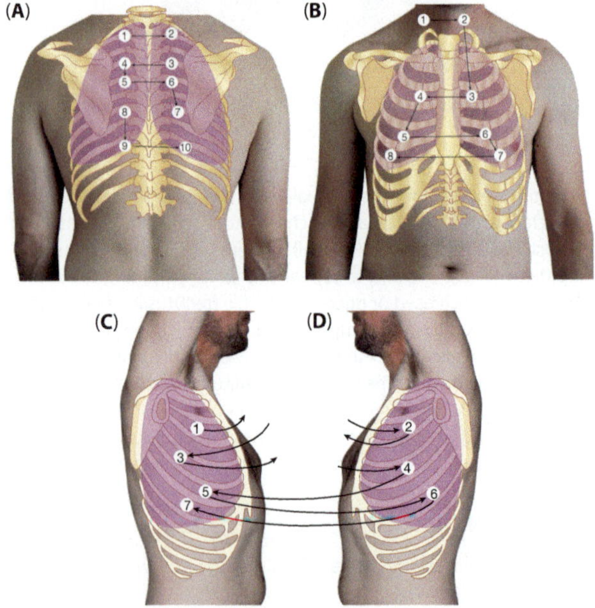

FIGURE 4.5 Landmarks for percussion and auscultation of lung fields. (**A**) Anterior. (**B**) Posterior. (**C, D**) Lateral.

- The landmarks used for percussion are illustrated in **Figure 4.5**; note that percussion is done in the same areas of the chest wall as auscultation.

AUSCULTATION

- Using a stethoscope, auscultate breath sounds.
- Instruct the individual to sit comfortably upright and take a deep breath in and out with the mouth open. Listen to at least one full breath in each auscultatory site. Caution the patient to do this leisurely so as not to get fatigued or hyperventilate and to take breaks as needed for comfort. Auscultate in a systematic manner from apex to base, comparing breath sounds from side to side.
- The auscultatory sites of the posterior, lateral, and anterior chest wall are the same as those used for percussion (see Figure 4.5). To assess breath sounds in all the lobes of the lungs, being systematic is a priority. Note the anatomic location of the lobes of the lungs, as shown in **Figure 4.6**.

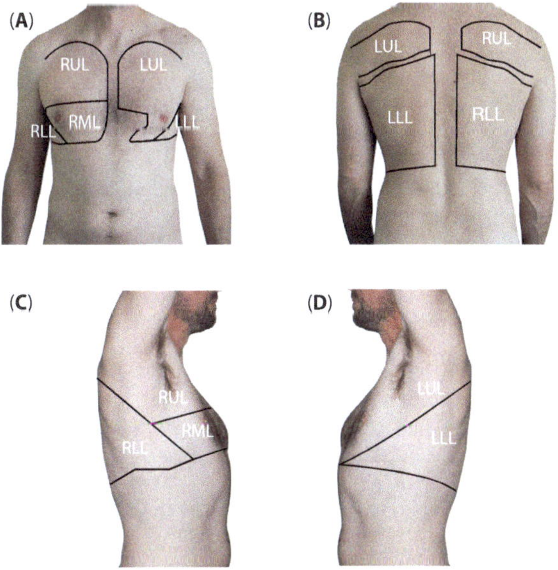

FIGURE 4.6 Lobes of the lungs. (**A**) Anterior lung fields. (**B**) Posterior lung fields. (**C**) Lobes of the right lung. (**D**) Lobes of the left lung. LLL, left lower lobe; LUL, left upper lobe; RLL, right lower lobe; RML, right middle lobe; RUL, right upper lobe.

- Auscultate to assess the characteristics of the breath sounds. Normal breath sounds include:
    - **Tracheal breath sounds**: Loudest and high pitched, usually heard over the upper aspect of the trachea and best heard on the anterior aspect of the neck
    - **Bronchial breath sounds**: Louder and higher in pitch, usually heard over the lower aspect of the trachea and best heard over the manubrium
    - **Bronchovesicular breath sounds:** Intermediate intensity and pitch, usually heard over the major bronchi in the midchest area anteriorly or between the scapulae posteriorly
    - **Vesicular breath sounds**: Soft in intensity and low pitched, usually heard over peripheral fields bilaterally
- Abnormal breath sounds include:
    - **Crackles**: Fine crackles are discontinuous high-pitched sounds that have a popping quality; these are usually inspiratory. Coarse crackles are discontinuous low-pitched, louder and longer. Crackles are heard as air passes through fluid-filled airways.
    - **Wheezes:** Continuous musical sounds, most likely to be heard during expiration. The tone of wheezing varies depending on area(s) of airways affected. If smaller airways are narrowed, resultant wheezes are musical in nature (polyphonic); if larger airways are narrow, then wheezes sound hoarse (monophonic).
    - **Rhonchi**: Continuous low-pitched rattling sounds heard when larger airways are obstructed with secretions. The rattling sounds may mimic snoring. The unique feature of rhonchi is that it clears with coughing or suctioning.
    - **Stridor:** Loud and high-pitched sound caused by disrupted airflow, typically heard during inspiration, and associated with upper airway obstruction. Stridor may indicate impending respiratory distress and/or failure.
    - **Pleural rub:** Creaking or grating sound that can be heard during both inspiration and expiration as a result of friction (lack of lubrication or irritation) between the pleura. Described as two pieces of leather rubbing together, the sound of a pleural rub is not likely to stop with coughing, but will stop when the patient holds their breath.
- If abnormal breath sounds are auscultated, the areas of abnormality can be further evaluated by auscultating for transmitted voice sounds:
    - **Bronchophony:** Ask the patient to say "99" while listening with the stethoscope. Normally the sound of "99" will sound

very faint and muffled. If the voice sounds become clear and distinct, bronchophony is present.

- **Egophony:** Ask the patient to repeatedly say the sound "ee" while listening with the stethoscope. Normally, it will sound muffled but unchanged. If the sound changes to "aaay" while the patient is saying "ee"' then egophony is present.
- **Whispered pectoriloquy:** For the whispered pectoriloquy test, ask the patient to whisper and repeat a few numbers or short phrases. For example, "1, 2, 3, 1, 2, 3, 1, 2, 3. . . ." Auscultate while the patient is whispering. Normally, the whispered voice will be distant, muffled, and not intelligible. If there is consolidation in an area of the lung, the whispered voice will sound unusually clear and loud.

PEDIATRIC CONSIDERATIONS

- For infants and children, the order of physical exam can be modified depending on their state of wakefulness and/or cooperativeness. The respiratory rate and rhythm can be assessed while the infant is sleeping in a parent's arms.
- The respiratory rate of infants can vary with temperature, activity, feeding, and even with sleep. When calculating respiratory rate, be sure to count for a full minute to calculate the normal respiratory rate because of these variations.
- When performing a physical exam on an infant, at some point during the exam be sure to examine the baby on the exam table, with only their diaper on so that their whole body can be viewed to get a better understanding of the infant's respiratory effort. While the infant is lying down, inspect the child's chest for size and shape. Infants are likely to have periodic, irregular breathing. Assess that the infant's color does not change and that they are not using accessory muscles to breathe.

CONSIDERATIONS FOR THE OLDER ADULT

- As a person ages, the amount of mucus produced throughout the body decreases and this can be evident with dry mucous membranes in the nares, throat, and respiratory tract.
- Because of changes in the respiratory system of the older adult, expect to find an increased AP diameter of the chest wall and slight hyperresonance of the lung fields with percussion. There is also a decreased amount of chest expansion and more reliance on the diaphragm for breathing.

RED FLAGS IN OBJECTIVE EXAM

- The initial assessment of an individual to determine physiology stability includes measurement of vital signs; assessment of the rate, rhythm, depth, and effort of breathing; and observation for signs of respiratory distress. **Box 4.3** lists key findings that indicate acute respiratory distress.

BOX 4.3 Red Flags in Objective Exam That Are Indications of Acute Respiratory Distress

- Labored or rapid breathing
- Absent or diminished breath sounds
- Suprasternal, substernal, or intercostal chest wall retractions
- Hypoxia, cyanosis
- Inadequate chest rise
- Loss of consciousness
- Additional population-specific signs:
  - In infants, nasal flaring, grunting, head bobbing
  - In children, drooling and stridor, extreme sleepiness
  - In older adults, confusion with tachypnea and hypotension

EVIDENCE-BASED RESOURCES

- **American Academy of Pediatrics:** https://pediatrics.aappublications.org/content/pediatrics/134/5/e1474.full.pdf
- **American Academy of Sleep Medicine:** https://aasm.org/clinical-resources/practice-standards/practice-guidelines
- **American College of Chest Physicians:** www.chestnet.org/Guidelines-and-Resources/CHEST-Guideline-Topic-Areas/Clinical-Pulmonary
- **American College of Physicians:** www.acponline.org/clinical-information/guidelines
- **American Thoracic Society:** www.thoracic.org/statements
- **Centers for Disease Control and Prevention:** Information for Healthcare Professionals About Coronavirus (COVID-19): www.cdc.gov/coronavirus/2019-nCoV/hcp/index.html

(*continued*)

EVIDENCE-BASED CONSIDERATIONS (*CONTINUED*)

- **Infectious Disease Society of America:** www.idsociety.org/practiceguidelines#/name_na_str/ASC/0/+/?Organ-System=Respiratory
- **Global Initiative for Asthma:** https://ginasthma.org
- **Global Initiative for Chronic Obstructive Lung Disease & COVID-19 Guidance:** https://goldcopd.org
- **World Health Organization:** www.who.int/respiratory/publications/strategy/en/index5.html

ABNORMAL FINDINGS

VARIATIONS IN PATTERNS OF BREATHING

- **Tachypnea**: Abnormally increased respiratory rate associated with shallow breaths.
- **Hyperpnea**: Increased rate and depth of breathing associated with elevated metabolic demand.
- **Bradypnea**: Abnormally slow respiratory rate, may affect alveolar ventilation.
- **Sighing respiration**: Normal respiratory rate with occasional deep, long breath; typically, non-pathologic and associated with emotional state.
- **Cheyne–Stokes breathing**: Abnormal breathing pattern; periods of progressively deeper breaths followed by gradual decrease that results in temporary period of no breathing; the pattern repeats, with each cycle usually taking 30 seconds to 2 minutes.
- **Biot's breathing**: Clusters of respirations that alternate with periods of no breathing due to damage to the breathing center of the brain.
- **Agonal breathing**: Occasional reflex-driven gasps, associated with anoxia, cardiac arrest, cerebral ischemia, or hypoxia.
- **Apnea**: Absence of breathing that signals a life-threatening situation resulting in death if intervention is not immediate.

COMMON RESPIRATORY DISORDERS

Acute Bronchitis

Lower respiratory tract infection most often of viral origin.

History

- Initial common cold symptoms progress to productive cough, dyspnea, pleuritic pain when coughing; cough persists 2 to 6 weeks

Physical Examination

- Mildly ill appearance
- Fever: <100.0 °F first few days of illness; resolves
- Lung exam may be normal or with wheezes and rhonchi, which clear with coughing

Consideration

- Differentiate from pneumonia: Not typical for healthy, immune-competent adult <65 years of age with normal vital signs and lung exam to have pneumonia

Asthma

Disease of chronic airway inflammation with many variations.

History

- Wheezing, dyspnea, chest tightness, cough that vary over time and in intensity
- May be worse at night, on awakening; often triggered by exercise, laughter, allergens, or cold air; may occur with or worsen during viral infections

Physical Examination

- Most common findings during exacerbations: wheezing, especially with expiration
- HEENT and skin exams may show evidence of allergies and/or eczema

Considerations

- Personal and family history of allergies, eczema increase risk
- Spirometry gives evidence of the variable expiratory airflow limitation through measurement of lung volumes and flow rates
- Important to assess pregnant women and those planning to become pregnant for history of asthma

Bronchiolitis

Acute viral infection that most commonly presents in children under 2 years of age.

History

- Most often occurs during winter season
- History often includes prodromal viral upper respiratory infection followed by increased respiratory effort and wheezing; presence of rhinorrhea, cough

Physical Examination

- Tachypnea, wheezing, crackles
- Increased respiratory effort: grunting, nasal flaring, intercostal and substernal retractions

Considerations

- Less common in adults
- Most cases caused by respiratory syncytial virus
- Underlying conditions, prematurity, tobacco exposure increase risk

COPD

Chronic inflammatory lung disease that causes obstructed airflow and decreased elasticity of the lungs.

History

- Primary risk factor: Current or former tobacco smoking
- Chronic cough, dyspnea, sputum production, recurrent lower respiratory tract infections, chest tightness (especially after exercise)

Physical Examination

- Exam findings vary with disease stage: Inspiratory and expiratory wheezes; decreased lung sounds; limited chest expansion; fatigue, weight loss, anorexia

Considerations

- Spirometry required for diagnosis: Persistent airflow limitation is confirmed when FEV1/FVC less than 0.70
- Goals of COPD assessment: Determine severity, impact of disease, risk of future exacerbations to guide therapy

COVID-19

Infectious disease caused by a novel (or new) coronavirus that has not previously been seen in humans.

History

- Cough; shortness of breath; fever, chills; muscle pain; sore throat; new loss of taste or smell (anosmia); headache; GI symptoms like nausea, vomiting, or diarrhea

Physical Examination

- Fever, fatigue, dry cough, dyspnea, abnormal chest x-ray, hypoxia

Considerations

- Atypical presentations in older adults and persons with medical comorbidities
- CT scans should not be used to screen for COVID-19 or as a first-line test to diagnose coronavirus disease

Cystic Fibrosis

Inherited disorder caused by gene defect.

History

- Infants will have positive newborn screening; may have meconium ileus, respiratory symptoms
- Pediatric and adults: Persistent, productive cough; wheezing; dyspnea; recurrent lung infections; pancreatic insufficiency; diabetes; infertility; anemia

Physical Examination

- Clinical features vary; respiratory: Chronic, productive cough; sinusitis; recurrent pneumonia, wheezing; clubbing
- GI: Malabsorption, abdominal distention, palpable masses
- GU: Frequent UTIs, amenorrhea in women, undescended testicles in men

Considerations

- CF is a complex, progressive disease with a varying course from mild symptoms to severe progressive airway and end-organ damage.
- Improved therapies for airway clearance, pancreatic enzyme supplements, and medications have improved life expectancy.

Influenza

Highly contagious viral respiratory infection.

History

- Cough, fever, sore throat, body aches, headache

Physical Examination

- Physical exam is nonspecific, except for likelihood of fever.
- Abnormal breath sounds generally indicate other illnesses, or complication of influenza.

Considerations

- Diagnostic testing is not necessary to make the diagnosis of influenza, especially in the midst of a community outbreak.
- Improved therapies for airway clearance, pancreatic enzyme supplements, and medications have improved life expectancy.

Lung Cancer

Malignancy that forms in the tissues of the lungs.

History

- Cough; hemoptysis; shortness of breath; chest pain; weight loss; hoarseness; bone pain; headaches; vision changes; confusion, weakness, nausea, constipation; clubbing

Physical Examination

- Lethargic, pale, with low-grade fever, tachypnea, hypoxia, jaundice, clubbing, swelling, weakness, lymphadenopathy
- Lungs: Decreased or absent breath sounds, dullness to percussion
- GI: Hepatomegaly, discomfort with exam

Considerations

- Screening guidelines vary
- Individuals who have symptoms of lung cancer should have diagnostic evaluation rather than screening

Obstructive Sleep Apnea

Syndrome of repeated episodes of reduced airflow during sleep.

History

- Loud snoring; frequent arousals; disruption of sleep
- Fatigue

Physical Examination

- Most common physical finding: Obesity, especially significant in undiagnosed patients with unexplained daytime sleepiness

Consideration

- Test: PSG observed in a sleep lab

Pertussis

Bacterial infection of the respiratory tract, also known as whooping cough.

History

- Begins with rhinorrhea and mild cough, progresses to severe coughing spasms, characteristic whoop sound to fill lungs, and post-cough vomiting.

Physical Examination

- Assess for paroxysms of coughing, especially in unvaccinated individuals.

Consideration

- Three stages: (1) catarrhal, 1 to 2 weeks; (2) paroxysmal, 1 to 6 weeks; (3) convalescence, 2 to 3 weeks

Pneumonia

Bacterial infection of the lower respiratory tract.

History

- Cough, dyspnea, pleural pain
- Sweating and night sweats
- Fever greater than 100.6 °F
- Chills, myalgias

Physical Examination

- Assess for abnormal vital signs: Tachycardia, tachypnea, fever.
- Assess for abnormal lung findings: Crackles, egophony, tactile fremitus.

Considerations

- Consider chest x-ray for suspected pneumonia.
- CURB-65 Pneumonia Severity Scale helps to determine treatment.

Tuberculosis

Infectious disease primarily caused by mycobacterium tuberculosis.

History

- Cough, possibly productive of blood or sputum
- Chest pain
- Fatigue
- Weight loss or in children, growth delay
- Anorexia
- Chills, fever
- Night sweats

Physical Examination

- Cannot be used solely to confirm or rule out active TB.
- Assess for malaise, fever, cutaneous lesions, lymphadenopathy, dyspnea, wheezing, respiratory distress, cough, hemoptysis, hepatosplenomegaly.

Consideration

- No single symptom, physical finding, or chest x-ray result can diagnose active TB alone.

PHYSICAL EXAMINATION DOCUMENTATION

Documentation should include results of inspection, palpation, percussion, and auscultation.

EXAMPLE OF NORMAL FINDINGS

Respirations easy without retractions; regular rate, and rhythm. No lesions, masses, or skin discolorations of anterior or posterior chest wall noted. AP less than transverse diameter. Chest expansion symmetric. Tactile fremitus equal bilaterally. No tenderness with palpation of thorax. Lung fields resonant to percussion throughout. Breath sounds full, equal, and clear bilaterally; no adventitious sounds auscultated.

EXAMPLE OF ABNORMAL FINDINGS

Respiratory rate 28 breaths/minute, shallow, rapid breathing with slight intercostal retractions; sitting in the upright position and leaning forward. No audible adventitious breath sounds; no nasal flaring, no suprasternal or substernal retractions noted. Mucosa pale pink. O_2 sat with pulse oximeter at 94%. Chest expansion symmetric. No skin discolorations of chest wall; no palpable tenderness. Tactile fremitus equal bilaterally. Negative egophony. Hyper-resonance to lower lung fields bilaterally to percussion. Breath sounds diminished, equal with scattered expiratory wheezes noted at the bases bilaterally.

REFERENCES

References for this chapter draw from Chapter 7, "Evidence-Based Assessment of Lungs and Respiratory System," of the textbook *Evidence-Based Physical Examination: Best Practices for Health and Well-Being Assessment*. The references may be accessed in the digital version of the handbook at https://connect.springerpub.com/content/book/978-0-8261-6466-7/chapter/ch04

5

Evidence-Based Assessment of Skin, Hair, and Nails

CLINICAL CONSIDERATIONS

- Be sure to ask about the patient's occupational history (e.g., exposure to chemicals, water, sun).
- Be consistent in the order in which the comprehensive skin exam is conducted. This will ensure a skin region is not missed.
- Integrate an exam of the surrounding skin when examining a specific body area.
- Include palpation of the skin in an attempt to feel abnormal areas on the skin that may be visually missed.
- During a total body skin exam, include an assessment of the mucous membranes of the oral cavity.
- There is assessment value in the use of smell during a skin exam to identify varied skin disorders.

SUBJECTIVE HISTORY

COMMON REASONS FOR SEEKING CARE

Rash; abnormal lesion(s); changes in hair/nails

HISTORY OF PRESENT ILLNESS

- **Onset:** When did the rash start? When the lesion was first noticed? Did this rash/lesion occur suddenly, or has it been developing gradually?
- **Location:** Where is the rash located? Have you noticed anything else on the rest of your skin? Are the hair changes on one side or both sides of your head?

- **Duration:** How long has the rash/lesion been present? Over what period of time has the rash/lesion developed?
- **Characteristics:** Are there any symptoms with this rash/lesion? Itching? Drainage? Tenderness or pain? Bleeding? Changes in color? Variations related to weather/season? Fever? Does anyone you have been in contact with have a similar skin disorder? Have the rash/hair/nail changes happened in the past? Have you had any changes to your hair (loss, growth [slow or excessive], texture, or color)? Are your nails brittle or thin? Are your nails thickening or changing in color? Have you noticed any discoloration in your nails?
- **Aggravating factors:** What action or activities make the rash worse? Have you started using new skin care products or new household cleaning products? Are you aware of any exposures? Hot tubs, pools, lakes, and so on? Are you aware of any exposure to toxins or chemicals (environmental or occupational)? Do you use any commercial hair products? Do you pull your hair? Do you bite your nails or pick your skin? Have you injured your nails or fingers? Are your hands/feet frequently in water?
- **Relieving factors:** How have you been treating the problem (e.g., medications such as steroids, antifungals, lotions)?
- **Treatment:** What medications or treatments have been tried to help with the rash/hair/nail changes?
- **Severity:** How severe are the symptoms on a scale of 0 to 10? Do the symptoms limit participation in activities or alter the quality of life? Are there associated symptoms? Are the symptoms worsening? How has this skin condition affected the patient (physical, psychological, or social)?

HEALTH HISTORY

Past Medical History

- History of allergic reactions, asthma, or allergic rhinitis
- Previous diagnoses of skin cancer, dysplastic nevi, or suspicious lesions
- History of any serious sunburns or childhood sunburns
- History of any chronic illnesses, mental health disorders, or autoimmune disorders
- History of tanning-bed use, nail salons
- Previous diagnoses of alopecia, onychomycosis
- Any contact with a person who has a similar rash/lesion
- History of pregnancy or traumatic event(s)
- History of recent travel (If so, where, when, how long did they stay?)
- Sunscreen use (frequency, SPF)

Medications

- Prescribed medications (oral and topical), including dose and frequency, specifically chemotherapy, psoralens, retinoids, tetracyclines, allopurinol, anti-seizure medications, or anti-malarials
- OTC medications or supplements, including dose and frequency
- Recent or new antibiotic and/or medication use

Allergies

- Allergies to medications or seasonal, environmental, and/or food allergies; if yes to being allergic to any substance or environmental trigger, clarify reaction, specifically previous reactions causing skin rashes, itching, or hives

Immunizations

- Risks for vaccine-preventable illnesses: Vaccine status, including childhood vaccines (MMR, varicella, zoster, meningococcal, and human papillomavirus)

Pediatric Considerations

- Is the infant breast or formula fed? If formula, what type?
- Have foods been introduced? If so, what has been introduced and when?
- What is the skin cleansing routine with diaper changes? What type of diapers are used?
- What types of soaps, oils, and lotions are applied to the infant/child's skin?
- What types of food does your child eat? What are their usual eating habits?
- Are you aware of any infectious diseases to which your child may have been exposed?
- Has your child had any recent skin injuries? Frequent/recent falls or abrasions? Unexplained injuries?
- Does your child pull or twist their hair?
- Does your child bite or pick their nails or surrounding skin?

Considerations for the Older Adult

- Do you have increased or decreased sensation to touch?
- What is your level of lifetime sun or irritant exposures? Occupational exposure?
- Do you fall frequently?
- Do you have any limitations in your mobility?

- Are you taking any anticoagulants?
- Are you incontinent of bowel or bladder?
- Does your skin ever rip or tear?

FAMILY HISTORY

- Skin disorders (skin cancer, psoriasis, eczema, hives, hay fever, allergies, asthma, autoimmune disorders)
- Hair loss (receding hairline, baldness)
- Any chronic diseases, mental health disorders, or cancers

SOCIAL HISTORY

- Do you use alcohol, tobacco, or recreational drugs? If so, what type and how frequently?
- Have you ever been diagnosed with a sexually transmitted infection or disease?
- Do you consistently wear condoms during sexual encounters?
- Do you practice any cultural or special rituals that may affect your skin, hair, or nails?
- Have you experienced any recent stress?
- Do you paint your nails or apply artificial nails?
- Do you dye your hair or get permanents?

Occupation

- Are you required to wear a specific type of helmet, hat, goggles, gloves, or shoes?
- Do you use personal protective equipment at work?
- Does your work require you to perform repetitive tasks?
- Do you work with or around chemicals? If so, which ones?
- Do you work outdoors?
- Do you wear sunscreen or sun-protective clothing?
- Does your occupation place you at risk for chemical exposure to skin, hair, and nails? If so, how?
- Can you describe your current living situation (who do you live with and type of residence)?
- Do you recall what you have eaten and drunk in the past 24 hours? Describe.
- Do you ever twist or pull your hair, bite nails, or pick your skin?

REVIEW OF SYSTEMS

- **General:** Fatigue, malaise, fever, weight loss or gain, pain anywhere in the body

- **HEENT:** Hair loss or excessive growth, change of hair texture, ringing in the ears, decreased hearing, changes in vision, photosensitivity, blurred vision, dry eyes, runny nose, altered smell, sinus congestion, sore throat, hoarseness, dry mouth, changes in teeth or gums, enlarged lymph nodes on the head or neck
- **Respiratory:** Shortness of breath, cough (productive or dry), painful or altered breathing
- **CV:** Chest pain, shortness of breath, palpitations, arrhythmias, hair loss on the lower extremities, swelling of hands, legs, or feet
- **GI:** Abdominal pain, bloating or distention, changes in bowel movements, heartburn, nausea, vomiting
- **GU:** Painful urination, urinary frequency, urinary retention, urinary urgency, incontinence, difficulty starting urine stream, blood in urine, vaginal or penile discharge, pain or swelling
- **MSK:** Single or multiple joint pain, swelling of joints, decreased movement or strength, muscle pain and/or muscle weakness, skin changes over bony prominences
- **Neurological:** Headaches, change in thinking or cognition, memory loss, tingling or numbness
- **Hematologic:** Easy bruising, bleeding, spider veins, prominent or painful blood vessels
- **Integumentary:** Changes in skin color; texture; thickness or thinning; excessive sweating or dryness; new lesions or rashes; temperature change; scar changes or nail changes; any loss of tissue in face, arms, legs, or buttocks
- **Mental health:** Increased or persistent anxiety and/or depression; scratching or picking of skin or nails; pulling of the hair; self-harm behaviors

RED FLAGS IN SUBJECTIVE HISTORY

- Immunosuppressed patient
- Severe pain
- Very old or very young age
- Associated photophobia, headache
- Start of a new medication

PHYSICAL EXAMINATION

GENERAL SURVEY

- **Vital signs:** Temperature, pulse rate, respiratory rate, blood pressure
- Toxic vs. nontoxic appearance
- Hygiene and odors

INSPECTION

- Inspect the skin in a head-to-toe sequence with the breast and genitalia examined last. Use the same assessment technique and order to maintain consistency and avoid omitting any portion of the patient's skin.
- Start with a general survey of the skin, including color, pigmentation, vascularity, bruising, lesions, color variations, and general hygiene.
- Inspect and measure all skin lesions (**Tables 5.1 and 5.2**). A dermatoscope can be helpful if it is available and the clinician is adequately trained in its use.
- Describe the findings, noting number, location, size, color, shape, morphology, distribution, and configuration.
- Note distribution, texture, and quantity of hair.
- Inspect the fingernails and toenails, noting color and shape. Nail polish should be removed.

PALPATION

- Palpate the skin and note the temperature, texture, moisture, and turgor.
- Palpate appropriate lesions, assessing the texture of the lesion, presence of tenderness or pain, temperature of lesion and surrounding skin, fluidity, and blanching capacity.
- Palpate fingernails and toenails for texture and note CRT.

PEDIATRIC CONSIDERATIONS

Preterm Infants

- Preterm infants' skin often appears ruddy, gelatinous, and almost transparent due to the decreased presence of stratum corneum and the small amount of fat present.
- Fine, silky hair called *lanugo* is more common in preterm infants and is usually present on the back and shoulders.
- The preterm and full-term infant's nails are soft and flexible.

Infants, Children, and Adolescents

- Approximately 50% of newborns experience physiologic jaundice, which is a normal phenomenon resulting from increased hemolysis of red blood cells following birth.
- Seborrheic dermatitis (cradle cap) appears as a scaly crust.
- There may be harmless markings on newborns such as tiny, white facial papules (milia), vascular markings (salmon patches/stork bites), and mongolian spots (congenital dermal melanocytosis).

TABLE 5.1 Primary Skin Lesions

Lesion	Description	Examples	Visual With Diagnosis
Macule	• Flat, nonpalpable • Smaller than 1 cm	• Freckles • Flat moles (nevi) • Measles • Petechiae*	Leukocytoclastic vasculitis 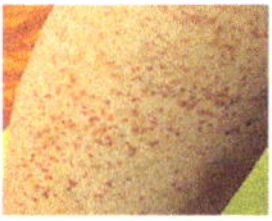
Patch	• Flat, nonpalpable • Larger than 1 cm	• Vitiligo • Mongolian spots • Port-wine stains • Chloasma • Café au lait patch	Tinea versicolor 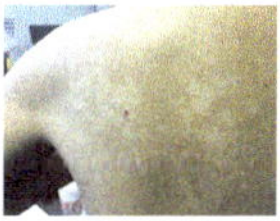
Papule	• Elevated, solid palpable • Smaller than 0.5 cm	• Purpura** • Elevated moles • Warts • Insect bites • Lichens planus	Bedbug bites 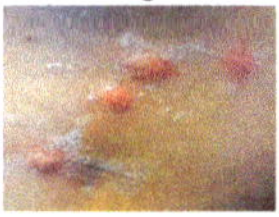
Plaque	• Groups of papules • Larger than 5 cm	• Psoriasis • Seborrheic and actinic keratosis • Lichen planus	Psoriasis 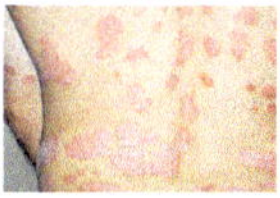
Pustule	• Elevated, pus-filled vesicle or bullae • Size varies	• Acne • Impetigo • Carbuncles	Pustules from fire ant bites 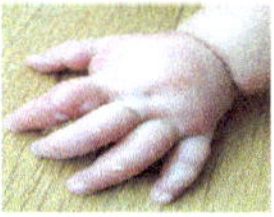
Cyst	• Elevated, encapsulated, fluid- or semisolid-filled, or solid mass in dermis or subcutaneous layers • 1 cm or larger	• Sebaceous cyst • Epidermoid cyst • Acne	Inflamed sebaceous cyst 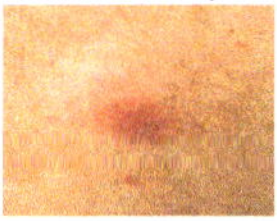

*Petechiae are unique in this list because they are nonblanching vascular lesions. They can be considered a subcategory of macules.
**Also a nonblanching lesion.

(continued)

TABLE 5.1 Primary Skin Lesions (*continued*)

Lesion	Description	Examples	Visual With Diagnosis
Vesicle	• Elevated, fluid-filled, round- or oval-shaped with thin, translucent walls • Smaller than 0.5 cm	• Herpes simplex or zoster • Early chicken pox • Poison ivy • Small burn blister	Herpes zoster 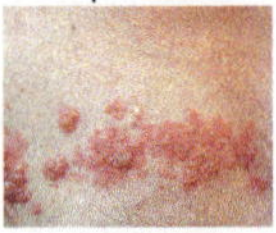
Bullae	• Elevated, fluid-filled, round- or oval-shaped with thin, translucent walls • Larger than 0.5–1 cm	• Contact dermatitis • Friction or fracture blister • Large burn blister • Pemphigus vulgaris	Fracture blister 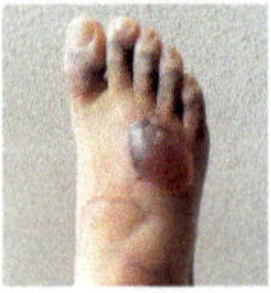
Nodule	• Elevated, solid, hard or soft, palpable mass deeper in the dermis • Smaller than 2 cm	• Small lipoma • Squamous cell carcinoma • Fibroma • Nevi • Erythema nodosum	Nodular melanoma 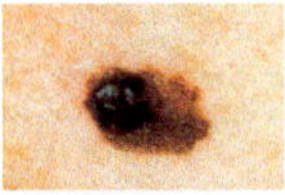
Tumor	• Elevated, solid, hard or soft, palpable mass deeper in the dermis with irregular borders • Larger than 2 cm	• Lipomas • Carcinoma • Hemangioma • Benign tumor	Basal cell carcinoma 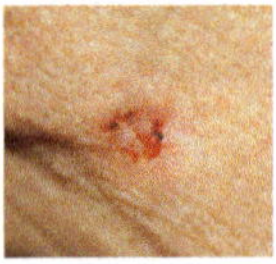
Wheal	• Elevated, often reddish area with irregular borders caused by diffuse fluid in tissues (cutaneous edema) • Size varies	• Insect bites • Hives (urticarial) • Allergic reaction	Urticarial drug reaction 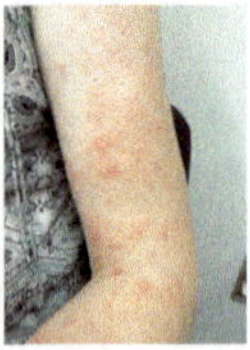

TABLE 5.2 Secondary Skin Lesions

Lesion	Description	Examples	Visual With Diagnosis
Atrophy	• Thinning or wasting of skin due to loss of collagen and elastin	• Striae • Aged skin	PUPPP rash 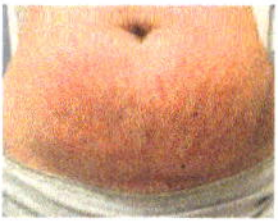
Excoriation	• Absence of superficial epidermis, causing a moist, shallow depression	• Scratch marks • Abrasion • Scabies	Abrasion (bike wreck on asphalt) 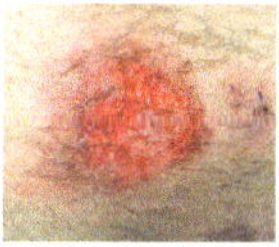
Keloid	• Elevated area of excessive scar tissue that extends beyond the site of original injury (caused by excessive collagen formation during healing)	• Keloid for ear piercing or following surgery	Keloids from folliculitis barbae 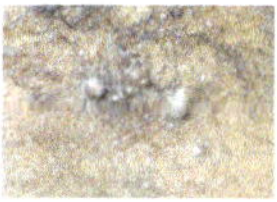
Scale	• Flakes of greasy keratinized skin tissue • May be white, gray, or silver • Texture may be fine or thick • Varies in size	• Dry skin • Dandruff • Psoriasis • Eczema	Psoriasis 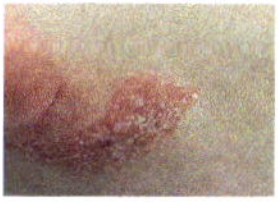
Crust	• Dried blood, serum, or pus on the epidermis from ruptured vesicles or pustules • Slightly elevated • May be red, brown, orange, or yellow • Size varies	• Eczema • Impetigo • Herpes • Scabs following an abrasion	Early impetigo 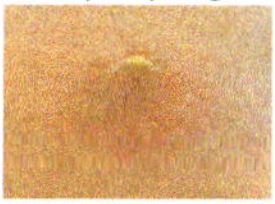

(continued)

TABLE 5.2 Secondary Skin Lesions (*continued*)

Lesion	Description	Examples	Visual With Diagnosis
Fissure	• Linear crack or break with sharp edges extending into the dermis • May be moist or dry	• Cracks at corner of the mouth, on the fingers, or on the feet (athlete's foot)	Fissure caused by finger eczema 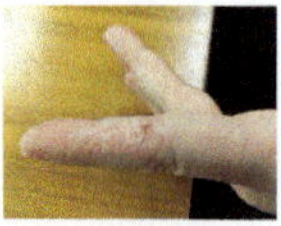
Lichenification	• A rough, thickened, hardened area of the epidermis resulting from chronic irritation such as scratching or rubbing (often involves flexor surfaces)	• Chronic dermatitis	Chronic dermatitis 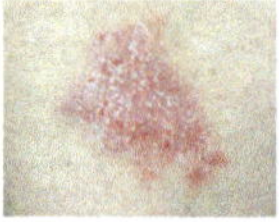
Scar	• Elevated, irregular area of connective tissue left after a lesion or wound has healed • New scars may be red or purple • Old scars may be silvery or white	• Healed surgical wound or injury • Healed acne	Surgical scar: knee replacement 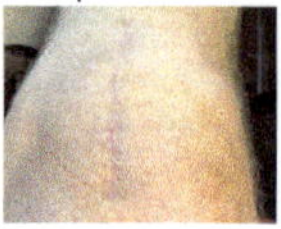
Ulcer	• Irregularly shaped area of skin loss that extends into the dermis or subcutaneous tissue; concave • Depth varies	• Stasis and decubiti ulcers • Aphthous ulcers	Aphthous ulcer 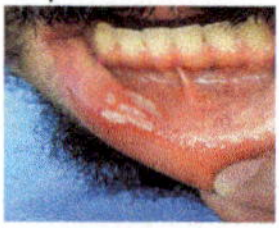

- Bruising to lower legs may be present as the child becomes mobile.
- There are a variety of different rashes that typically occur only in childhood (**Table 5.3**).

TABLE 5.3 Common Childhood Rashes

Disease State	History and Physical Findings	Visual
Fifth's disease • Also called *erythema infectiosum* • Caused by parvovirus B19 • Transmitted through respiratory secretions and blood	• Incubation period is 4–14 days • Often have fever, rhinorrhea, myalgias, and a headache • Facial rash that has a "slapped cheek" appearance • Can get a second itchy rash a few days after the facial rash that appears on the chest, back, buttocks, or arms and legs	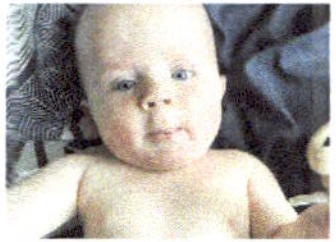
Hand, foot, mouth disease • Caused by a virus called *Coxsackievirus A16* • Transmitted through respiratory secretions, fecal–oral route, or vesicle fluid	• Usually affects infants and children 5 years old or younger • Typically occurs in summer and early fall • Starts with fever, malaise, sore throat, and anorexia • Painful macular or vesicular lesions can develop in the mouth several days after the fever starts • Rash on the palms of the hands and soles of the feet may also develop over 1 or 2 days as a macular and/or vesicular red rash; it may also appear on the knees, elbows, buttocks, or genital area	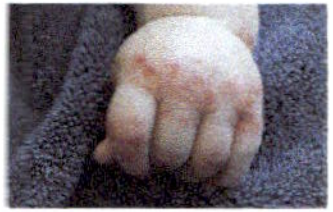 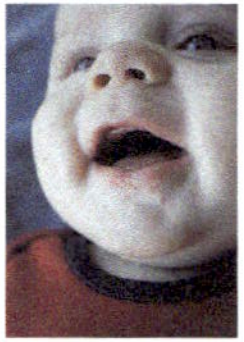

(continued)

TABLE 5.3 Common Childhood Rashes (*continued*)

Disease State	History and Physical Findings	Visual
Impetigo • Usually caused by *Staphylococcus aureus or Streptococcus pyogenes* • Bacteria is introduced through a break in the skin • There are three types of impetigo: bullous (large blisters), nonbullous (crusted), and ecthyma (ulcers)	• Most common in children between the ages of 2 and 6 • Lesions can be anywhere, but usually occur on the face, around the mouth and nose, and on the hands/feet • Lesions are vesicular, burst, and develop honey-colored crusts • Can be spread to other areas of the body by fingers, clothing, and towels • Bullous impetigo has larger blisters that are more likely to be on the trunk • Ecthyma impetigo can form deep, painful ulcers	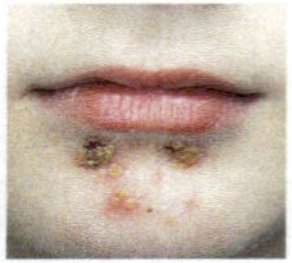
Infantile seborrheic dermatitis • Commonly referred to as *cradle cap* when it is found on the scalp • Noncontagious	• Affects the oily areas of the body, including the scalp, face, sides of the nose, eyebrows, ears, eyelids, and chest • Typically presents with erythema and greasy scales • Usually benign and self-limited • Typically resolves within several weeks to several months	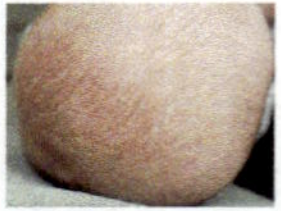
Measles (Rubeola) • Caused by the virus Rubeola • Spread to others through respiratory secretions • Highly contagious • Vaccination available	• Incubation period is 7–14 days after a person is infected • Maculopapular rash that starts on the head and moves down the body • Other symptoms include malaise, high fever, cough, rhinorrhea, conjunctivitis, koplik spots (tiny white spots inside the mouth) • Conjunctivitis, in addition to the rash, is the main symptom that distinguishes measles from influenza	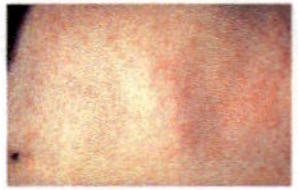

(*continued*)

Molluscum contagiosum • Caused by a virus called the *poxvirus* • Transmitted from direct person-to-person physical contact and through contaminated fomites	• White-, pink-, or flesh-colored papules that are umbilicated • They often have a pearly appearance • Usually smooth and firm • Lesions range from about 2–5 mm in diameter • They may become pruritic, painful, erythematous, and/or swollen • May occur anywhere on the body, including the face, neck, arms, legs, abdomen, and genital area • They can occur alone or in groups	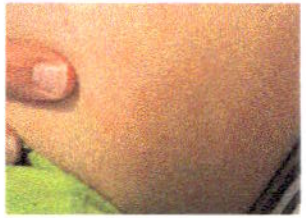
Mumps • Caused by the mumps virus, which belongs to a family of viruses known as *paramyxoviruses* • Transmitted through direct contact with saliva or respiratory droplets from the mouth, nose, or throat • Vaccination available	• Symptoms typically appear 16–18 days after infection • Puffy cheeks and a tender, swollen jaw due to swollen salivary glands on one or both sides (parotitis) • Other symptoms include fever, headache, myalgias, malaise, and anorexia • Can be asymptomatic in some	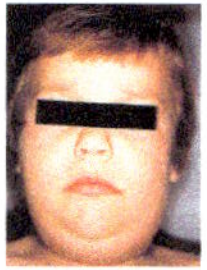
Roseola • Caused by a virus called *human herpesvirus 6* • Transmitted by oral and respiratory secretions and direct person-to-person contact • Vaccination available	• Incubation period is 9–10 days • Common in children aged 3 months to 4 years (most commonly, 6 months to 1 year) • Initial symptoms include acute-onset high fever, eye redness, sore throat, irritability, rhinorrhea • Once the fever resolves (after 2–4 days), a pinkish-red, maculopapular rash presents	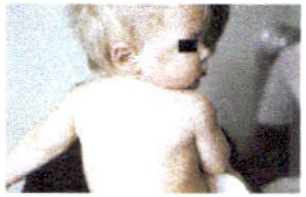

(continued)

TABLE 5.3 Common Childhood Rashes (*continued*)

Disease State	History and Physical Findings	Visual
Rubella • Also called *German measles* • Caused by the rubella virus (genus *Rubivirus* in the family *Togaviridae*) • Transmitted via direct or droplet contact with respiratory secretions • Vaccination available	• Rash starts on trunk and spreads peripherally • Symptoms that may occur 1–5 days before the rash appears include low-grade fever, headache, conjunctivitis, lymphadenopathy, cough, and/or rhinorrhea • Rash generally first appears on the face and then spreads to the rest of the body and lasts about 3 days • Can be asymptomatic • Typically, mild presentation	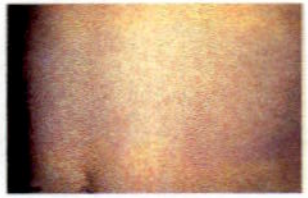
Scarlet fever • Also known as *scarlatina* • Caused by *group A hemolytic Sreptococcus*	• Most common in children 5–15 years • Most commonly seen in conjunction with strep pharyngitis • Typically starts with a high fever and sore throat • Rash appears after 1–2 days • Maculopapular exanthematous rash that looks like a sunburn and feels like sandpaper • Rash initially appears on the neck and chest, then spreads over the body • Pastia's sign (linear bright red coloration of the creases in the axillary and inguinal folds) • Tongue may appear white, with red, swollen papillae (white strawberry tongue), but by the fourth or fifth day, it becomes bright red (red strawberry tongue)	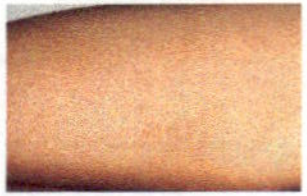

(*continued*)

• Rash caused by an erythrogenic exotoxin emitted by the streptococci	• Other symptoms include headache chills, flushed face, nausea, and vomiting • Rash usually fades in 4–5 days and is followed by diffuse desquamation	
Varicella • Caused by the varicella-zoster virus • Transmitted mainly through close contact with someone who has chicken pox • Highly contagious disease • Vaccination available	• Incubation period is from 10–21 days • Rash first appears on the chest, back, and face and then spreads over the entire body • Initial appearance of rash is vesicular, followed by simultaneous occurrence of papular and macular rashes with crusting • Rash is highly pruritic • Other symptoms include fever, malaise, anorexia, and headache • Last 5–6 days • Disease is contagious until crusting appears	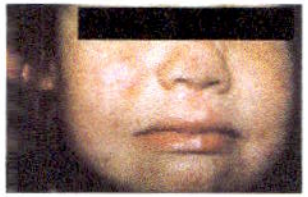

Sources: From Centers for Disease Control and Prevention (roseola, rubella, scarlet fever, varicella); Centers for Disease Control and Prevention and Heinz F. Eichenwald, MD (measles [rubeola]); Centers for Disease Control and Prevention, Patricia Smith, and Barbara Rice.

- The presence and characteristics of facial hair (males) and body hair (males and females) change considerably during adolescence. See **Table 5.4** for the Tanner stages.
- Increased perspiration, oiliness, and acne are common in adolescents due to increased sebaceous activity.

TABLE 5.4 Tanner Stages for Female and Male Development

Stage	Female	Male
1	Breast: Small nipples, no breasts Pubic hair: none	Penis: No change in size Testes: >2.5 cm Pubic hair: None
2	Breast: Starting to grow, areola becoming larger, breast tissue bud feels firm behind nipples Pubic hair: Initial growth of long pubic hairs; straight, without curls, and of light colors	Penis: No change in size Testes: Enlargement; pigmentation of scrotal sac Pubic hair: Long, downy, and variable in pattern
3	Breast: Further growth of breast and nipples, areola has become darker, breast tissue bud is larger Pubic hair: More widespread, hair is darker and curls may have appeared	Penis: Significant enlargement, especially in diameter Testes: Frther enlargement Pubic hair: lincrease in amount and curling
4	Breast: Nipples and areolas elevated and form an edge toward the breast, breast has grown a little larger Pubic hair: More dense hair growth with curls and dark hair	Penis: Further enlargement Testes: Further enlargement Pubic hair: Adult in type but not distribution Axillary/facial hair: Growth begins
5	Breast: Fully developed breast, nipples protruding and edge between areola and breast has disappeared Pubic hair: Adult hair growth; dense, curly hair extending toward inner thighs	Penis: Adult size Testes: Adult size Pubic hair: Adult in distribution Axillary/facial hair: Further growth Overall growth (height/weight/muscle) velocity: Peaks

CONSIDERATIONS FOR THE OLDER ADULT

- The clinician must be cognizant of signs of maltreatment by assessing for bruising, lacerations, pressure ulcers, dehydration, and poor hygiene.
- Skin may appear pale and to hang from the frame.
- Normal older adult skin variations may include solar lentigo (liver spots), seborrheic keratosis, and acrochordon (skin tag).
- Skin tears may also be present due to the fragility of the skin.
- The hair may be thin, gray, and coarse with symmetric balding in men.
- The amount of body hair decreases (body, pubic, and axillary hair).
- Men have an increase in the amount and coarseness of nasal and eyebrow hair, and women may develop coarse facial hair.

RACIAL AND ETHNIC CONSIDERATIONS

- Hispanics, Asians, American Indians (including Pacific Islanders), Africans, and Black Americans have unique skin presentations. A predisposition to scarring and pathogenesis of skin disorders are unique and common to these groups.
- There is a greater susceptibility to forming melasma, keloids, and dyschromia in these races versus Caucasians. These benign lesions tend to be larger than the site of trauma and are often distressing to patients who form them.
- Skin cancer occurs at a lower rate in ethnic skin compared to whites; however, the morbidity and mortality is significantly higher in persons of color due to late diagnosis.

RED FLAGS IN OBJECTIVE EXAM

- Toxic appearance
- Unstable vital signs
- Fever and a petechial/purpura or erythematous rash
- Scalded skin appearance
- Rash covering more than 90% of the body
- Nonblanching rash
- Mucosal lesions
- Rash or lesion that does not go away
- ABCDE for a mole

EVIDENCE-BASED RESOURCES

- **American Academy of Dermatology:** www.aad.org/member/clinical-quality/guidelines

(continued)

EVIDENCE-BASED RESOURCES (*CONTINUED*)

- **The American Cancer Society:** www.cancer.org/cancer.html
- **Choosing Wisely® initiative:** www.choosingwisely.org
- **Cochrane US:** https://us.cochrane.org
- **U.S. Preventative Services Task Force:** www.uspreventiveservicestaskforce.org/uspstf

ABNORMAL FINDINGS

The abnormal findings and differential diagnoses listed in this section are in alphabetical order, not order of prevalence. The list is not exhaustive.

COMMON DISORDERS

Acne

Chronic inflammatory dermatosis affecting the pilosebaceous follicles of the skin.

History

- Typically in adolescents but can occur at any age
- History of PCOS
- May report pain, tenderness, and/or erythema in affected areas

Physical Examination

- Closed and open comedones (noninflammatory acne); papules, pustules, nodules, or cysts (inflammatory acne)
- May affect only the face, but the chest, back, and upper arms are frequently involved due to the density of sebaceous glands
- Postinflammatory hyperpigmentation and/or atrophic scars (moderate to severe acne)

Considerations

- May have a psychological impact.
- Assessment and examination should focus on the extent and severity of acne lesions, number of lesions, anatomic location of acne, scarring, and quality of life and other psychosocial metrics.
- Grading and classification systems may also be useful in acne patient care by specifically classifying acne (mild, moderate, or severe), directing treatment options, and assessing patient response to therapy.

Actinic Keratosis

Premalignant skin lesions that form from an abnormal production of keratinocytes after excessive prolonged ultraviolet exposure.

History

- Frequently seen in people over 50 with excessive sun exposure
- History of sunburns
- Immunosuppression

Physical Examination

- Erythematous, hyperkeratotic scaly macules, papules, and plaques on sun-damaged skin (**Figure 5.1**)
- Typically located on the face, ears, scalp, neck, and extremities
- The average number of lesions identified is six to eight
- Lesions range in color from white, yellow, pink, or red
- Feel rough on palpation

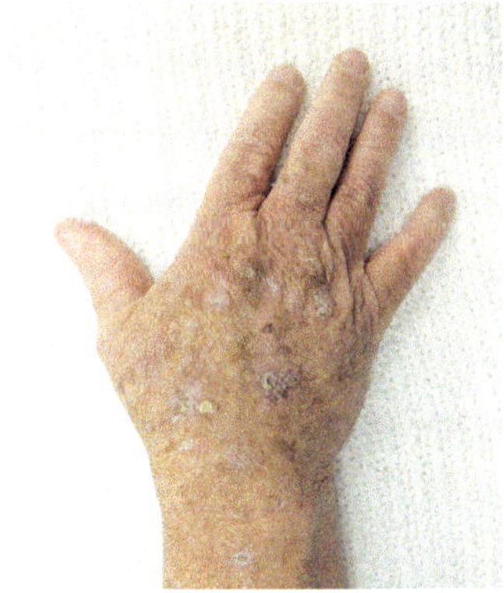

FIGURE 5.1 Actinic keratosis on the back of hand.
Source: Image courtesy of James Heilman, MD.

Considerations

- Without treatment, can progress to squamous cell carcinoma
- Also known as *solar keratosis*

Basal Cell Carcinoma

Evolves from the basal cells found in the lower layer of the epidermis.

History

- Most commonly develops on sun-exposed skin areas; history of sun damage.
- Is slow growing; bleeds with trauma.
- Fair skin patients are disproportionately affected.

Physical Examination

- A nonhealing sore that is friable and umbilicated
- Waxy papules with central depression, pearly, erosion, or ulceration (see "Tumor" in Table 5.1)
- Crusting
- Rolled border
- Translucency
- Surface telangiectasia

Consideration

- The most common malignancy in humans but usually does not metastasize.

Bed Bug Bites

Small, parasitic insects that feed on the blood of people and animals while they sleep.

History

- Bite marks appear anywhere from one to several days after the initial bite
- Bites are mildly erythematous and pruritic
- Can cause insomnia and anxiety
- History of recent travel
- Contact with similar bites
- Identified bugs in sleeping environment
- No systemic symptoms

Physical Examination

- Bite marks can occur in a random distribution, a straight line, or in groups of three (see "Papule" in Table 5.1)
- Can cause additional skin problems that arise from intense scratching of the bites

Consideration

- Can be difficult to eradicate from housing

Cellulitis

A bacterial infection of the deeper dermis and subcutaneous tissues predominantly caused by group A *Streptococcus*, *Staphlococcus aureus* in adults, and *Haemophilus influenza* type B in children less than 3 years old.

History

- Those with a history of lymphedema, venous insufficiency, a previous history of cellulitis, tinea pedis, and obesity are at increased risk
- History of diabetes and peripheral vascular disease

Physical Examination

- Trauma to the skin
- Erythema
- Calor
- Edema of the skin
- Pain
- Fever
- Leukocytosis

- Mildly elevated sedimentation rate
- Unilateral
- Has indistinct borders

Considerations

- Cellulitis typically affects the skin on the lower legs, but can occur on any skin surface area (**Figure 5.2**).
- Can progress quickly to fulminant sepsis with necrotizing fasciitis especially in patient with comorbidities.

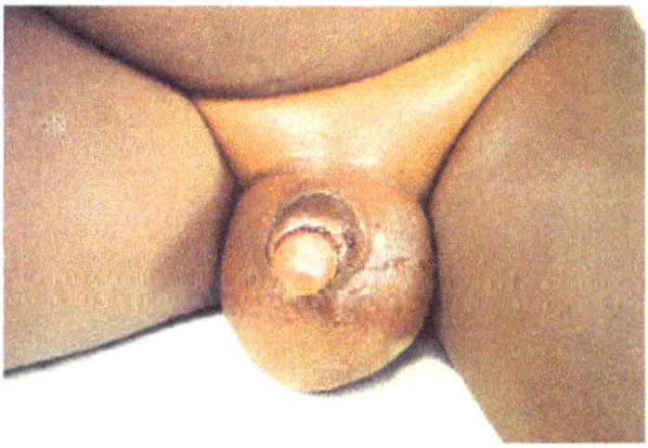

FIGURE 5.2 Cellulitis on the scrotum of an infant.
Source: Centers for Disease Control and Prevention/ Robert S. Craig.

Contact Dermatitis

An eczematous inflammatory skin condition.

History

- Painful or itchy skin
- Exposure to an allergen or irritants (poison ivy is most common)
- Common allergens include jewelry metals (e.g., nickel), cosmetic products, fragrances, and preservatives
- Common irritants include detergents, soap, cleaners, and acid
- Certain professions are at higher risk, including construction workers, hair stylists, florists, landscapers, food handlers, healthcare clinicians, janitors, plumbers, and mechanics

Physical Examination

- Dryness and scaling
- Pruritic papules, vesicles, and/or bullae with an erythematous base; crusting and oozing may be present
- Chronic presentation may include lichenification, scaling, and fissuring
- Can occur on any part of the body that has come in contact with the offending agent

Considerations

- Irritant dermatitis accounts for 80% of contact dermatitis cases
- Skin areas more vulnerable to contact dermatitis include hands, face, eyelids, neck, scalp, lower extremities, feet, and the anogenital region
- Areas with thinner epidermis are at increased risk

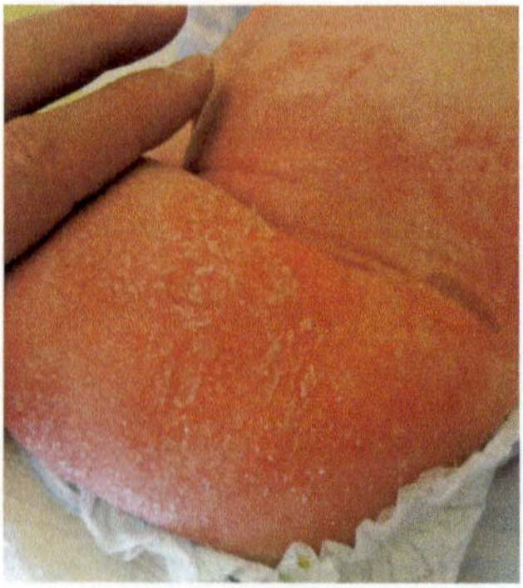

FIGURE 5.3 Atopic dermatitis (eczema) on the abdomen and thigh of an infant.
Source: Image courtesy of GZ.

Eczema (Atopic Dermatitis)

An inflammatory skin disorder characterized by pruritus and exacerbation and remission of dry, itchy, erythematous skin with no known etiology.

History

- Occurs most commonly in infants 3 to 6 months of age (**Figure 5.3**)
- Often has a history of asthma, allergic rhinitis, urticaria, or acute allergic reactions to certain foods
- Pruritis

Physical Examination

- Scaly, erythematous patches
- Xerosis
- Lichenification
- Excoriation
- Possible erosions commonly appear in creases of the elbows or knees or the nape of the neck

Considerations

- Scratching and rubbing further irritate the skin, increase inflammation, and make itchiness worse
- Treatment for the condition aims to heal the affected skin and prevent flare-ups of symptoms

Epidermoid Cyst (A Sebaceous Cyst)

A benign encapsulated, subepidermal keratin-filled nodule.

History

- Most commonly located on the face, neck, and trunk; however, epidermoid cysts can develop anywhere
- Slow growing
- History of chronic sun damage
- Asymptomatic

Physical Examination

- 0.5 cm to several centimeters, non-fluctuant, compressible, smooth, shiny, mobile nodule

- A central, dark comedone opening is frequently present
- If the cyst ruptures, it may look like a furuncle with tenderness, erythema, and swelling (see "Cyst" in Table 5.1)
- A foul-smelling, yellowish cheese-like discharge

Considerations

- May transform into SCC or BCC.
- Can be caused by imiquimod and cyclosporine.

Erythema Migrans

A bulls-eye rash associated with the first stage of Lyme disease.

History

- History of tick bite or being outdoors
- Appears 3 to 30 days after the bite occurred (average is about 7 days)
- Rarely itchy or painful
- Can also be associated with fever, myalgias, lymphadenopathy, fatigue, and malaise

Physical Examination

- Typically the rash occurs at the site of the tick bite.
- Has a distinct bulls-eye appearance (**Figure 5.4**).
- Expands in size gradually over a period of days reaching up to 12 inches or more (30 cm) across.
- May have mild calor.

Considerations

- Caused by the bacterium *Borrelia burgdorferi.*
- Approximately 70% to 80% of people with Lyme disease will have this rash.

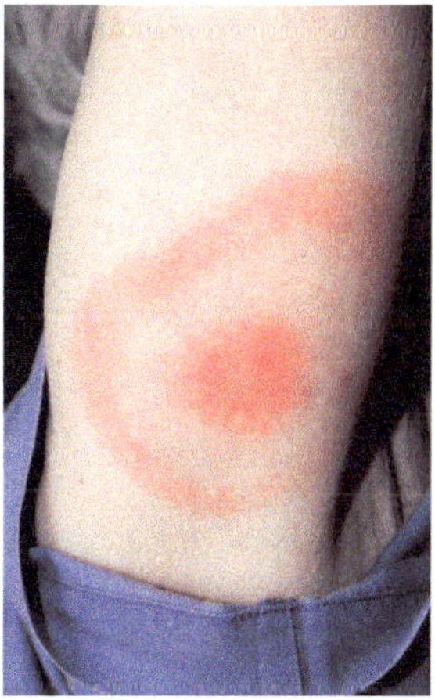

FIGURE 5.4 Erythema migrans.
Source: Centers for Disease Control and Prevention.

Folliculitis

An infection of the hair follicles caused by damage to the hair follicle or from blockage of the follicle.

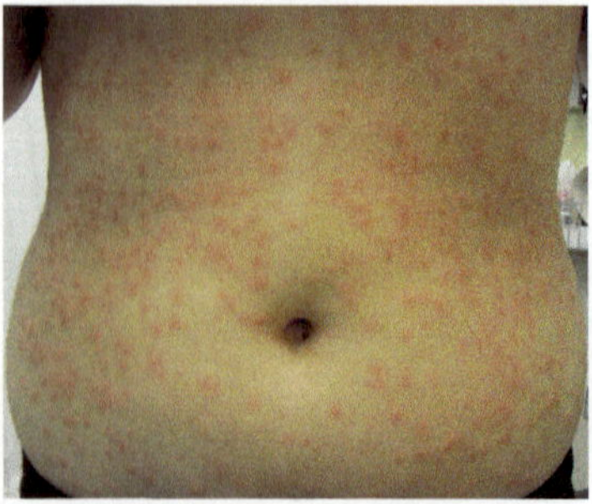

FIGURE 5.5 "Hot tub" folliculitis.
Source: Image courtesy of James Heilman, MD.

History

- Use of razor in affected area.
- Can cause itching or soreness.
- History of hot tub, whirlpool, or swimming pool use.

Physical Examination

- Can occur anywhere on the skin.
- Papules or pustules form around a hair follicle; can look similar to acne (**Figure 5.5**).

Consideration

- Typically due to *S. aureus* bacteria but can also be caused by *Pseudomonas aeruginosa.*

Herpes Zoster (Shingles)

A cutaneous viral infection caused by the reactivation of the varicella-zoster virus, the same virus that causes varicella.

History

- Older adults
- Immunosuppression
- History of spinal surgery
- Tingling, pruritus in the area prior to the eruption of the rash
- Burning, throbbing, or stabbing ("knife-like") pain in the dermatomal area
- Fatigue, malaise, headache

Physical Examination

- Low-grade fever
- Dermatomal rash (thoracic and lumbar areas are the most common sites)
- Unilateral lesion eruption that is initially erythematous and maculopapular then becomes clusters of clear vesicles
- Regional lymphadenopathy
- The lesions crust within 7 to 10 days of eruption (see "Vesicle" in Table 5.1).

Consideration

- Vaccine is available but efficacy decreases with age

Melanoma

A malignancy of the pigment-producing melanocytes in the basal layer of the epidermis.

History

- Reports a spot or sore that burns, itches, stings, crusts, or bleeds or any mole or spot that changes in size or texture, develops irregular borders, or appears pearly, translucent, or multicolored
- A new mole or lesion in adulthood (aside from pregnancy)

Physical Examination

- Lesion that is typically black or brown, but can be skin-colored, pink, red, purple, blue, or white (see "Nodule" in Table 5.1).
- Lesion typically has one or more of the following: **A**symmetry, **B**order irregularity, **C**olor variegation, **D**iameter larger than 6 mm, and **E**volution or timing of the lesion's growth.
- Most commonly located in sun-exposed areas.
- Satellite lesions are present, which are new moles that grow near an existing mole.
- Spread of pigment from the border of a spot into surrounding skin.
- A mole that looks different from surrounding moles (ugly duckling).

Considerations

- Melanoma is often diagnosed in later stages in Hispanics and African Americans leading to poorer survival rates.
- In African Americans, Asians, Filipinos, Indonesians, and Native Hawaiians, melanoma can occur on nonexposed skin with less pigment, with 60% to 75% of lesions presenting on the palms, soles, mucous membranes, and nails.

Onychomycosis

A disease of the nail(s) caused by yeast, dermatophytes, and nondermatophyte molds.

History

- History of diabetes, HIV
- Immunosuppression
- Obesity

- Smoking
- Older age

Physical Examination

- Typically affects the toenails but can also occur on the fingernails
- Discoloration of the nail(s) (whitish, yellow, brown in color; **Figure 5.6**)
- Thickened and brittle nail(s); distortion of shape (ragged, crumbly)
- Onycholysis
- Can have an associated foul odor, pain, or paresthesia
- Microscopy consistent with fungus

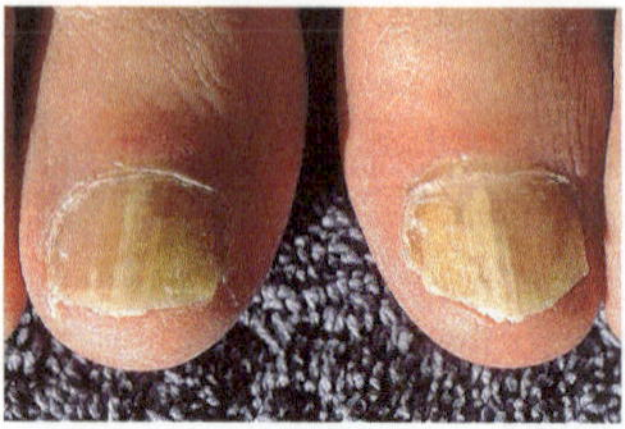

FIGURE 5.6 Onychomycosis of the toenails.
Source: Centers for Disease Control and Prevention/Edwin P. Ewing, Jr, MD.

Considerations

- Candida is the most common type of yeast species involved
- Difficult to treat

Pityriasis Rosea

Pityriasis rosea is an acute exanthematous disease that is associated with the endogenous systemic reactivation of HHV-6 and/or HHV-7.

History

- Usually develops in healthy people who are 10 to 35 years old
- Mild and self-limiting; rash usually disappears on its own without treatment
- Duration may vary from 2 weeks to a few months

Physical Examination

- Begins with a single, circular, erythematous patch called a *herald patch* (**Figure 5.7**)
- Herald patch is followed by a secondary eruption with smaller patches on the cleavage lines of the trunk (configuration of a "Christmas tree")

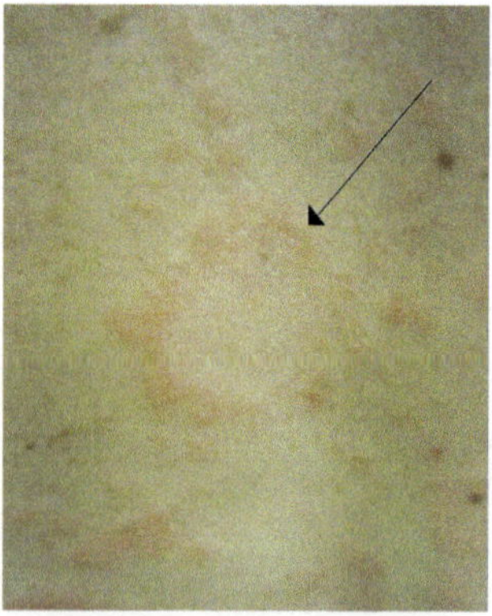

FIGURE 5.7 Pityriasis rosea and associated erythematous "herald patch."
Source: Image courtesy of James Heilman, MD.

Consideration

- Not thought to be contagious

Psoriasis

A complex, inflammatory, multisystem disease characterized by hyperproliferation of the keratinocytes in the epidermis. Most common type is plaque psoriasis.

History

- Pruritic skin lesions are often the most prominent and the only recognized feature of the disease
- Lesions can be painful
- Periods of exacerbations and remissions
- Family history of a psoriasis
- Recent streptococcal throat infection, viral infection, immunization, or trauma
- Joint pain

Physical Examination

- Reddish pink, well-demarcated macules, papules, and plaques with a silvery scale (see "Plaque" in Table 5.1)
- Presence of Auspitz sign (pinpoint bleeding with removal of scales) is a hallmark sign
- Usually form on the scalp, elbows, knees, lower back, but they can develop anywhere
- Worsening of a long-term erythematous scaly area
- Dystrophic nails
- Ocular symptoms: conjunctivitis and blepharitis

Considerations

- Appears to be induced by genetic, environmental, and immunologic factors
- Psoriasis flares may result from systemic, psychological, infectious, and environmental influences

Rosacea (Acne Rosacea)

A common, chronic, and relapsing inflammatory skin condition involving the face and less often the neck and chest.

History

- Can be triggered by ultraviolet light (most common), stress, exercise, wind, heat, spicy foods, dairy, and alcohol
- Fair-skinned European and Celtic individuals; most common in women aged 30 to 50 who are fair-skinned
- History of facial flushing

Physical Examination

- Nontransient erythema, telangiectasia, roughness of the skin, or papulopustular lesions
- Can resemble acne; comedomes are absent
- Neck and upper chest may also have erythema or flushing
- Thickening of the skin of the nose (rhinophyma; **Figure 5.8**)
- Ocular involvement may be present

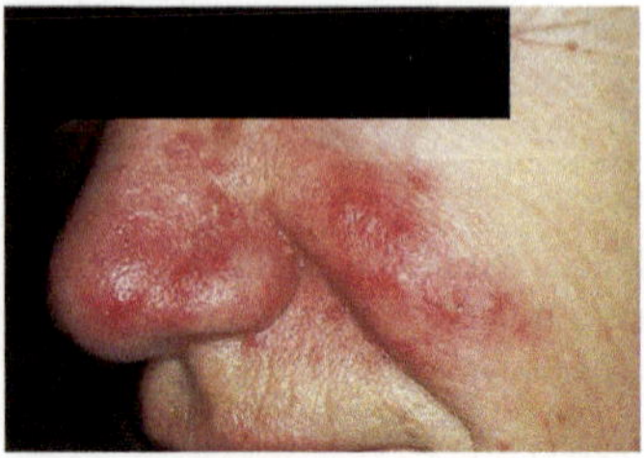

FIGURE 5.8 Rosacea.
Source: Image courtesy of Michael Sand, Daniel Sand, Christina Thrandorf, Volker Paech, Peter Altmeyer, and Falk G. Bechara.

Consideration

- Cause of rosacea is unknown.

Scabies

A skin infestation caused by *Sarcoptes scabiei*, tiny parasites that burrow into the skin and lay eggs.

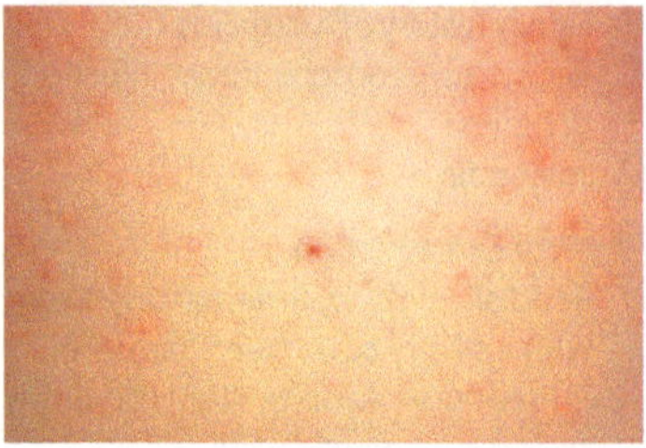

FIGURE 5.9 Scabies.
Source: Centers for Disease Control and Prevention/Joe Miller.

History

- Can take 2 to 6 weeks to appear after exposure
- Institutionalized individuals are higher risk
- Intense, pruritic rash; pruritus worsens at night

Physical Examination

- Maculopapular rash that can be found anywhere but tends to occur between the fingers and toes, under jewelry or watches on the wrist, and in armpits, skin folds, and genitalia
- Lesions can arrange in linear patterns
- Can also resemble pimples, eczema, and insect bites (**Figure 5.9**)
- Infants and young children may appear irritable, not wanting to eat or sleep, and have the rash in less common areas including on their palms or the soles of their feet, face, scalp, and neck

Considerations

- Highly contagious
- Spread by direct, prolonged, skin-to-skin contact with another person who harbors the mites but can also be spread indirectly by sharing articles such as clothing, towels, or bedding used by an infested person

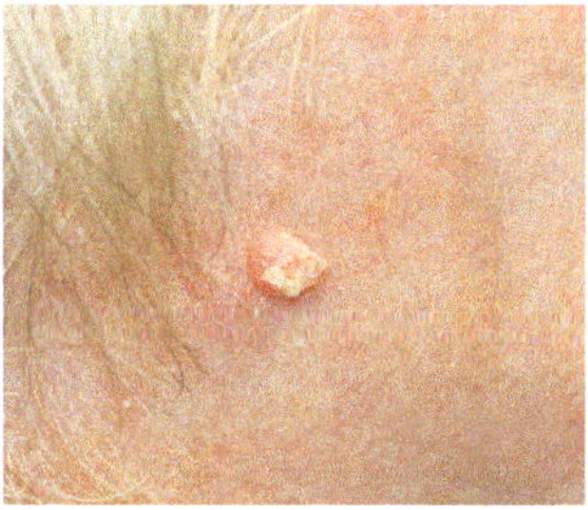

FIGURE 5.10 Squamous cell carcinoma.
Source: National Cancer Institute/Kelly Nelson, MD.

Squamous Cell Carcinoma

Arises from the epidermal keratinocytes.

History

- History of radiation
- Elderly
- Fair skin
- History of sun damage or actinic keratosis
- Can itch, feel sore or tender, and/or feel numb

Physical Examination

- Most common on sun-exposed areas of the skin
- Generally slow growing
- A raised, firm, skin-colored or pink, hyperkeratotic papule, or plaques (**Figure 5.10**)
- Lesion can be isolated or there can be multiple lesions; most occur on the head and upper extremities
- A nonhealing sore or patch of rough skin
- Firm, dome-shaped growth; tiny, rhinoceros-shaped horn growing from the skin; wart-like growth
- Black line under the nail

Considerations

- Second most common form of cancer
- Poses a substantial risk for morbidity, mortality, and impact on quality of life
- Most common skin cancer in Blacks

Tinea Corporis

A dermatophyte (fungal) infection of the face, trunk, and/or extremities.

History

- Highest prevalence in children
- Contact sports participation especially common in wrestlers
- History of diabetes or obesity
- Living or spending time in tropical, humid areas
- Lesions may be pruritic or asymptomatic, occasionally burn, and vary in number

Physical Examination

- A red, scaly patch with distinct annular borders and central clearing; at the lesion's border, inflammation, scale, crusts, papules,

vesicles, and bullae can develop (**Figure 5.11**).
- The size of lesions ranges from 1 to 5 cm, but varying size and distribution may occur.
- Microscopy is consistent with fungus.

Consideration

- Highly contagious

Tinea Versicolor

A benign fungal infection of the skin caused by the fungus *Malassezia furfur*.

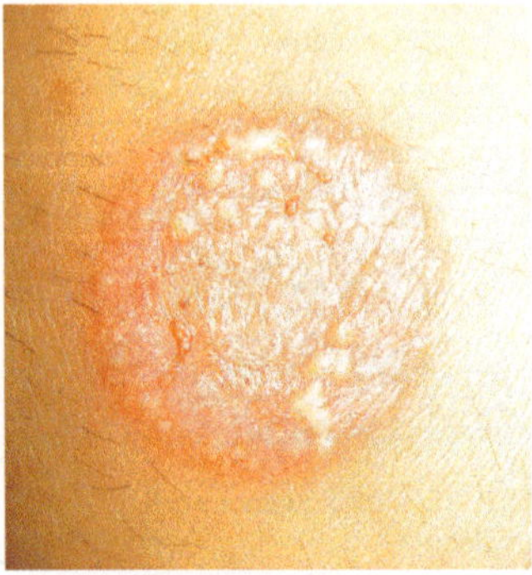

FIGURE 5.11 Tinea corporis.

History

- Often diagnosed in summer
- Teens and young adults are most susceptible
- People of all skin colors are susceptible
- Can be pruritic

Physical Examination

- Multiple tan, brown, salmon, pink, or white scaling patches on the trunk, neck, abdomen, and occasionally face (see "Patch" in Table 5.1); patches may coalesce
- Budding and hyphae noted on a KOH wet mount

Urticaria (Hives)

A skin infection caused by the release of histamine and other inflammatory mediators from mast cells and basophils in the dermis.

History

- May be acute or chronic and is often self-limited.
- May cause significant pruritus (as a result of the histamine released in the dermis) and discomfort.
- Usually resolves within 24 hours; however, they may persist depending on underlying etiology.

Physical Examination

- Raised wheals that blanch with palpation (see "Wheal" in Table 5.1).
- May appear on any part of the body.
- Can be linear, annular (circular), or arcuate (serpiginous).
- Lesions are typically temporary on the affected skin and are usually mobile.

Considerations

- Most frequently identified cause of urticaria is infection.
- Urticaria that is recurrent is frequently associated with sun exposure, exercise, emotional or physical stress, and exposure to water.

Verruca Vulgaris (Warts)

Benign epidermal growths that are caused by various types of HPV.

History

- Common in children; will often resolve on their own.
- Are often asymptomatic.
- Can be painful.

Physical Examination

- Hyperkeratotic papules with a rough irregular surface; may vary in size (1 mm to larger).
- May occur anywhere on the epidermis but commonly found on the fingers, hands, knees, and feet.
- Can contain black dots that look like seeds.
- Are common where the skin is broken.

Considerations

- Wart viruses are contagious and can spread by contact with the wart or something that touched the wart.
- There are several different types of warts.

PHYSICAL EXAMINATION DOCUMENTATION

EXAMPLE OF ABNORMAL FINDINGS

Documentation should include results of inspection and palpation. When describing a lesion/rash, note the following:

1. Primary morphology
2. Size
3. Demarcation
4. Color
5. Secondary morphology
6. Distribution

- **Skin**: Skin is clean, dry, and intact. Skin color and pigmentation are uniform. No lesions, rashes, or ecchymoses are present. Odor and hygiene are appropriate. Skin temperature is warm.
- **Hair**: Hair is thick and blond. Hair distribution is equal and even with no signs of hair loss, hair thinning, infection, or infestation.

- **Nails**: Nails are clean, smooth, and intact with the epidermis.
- **Skin lesion**: 6 mm well-demarcated red plaque with dry serum/ crusting, erosions, and scaling located on the extensor surface of the left leg.

REFERENCES

References for this chapter draw from Chapter 9, "Evidence-Based Assessment of Skin, Hair, and Nails, " of the textbook *Evidence-Based Physical Examination: Best Practices for Health and Well-Being Assessment*. The references may be accessed in the digital version of the handbook at https://connect.springerpub.com/content/book/97808-0-8261-6466-7/chapter/ch05

6

Evidence-Based Assessment of the Lymphatic System

CLINICAL CONSIDERATIONS

- The lymphatic system has many functions and plays a large role in immune system function.
- Palpable lymph nodes can be a normal part of an infectious process or be a sign of underlying pathology.
- Multiple disease processes can cause lymphadenopathy.
- Lymph nodes greater than 1 cm in diameter or in the supraclavicular region should be further investigated.
- In both adults and children, enlarged lymph nodes that are present less than 2 weeks or more than 12 months without changing in size have a very low likelihood of being neoplastic.
- Lymph nodes do not pulsate.
- Both edema and lymphedema can exist in the same patient.

SUBJECTIVE HISTORY

COMMON REASONS FOR SEEKING CARE

Enlargement of lymph nodes (generalized or regional lymphadenopathy)

HISTORY OF PRESENT ILLNESS

- **Onset:** When did you first notice the lymph node(s)? Was it a sudden versus insidious onset?
- **Location:** Is it one lymph node versus one region of lymph nodes versus multiple regions of lymph nodes that are affected? Are the lymph nodes unilateral versus bilateral?

- **Duration:** Is the enlargement of the lymph node(s) recent, intermittent, and/or chronic? How long have they been there?
- **Character:** Are the lymph node(s) painful? What is their approximate size? Are they mobile or fixed? Are they soft or hard? Matted, or discrete? Is there any surrounding redness or red streaks present?
- **Associated symptoms:** Do you have any other symptoms of fever, chills, fatigue, night sweats, sore throat, abdominal pain, nausea/vomiting, arthralgias, or rashes?
- **Aggravating factors:** Have you had any recent infections/illnesses?
- **Relieving symptoms:** Have you tried any pharmacologic treatment, including OTC pain relief or nonpharmacologic treatment, including application of heat or cold to the affected areas?

HEALTH HISTORY

PAST MEDICAL HISTORY

- Chronic diseases (cancers, congenital disorders, autoimmune disorders, CVD, renal diseases, HIV)
- Anemia
- Surgeries (including lymph node dissection/removal)
- Blood transfusions
- Radiation therapy
- Recent injury, trauma, or skin infection
- Recent strep throat or mononucleosis
- Allergies
- Allergic reactions
- Chronic venous insufficiency
- Tuberculosis

Medications

- Prescribed and OTC medications or supplements, including dose and frequency
- Medications that weaken the immune system (e.g., chemotherapy, TNF inhibitors, and corticosteroids)

Immunizations

- Risks for vaccine-preventable illness: Vaccine status; risks for tuberculosis, recent PPD

FAMILY HISTORY

- Cancer
- Infectious disease
- Immune disorders
- Anemia
- TB/positive TB reading

SOCIAL HISTORY

- Smoking history or history of tobacco use
- IV drug use/drug use prescribed, not prescribed
- Recent travel out of the country
- Sleep history
- Sexual history (including risk factors for HIV exposure)
- Animal or food contact
- Exposure to cat feces
- Insect bites
- Stress and coping

REVIEW OF SYSTEMS

- **General:** Weight loss or gain, fatigue, fever, pain
- **HEENT:** Headache, ear pain, nasal congestion, sinus pain, sore throat
- **CV and respiratory:** Shortness of breath at rest or with exertion, cough, chest pain, orthopnea
- **GI/GU:** Abdominal pain, nausea, vomiting, difficulty swallowing, black or tarry stools, dysuria, vaginal/penile discharge, dyspareunia
- **Neurologic:** Weakness, numbness, dizziness
- **Endocrine:** Changes to skin, hair; temperature intolerance
- **Hematologic:** Bruising, bleeding, jaundice, paleness
- **Skin:** Itching, rashes, lesions changing shape, size, or color, nonhealing sores/wounds
- **Psychiatric:** Depression, sadness, worry, insomnia; changes in memory, concentration, or mood

RED FLAGS IN SUBJECTIVE HISTORY

- Unintentional weight loss
- Unexplained fevers
- Night sweats

- Lymphadenopathy without known infection that is persistent, enlarging, or present in multiple locations

PHYSICAL EXAMINATION

GENERAL SURVEY

- **Vital signs:** Temperature, pulse rate, respiratory rate, blood pressure
- Height, weight, body mass index as compared to previous visits (if available)
- Toxic versus nontoxic appearance

INSPECTION

- Do a complete visual inspection, including axillae and groin (**Figure 6.1**).
- Lymph nodes and lymphatic organs should never be visible on inspection.
- Note any edema or redness, including erythematous lines along nodal tracks, lesions/rashes, or indications of trauma on the skin.
- Note any areas of localized edema in the limbs.

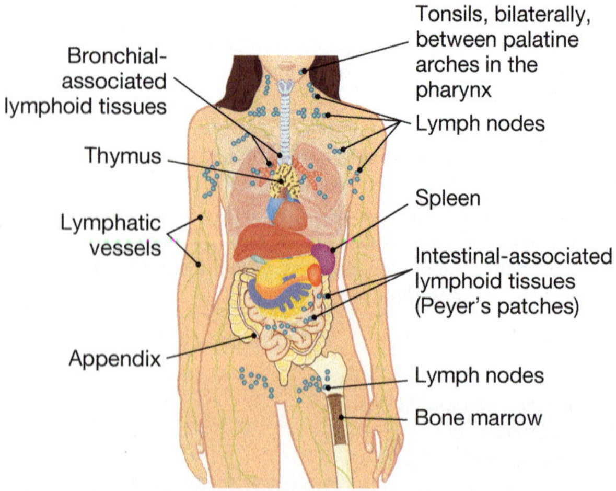

FIGURE 6.1 Lymphatic organs.

PALPATION

- Clinician's hands should be clean, dry, and warm, and fingernails should be short.
- Clinician's fingers should be placed firmly in alignment and against one another to provide a large surface area and better coverage for detection of enlargement or abnormalities. Pads of the fingers should be used for palpation.
- Palpation should be completed using a fluid, circular motion. Soft palpation should be followed by a deeper palpation in order to feel for any hidden enlargement. Too much pressure can cause a mobile lymph node to move out of the examiner's line of palpation.
- Care should be taken to ensure the entire surface area of the lymphatic region is palpated. Remember what part of the body a particular lymph node drains so the clinician can also examine this particular area for local signs of infection or abnormality. It is important to palpate the surrounding tissues since lymph nodes are often found in chains.
- If a lymph node is palpated, the clinician should note the size, consistency, discreteness, mobility, tenderness, warmth, and border edges of the lymph node.

Head and Neck

- Ask the patient to remove all clothing from the regions of the head, neck, and upper shoulders.
- Ask the patient to tilt head slightly down and relax the neck and shoulder muscles. Using both hands, palpate the occipital and posterior cervical lymph nodes.
- Have the patient return their neck to its upright position and ask the patient to raise their chin. Palpate the submental, submandibular, retropharyngeal, tonsillar, preauricular, postauricular, and anterior cervical lymph nodes (**Figure 6.2**).
- Ask the patient to move their shoulders slightly forward and palpate the supraclavicular fossa for supraclavicular lymph nodes (**Figure 6.3**). Then palpate below the clavicles to feel for any infraclavicular lymph nodes.
- Evaluate for symmetry. Clinically significant lymph nodes often present asymmetrically.

Axillae

- Make sure clothing has been removed from the area. Have the patient lay supine and raise their arm over their head. Axillary palpation can occur with the patient sitting in an upright position, but this method can be limiting (**Figures 6.4 and 6.5**).

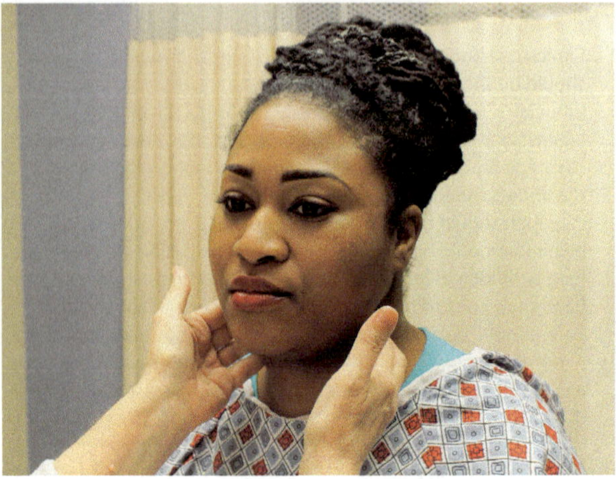

FIGURE 6.2 Proper hand placement for palpation of anterior cervical lymph nodes.

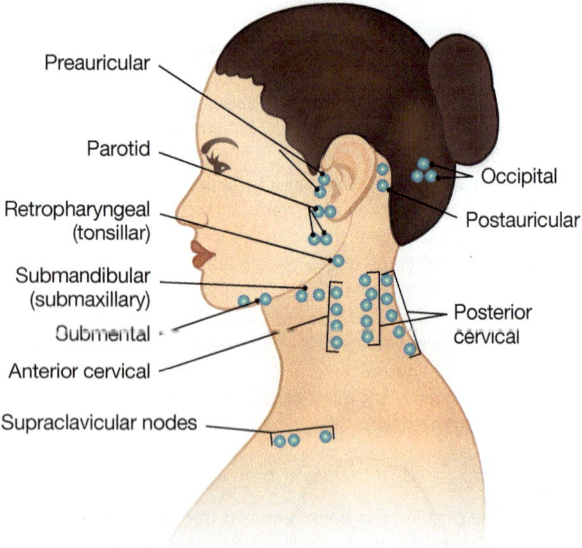

FIGURE 6.3 Lymph nodes of the head and neck.

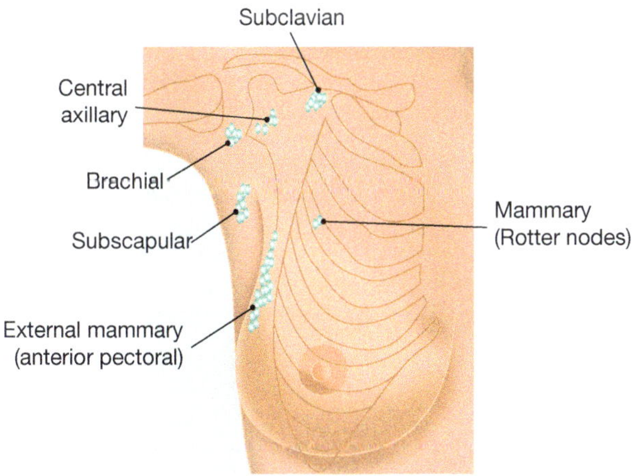

FIGURE 6.4 Axillary lymph nodes.

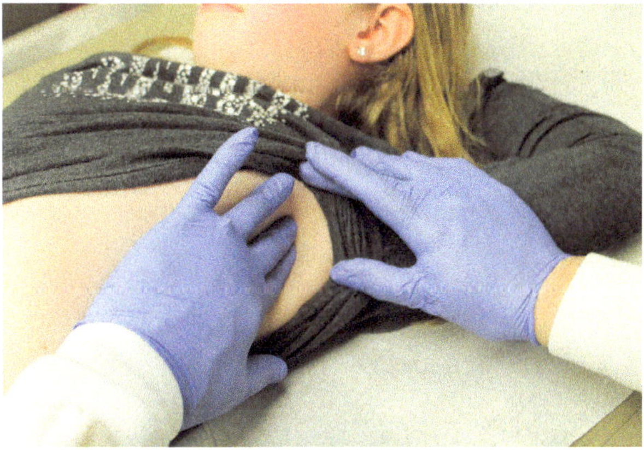

FIGURE 6.5 Palpation of axillary lymph nodes in supine position.

- Use the same circular motion; ensure the entire surface has been palpated then move the hand slowly down toward the elbow until the epitrochlear notch has been located. Epitrochlear nodes are found on the medial aspect of the elbow, about 4 to 5 cm above the humeral epitrochlea. Repeat on the other side.

Inguinal

- Have the patient lay supine. Remove all clothing from the area but maintain a modest environment for the patient by keeping them covered before and after the exam.
- Locate the iliac crest. Move hand toward midline then palpate downward in a diagonal line, remaining parallel to the crease separating the upper thigh from the abdomen (**Figures 6.6 and 6.7**).
- Cover the entire region using a firm, circular motion. Repeat on the other side. With the patient already lying supine, palpate for the spleen if needed.

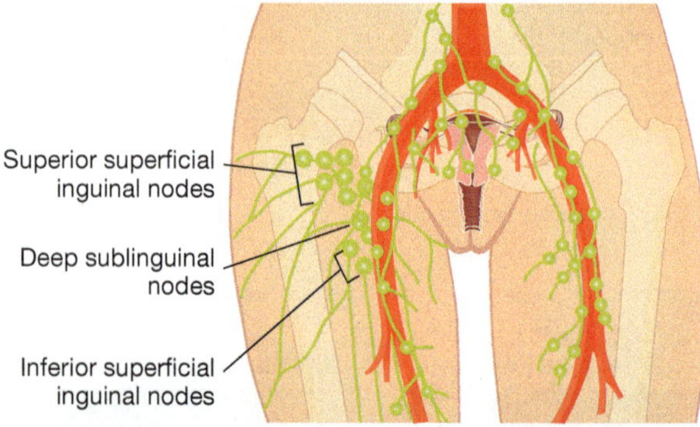

FIGURE 6.6 Inguinal lymph nodes.

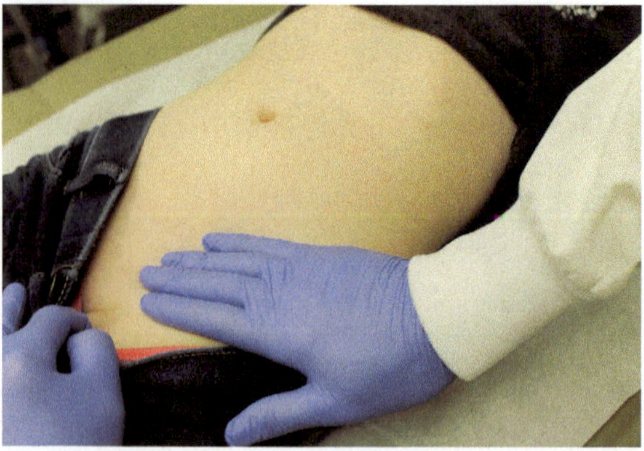

FIGURE 6.7 Palpation of inguinal lymph nodes with the patient in the supine position.

RED FLAGS IN OBJECTIVE EXAM

Lymph nodes with the following characteristics:

- Hard
- Fixed
- Matted
- >1 cm in size
- Located in supraclavicular, infraclavicular, iliac, popliteal, or epitrochlear regions
- Generalized
- Unilateral
- Symptoms:
  - Weight loss
  - Fever
  - Night sweats

PEDIATRIC CONSIDERATIONS

- Roughly 50% of healthy children have palpable lymph nodes at any one time that are either benign or infectious in etiology with up to 90% of children aged 4 to 8 having palpable cervical lymph nodes. The lymphadenopathy is typically self-limiting and does not require further work-up or treatment.
- Similar to adults, large and supraclavicular lymph nodes in children need further investigation in addition to the presence of systemic symptoms.

CONSIDERATIONS FOR THE OLDER ADULT

In elderly patients, malignant disease is the most common cause of persistent lymphadenopathy.

ABNORMAL FINDINGS

COMMON LYMPHATIC DISORDERS

Cat Scratch Disease

A bacterial infection caused from the organism *Bartonella henselae.*

History

- Scratch or bite from a cat/kitten
- Anorexia, fever, malaise, headache

Physical Examination

- Fever
- Erythema, edema, and/or purulent discharge at the site of the bite or scratch
- Persistent regional lymphadenopathy (e.g., if bite is on arm, axillary lymphadenopathy)
- Positive *B. henselae* IFA blood test

Considerations

- Disease spreads to the human when an infected cat licks a person's open wound or bites or scratches hard enough to break the surface of the skin.
- It can have serious complications if not caught early.

HIV/AIDS

A virus that enters the body and invades helper T cells.

History

- Symptoms vary based on disease stage; some individuals are asymptomatic
- History of high-risk sexual activity (e.g., multiple partners, unprotected, prostitution)
- History of IV drug use

Physical Examination

- Stage I—Acute HIV: Flu-like symptoms; positive HIV test
- Stage 2—Chronic HIV: Often asymptomatic and can last up to 10 years
- Stage 3—AIDS:
  - Rapid weight loss; lymphadenopathy; chronic diarrhea; mouth, anus, and/or genital sores; night sweats
  - Opportunistic infections (e.g., pneumonia, tuberculosis)
  - Cancers (Kaposi's sarcoma, cervical cancer)
  - Memory loss, depression, and other neurological disorders
  - Decreasing CD4+ lymphocytes and increasing viral load levels (CD4+ count is <200 cells/mm^3)

Considerations

- It is a retrovirus, a type of virus that integrates its viral DNA into the DNA of the host cell by converting its RNA to DNA.
- HIV destroys the T cells, making it hard for the body to fight infection or infection-related cancers.

Lymphadenitis

An inflammation or infection of one or more lymph nodes.

History

- Often has a history of fever and malaise
- Reports pain/tenderness in lymph node

Physical Examination

- Often unilateral
- Lymph node enlargement, node filled with exudate
- Can have erythema or red streaking over lymph nodes

Considerations

- It most often results from an acute streptococcal or staphylococcal infection.
- Pain and tenderness typically distinguish lymphadenitis from lymphadenopathy.

Lymphangitis

An inflammation or infection of the lymphatic vessels that commonly develops after cutaneous inoculation of microorganisms into the lymphatic vessels through a wound in the skin.

History

- History of fever and malaise
- History of abrasion, wound, or co-existing infection (cellulitis) of the skin

Physical Examination

- Fever
- Enlarged lymph nodes (often in the axillae, groin, or epitrochlear regions)
- Red streaking that extends proximally from a wound or site of infection toward regional lymph nodes
- Leukocytosis

Consideration

- It most often results from an acute streptococcal or staphylococcal infection of the skin. It can have serious complications if not caught early.

Lymphatic Filariasis

A parasitic disease that is transmitted through mosquitos, which impairs the normal function of the lymphatic system, causing edema and decreased immune function.

History

- Travel to endemic areas: Asia, Africa, the Western Pacific, Haiti, the Dominican Republic, Brazil, Guyana, and parts of the Caribbean
- Can be asymptomatic
- Increased infections in the skin and lymph systems

Physical Examination

- Gross edema of an entire limb or body area (most commonly affects the legs but can occur in arms, breasts, vulva, or scrotum)
- Hardening and thickening of the skin in the affected extremity
- Elevated levels of antifilarial IgG4 in serum
- Microfilariae in a blood smear by microscopic examination

Consideration

- *Wuchereria bancrofti* is responsible for 90% of cases.

Lymphedema

Edema or enlargement due to localized lymphatic fluid retention.

History

- History of congenital malformations and/or dysfunction to the lymphatic system
- History of injury, removal, or damage to the lymphatic vessels from surgery, radiation, infection, malignancy
- History of lymph node dissection
- A feeling of heaviness, fullness, or tightness or aching, tingling, or discomfort to the affected area
- History of recurring infections
- Noticeably tighter clothing or jewelry in the affected area
- Diuretics do not improve the swelling
- Elevation of the limb may improve swelling in the early stages but not as the condition progresses

Physical Examination

- Swelling of part or all of the arm or leg, including fingers or toes
- Restricted range of motion and decreased flexibility in nearby joints
- Changes in skin texture or appearance, such as tightness, redness, or hardening
- May or may not pit to palpation

Considerations

- Primary lymphedema: Congenital malformation or dysfunction of the lymphatic system
- Secondary lymphedema: From surgery, radiation, malignancy

Lymphoma

A form of cancer that originates in the lymphatic system.

History

- Lymphoma
- Personal history of the EBV
- Fever and night sweats, fatigue
- Severe pruritus
- Chest or abdominal pain

Physical Examination

- Generalized, painless lymphadenopathy (with the exception of the inguinal region)
- Fever, unexplained weight loss

Considerations

- Two main types: Hodgkin lymphoma and non-Hodgkin lymphoma, although many different subtypes exist
- Tumors develop from the T cells or B cells

Mononucleosis (or Mono)

A contagious illness caused by EBV that invades the body's B cells.

History

- Most common in children and young adults
- Reports extreme fatigue that can last for months
- Throat pain is often severe
- Headaches, myalgias

Physical Examination

- Fever (children may not have)
- Anterior/posterior cervical lymphadenopathy, although others can be enlarged
- White exudate on posterior pharynx and tonsillar; petechiae on the soft and hard palates
- Evanescent nonpruritic maculopapular rash (often occurs early in the illness)
- Palpebral edema
- Splenomegaly (50% of cases), hepatomegaly (10% of cases), jaundice (5% of cases)
- Elevated liver enzymes
- Positive mononucleosis spot blood test

Considerations

- Spread through saliva.
- Children typically don't have as dramatic a presentation, so it is often missed.

PHYSICAL EXAMINATION DOCUMENTATION

Documentation should include results of inspection and palpation.

EXAMPLE OF NORMAL FINDINGS

Anterior cervical lymph nodes are soft, mobile, and tender to palpation bilaterally. Size of lymph nodes are estimated at 8 to 10 mm. All other lymph nodes are nonpalpable, nontender.

REFERENCES

References for this chapter draw from Chapter 10, "Evidence-Based Assessment of the Lymphatic System," of the textbook *Evidence-Based Physical Examination: Best Practices for Health and Well-Being Assessment*. The references may be accessed in the digital version of the handbook at https://connect.springerpub.com/content.chapter/book/97808-0-8261-6466-7/chapter/ch06

7

Evidence-Based Assessment of Head and Neck

CLINICAL CONSIDERATIONS

- Assessment of the head and neck includes review of neurologic, musculoskeletal, and vascular systems.
- Signs and symptoms of thyroid dysfunction can be mild, nonspecific, and varied, and may include symptoms of depression and anxiety.
- Physical examination begins with a general survey, observation, and inspection of the head and neck.
- Expose the neck and clavicles to fully view the head and neck for symmetry, obvious masses, or lesions.
- Infants and children with craniofacial abnormalities may have an underlying genetic syndrome.
- More than 90% of individuals who present with a headache have a primary headache disorder, and their physical exam will be normal.

SUBJECTIVE HISTORY

COMMON REASONS FOR SEEKING CARE

- Headache
- Head injury or trauma; limited mobility of neck or jaw, neck pain
- Difficulty or pain with chewing or swallowing, sense of lump in throat with swallowing
- Constellation of symptoms: Constipation, fatigue, irritability, temperature intolerances, weight gain or loss, skin or hair changes, hoarseness or change in voice

HISTORY OF PRESENT ILLNESS

- **Onset:** When did symptoms start? In what way did symptoms begin? Did symptoms occur suddenly or gradually? Was any type of prodrome or aura experienced?
- **Location:** Where is pain or discomfort located? Is pain or discomfort unilateral or bilateral; in a generalized area or at a specific location of the head, face, or neck?
- **Duration:** How long do symptoms or episodes of having the symptoms last? Has pain or discomfort persisted since the onset? Are symptoms becoming progressively worse?
- **Characteristics:** How would you describe the pain? Is it sharp, dull, stabbing, burning, crushing, throbbing, or nauseating? Does the pain move or radiate when it occurs?
- **Aggravating factors:** What actions, activities, or body positions make the symptoms worse? Are symptoms worsened by lights or sounds?
- **Relieving factors:** What actions, activities, or body positions decrease the symptoms? If relieved, how long does the relief last?
- **Treatment:** What medications has the individual taken to help with the symptoms? Clarify dosage and frequency of any medications.
- **Severity:** How severe are the symptoms on a scale of 0 to 10 currently, and when the symptoms are at their worst? Do the symptoms limit participation in activities? Does pain force the individual to lie down, sit down, or slow down?

HEALTH HISTORY

Past Medical History

- Headaches
- Injury or trauma to the head or neck
- Recent motor vehicle accident
- Past surgical history
- Cancer, past history of radiation therapy
- HIV or other viral infections that cause damage to the immune system
- Elevated blood pressure, hypertension, heart disease
- Smoking history
- Depression, anxiety, or mental health disorder
- Osteoarthritis or rheumatoid arthritis
- Poor visual acuity, need for corrective lenses

Medications

- Prescribed and OTC medications or supplements, including dose and frequency

- Medications that weaken the immune system (e.g., chemotherapy, corticosteroids)

Allergies

Allergies to medications or seasonal, environmental, and/or food allergies. If yes, clarify reaction.

Immunizations

- Risks for vaccine-preventable illnesses; vaccine status, including HPV immunizations, needed or received

FAMILY HISTORY

- Migraine or recurrent headaches
- Neck or thyroid cancer
- Thyroid disorders or dysfunction
- Endocrine disorders or dysfunction
- Arthritis, inflammatory disorders
- Infectious diseases
- Immune disorders

SOCIAL HISTORY

- Use of tobacco, including cigarettes, smokeless tobacco, e-cigarettes or vaping, cigars
- Typical use of alcohol, episodes of binge drinking, alcohol misuse
- Use of prescription medications, OTC drugs, or illicit substances used for nonmedical purposes
- Environmental exposures at work or at home
- Health behaviors, including sleep and rest, coping with stress, nutrition, physical activity
- Sports participation (specifically, contact sports like football)
- Social support system

REVIEW OF SYSTEMS

- **General:** Fever, fatigue, weight changes, appetite changes
- **Lymph:** Lymph node swelling and/or tenderness, bruising, bleeding
- **EENT:** Ear pain, eye drainage or redness, nasal congestion, sinus pain, sore throat
- **Neurologic:** Weakness, numbness, loss of consciousness, headache, recent fall, dizziness
- **MSK:** Injury history, pain with movement; neck pain, stiffness, or swelling

- **GI:** Nausea, vomiting, constipation, abdominal pain
- **Mental health:** Sadness; insomnia; uncontrolled worry; changes in mentation, memory, or mood; current stress level and coping mechanisms; history of panic attacks
- **Endocrine (skin, hair, nails):** Changes in skin, hair, or nails; temperature intolerance; weight changes, fatigue

RED FLAGS IN SUBJECTIVE HISTORY

- Secondary headaches are those with an underlying cause (e.g., tumor, trauma, infection, or inflammation). Although fewer than 10% of headaches have a secondary cause, the higher likelihood of serious complications with secondary headaches warrants a comprehensive history and exam.
- **Box 7.1** includes a summary list of symptoms (using the mnemonic SNOOP) that indicate risk for secondary headache

BOX 7.1 Red Flags in Subjective History That Indicate Risk for Secondary Headache

S = Systemic symptoms
Unexplained fever, weight loss, myalgia, fatigue

N = Neurologic symptoms
Motor weakness, sensory loss, diplopia, tinnitus

O = Onset
Sudden "split second" or "thunderclap"

O = Older age
New onset of "migraines" in those over 50

P = Pattern change
Progressing to daily, precipitated by Valsalva, exacerbated by postural change

PHYSICAL EXAMINATION

INSPECTION

- Inspect the position of the head, symmetry of the cranium; note quality and condition of the hair and scalp.
- Inspect the face and facial expressions for symmetry; note alignment of the eyebrows, eyes, ears, nose, and mouth.
- Inspect the skin integrity of the head, face, and neck; inspect the neck for deformities, pulsations, areas of edema, and limitations in movement.

PALPATION

- Palpate the head for areas of edema or tenderness, including mastoid process; test sensation of light touch on forehead, cheeks, chin.
- Palpate while the individual clenches jaw; palpate the TMJ with opening, closing mouth,
- Palpate the submental, submandibular, retropharyngeal, tonsillar, preauricular, postauricular, and anterior and posterior cervical lymph nodes (see Chapter 6, "Evidence-Based Assessment of the Lymphatic System").
- Palpate the thyroid gland to assess for nodules; enlargement begins with identifying the structures (**Figure 7.1**) and the landmarks of the neck (**Figure 7.2**).
- An anterior or posterior approach can be used for thyroid palpation (**Figure 7.3**).
- To palpate the thyroid gland using a posterior approach (**Figure 7.3A**), ask the patient to tip their chin slightly forward; stand behind the individual and place fingers on the patient's neck just below the cricoid cartilage. Ask the patient to swallow while keeping fingers steady in this position, and the thyroid isthmus can be felt rising under the pads of the fingers as the person swallows. To palpate the lobes of the thyroid, the clinician can (a) ask the individual to tip their chin to their chest; (b) displace the individual's trachea slightly and gently to the right with their left hand; and (c) in this position, palpate the right thyroid lobes with their right hand. Repeat this technique on the other side, by displacing the trachea to the left with the right hand and palpating the left thyroid lobes.
- To use an anterior approach to thyroid assessment (**Figure 7.3B**), ask the patient to tip the head back slightly, and use the landmarks of

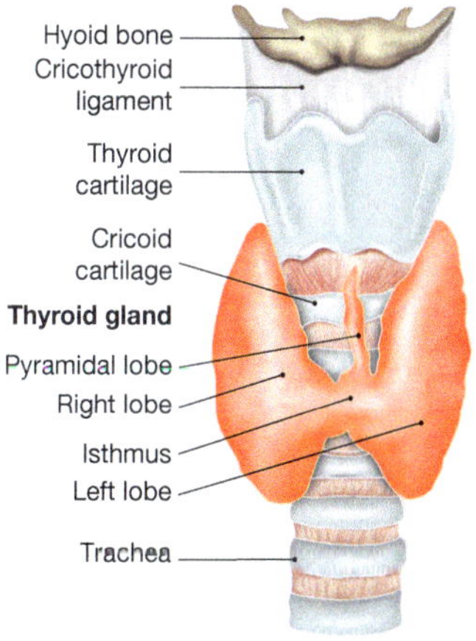

FIGURE 7.1 Midline structures of the neck within the anterior triangle.

the notched thyroid cartilage and the cricoid cartilage to locate the thyroid. Palpate the region below the cricoid cartilage to identify the contours of the thyroid. Simultaneously moving the sternocleidomastoid muscles further apart causes the skin to be taut over the thyroid gland and can enhance the anterior inspection and palpation techniques. To verify the location of the thyroid gland, ask the patient to swallow, and note movement of the thyroid isthmus. With palpation, the thyroid gland is normally soft, without distinctly palpable nodules.

PERCUSSION AND AUSCULTATION

Auscultation and percussion of the head and neck are not components of the routine head and neck exam for asymptomatic, healthy individuals.

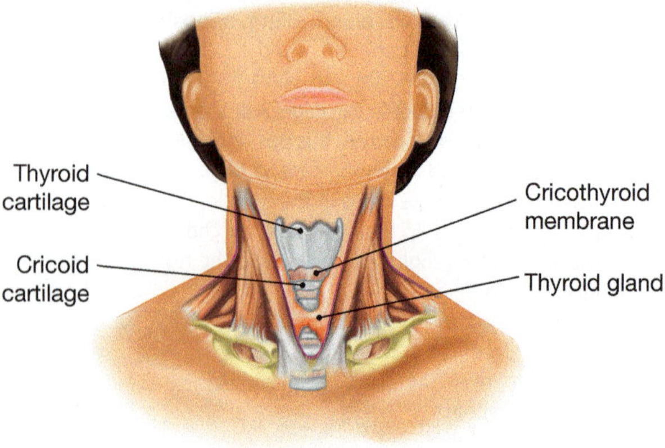

FIGURE 7.2 Anatomic structures and landmarks of the neck used to assess thyroid gland.

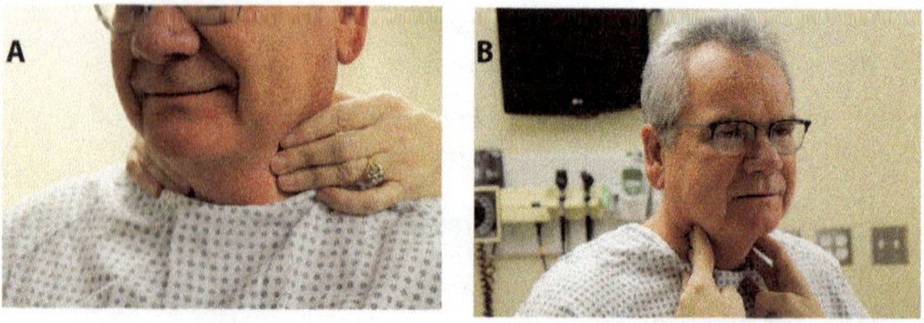

FIGURE 7.3 Palpation of the thyroid. (**A**) Posterior approach. (**B**) Anterior approach.

PEDIATRIC CONSIDERATIONS

- Inspect the head of a newborn, infant, or child to assess size, shape, and form, including presence of fontanels and suture ridges. An accurate head circumference measurement, using a nonstretchable measuring tape to measure above the eyebrows and ears, should be compared with expected size on the growth chart. Inspect for symmetry or asymmetry of an infant or child's head from above and from all angles. Confirm that the line of the eyes is horizontal and that the child's ears are in alignment, to confirm head symmetry.
- During the first days of life, expect that the newborn will have cranial molding. Inspect and palpate the head, noting overlapping suture ridges. A newborn's scalp is likely to be diffusely soft and swollen, a condition called *caput succedaneum.*
- Inspect and palpate the fontanels of infants and children under age 2. The small posterior fontanel is located where the two parietal bones join the occipital bone; the larger anterior fontanel is palpable where the two frontal and two parietal bones join (**Figure 7.4**). Although the posterior fontanel is often not palpable beyond 2 months of age, the anterior fontanel can be palpable up to the age of 2 years. Fontanels should be flat, not depressed or bulging, when palpated. Begin the exam while the infant is calm. Palpate the fontanels while the child is held in both supine and upright positions. Palpation of the anterior fontanel in the upright position may reveal a normal, slight pulsation. If the anterior fontanel has closed prematurely, percuss the skull near the junction of the frontal, temporal, and parietal bones to assess for Macewen's sign, an unusually resonant, "cracked-pot" sound that indicates increased intracranial pressure. Infants with an asymmetrical shape of the cranium that has resulted from positioning, a condition known as *plagiocephaly*, will have normal cranial suture lines and flat fontanels.

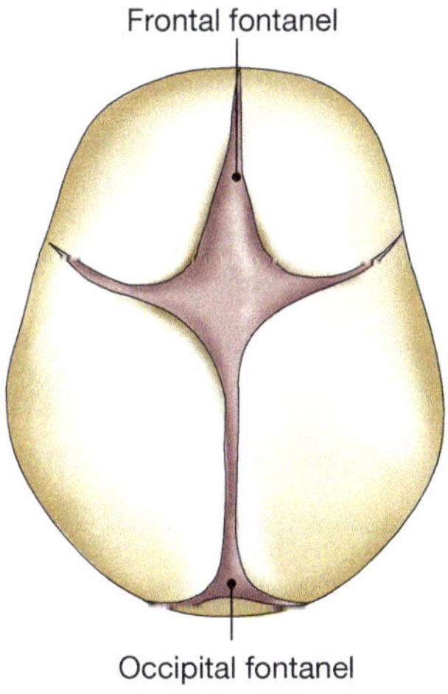

FIGURE 7.4 Anterior and posterior fontanels of the newborn's skull.

- Observe the infant or child's neck control, head movement, and position. Palpate the neck for masses and/or lymphadenopathy. To assess the neck of a newborn more easily, elevate the upper back of the infant to allow the head to extend slightly. Infants and children should have full and easy range of motion of the neck. Nuchal rigidity, or resistance to flexion of the neck, is associated with meningeal irritation. Postural torticollis, twisting of the neck muscles, is relatively common in newborns related to positioning in utero; associated physical exam reveals a preference for tilting the head in one direction.

RED FLAGS IN OBJECTIVE EXAM

- The initial assessment of an individual who has sustained a head injury should include evaluation of neurologic and mental status testing. Red flags indicating severe TBI are listed in **Box 7.2**.

BOX 7.2 Red Flags in Objective Exam That Are Indications of Severe TBI

- Progressive decline in consciousness, profound confusion
- Persistent mental status changes, incoherent speech
- Loss of coordination, seizures
- Pupil dilation
- Mastoid ecchymosis (Battle sign)
- Bruising around orbits of the eyes (Raccoon eyes)
- Clear fluid drainage from the eyes, ears, or nose
- Symptoms in children may include persistent crying, inability to be consoled, or unusual irritability

EVIDENCE-BASED RESOURCES

- **American Academy of Pediatrics:** www.choosingwisely.org/societies/american-academy-of-pediatrics
- **American College of Emergency Physicians:** www.choosingwisely.org/societies/american-college-of-emergency-physicians
- **American College of Radiology:** www.choosingwisely.org/societies/american-college-of-radiology

(continued)

EVIDENCE-BASED RESOURCES *(CONTINUED)*

- **American Medical Society for Sports Medicine:** www.choosingwisely.org/societies/american-medical-society-for-sports-medicine
- **American Thyroid Association:** www.thyroid.org/professionals/ata-professional-guidelines
- **Choosing Wisely Campaign:** www.choosingwisely.org/clinician-lists
- **Endocrine Society:** www.choosingwisely.org/societies/endocrine-society
- **U.S. Preventive Services Task Force:** www.uspreventiveservicestaskforce.org

ABNORMAL FINDINGS

HEADACHE

Primary headaches are those that have no identifiable cause on exam; the diagnosis of a primary headache is made based on recognizing a pattern (which is the reason that only the history is listed in this section). Migraine with and without aura, tension-type, and cluster headaches are primary headaches.

Migraine Headache

History

- Gradual in onset, builds in intensity
- Unilateral in most adults; bilateral in children and teens
- Lasts from 4 to 72 hours, may be recurrent
- Moderate to severe intensity; described as throbbing
- May have aura or prodrome
- Associated symptoms likely to include photophobia, phonophobia, nausea, or vomiting
- Preference for dark, quiet setting to relieve symptoms
- Triggers include stress, food, alcohol, hunger, weather, menstrual cycle, hormones, environment, and/or sleep disturbances

Tension-Type Headache

History

- Gradual onset
- Bilateral; generalized or localized

- Lasts from 1 hour to 1 week; can be infrequent, frequent, or chronic
- Described as pressure, heaviness, or band-like tightness
- No nausea or vomiting associated; may have fatigue, stress, anxiety
- May be related to stress and tension in neck and back
- Can be precipitated or co-occur with migraine

Cluster Headaches

History

- Quick onset, pain intense within minutes
- Unilateral, begins around the eye, temple
- Recurrent, short, painful attacks of 15 minutes to few hours
- Describes pain as severe or very severe burning, piercing, or stabbing
- Ipsilateral lacrimation and redness of the eye, congestion, pallor, sweating, or ptosis
- Can remain active despite headache pain
- Abrupt onset can happen at night; attacks occur one to eight times daily for weeks, followed by remission

HEAD INJURY OR TRAUMA

The initial assessment of an individual who has sustained a head injury should include evaluation of neurologic and mental status testing. See Box 7.2 for red flags indicating severe TBI.

Epidural Hematoma

History

- Experience of blunt trauma or traumatic injury of the skull
- Progressively worsening headache, vomiting
- Dizziness, drowsiness, confusion
- Typically have brief loss of consciousness after trauma, become alert, then rapidly deteriorate

Physical Examination

- Initial Glasgow Coma Scale score is predictor of outcome
- Abnormal neurologic exam
    - Pupils unequal, dilated
    - May become obtunded, have difficulty breathing
    - Risk of seizure
    - Can progress to loss of brain function and death

Considerations

- Neurosurgical emergency
- Occurs less often than subdural hematomas, and usually occur in young adults
- Occurs four times as often in males

Facial Fractures

History

- Generally trauma related (e.g., road traffic collisions, fights, and falls)
- Most common are injuries to nasal bone with profuse bleeding, swelling, bruising

Physical Examination

- Deformity, discoloration
- Profuse swelling and/or bleeding
- Anesthesia of skin at fracture site, may be exquisitely tender to touch
- Cranial nerve abnormalities may be associated with orbital fracture
- Broken or missing teeth with jaw fracture; trouble with chewing, eating, or speaking

Consideration

- Imaging recommendations depend on location and extent of injury

Skull Fractures

History

- Trauma, for example, blow to the head, falls, high-impact motor vehicle collisions
- Pain, bruising, and/or swelling at the area of impact

Physical Examination

- Neurologic changes: changes in level of consciousness, vision, balance
- Bleeding or clear fluid from nostrils or ears
- Bruising at the trauma site, under the eyes, or behind the ears (**Figure 7.5**)

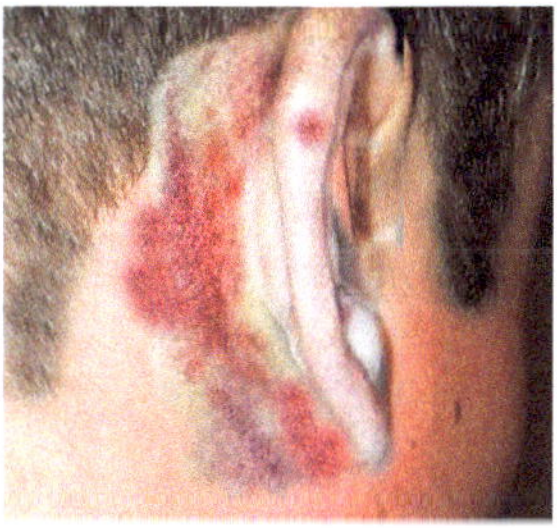

FIGURE 7.5 Battle's sign.
Source: Image courtesy of S. Bhimji. © 2019 StatPearls Publishing LLC.

Considerations

- Type of fracture determined by location of the fracture and the mechanism of injury
- Thin-slice CT has become an integral part of the diagnosis of subtle skull base fractures
- Four types: Depressed, linear, diastatic, and basal skull fractures

Acute, Mild Traumatic Brain Injury (Concussion)

History

- Recent motor vehicle accident, fall, occupational accident, assault, or sports injury
- Injury from direct external contact force or from acceleration/deceleration forces
- Headache, dizziness
- Emotionality, irritability
- Fatigue, drowsiness
- Difficulty concentrating

Physical Examination

- Incoordination, delayed verbal expression
- Inability to focus, blank stare or stunned appearance
- Disorientation, slurred and incoherent speech
- Memory deficits

Considerations

- Information from an observer or bystander can provide key information as individuals often experience posttraumatic amnesia.
- Use of a concussion assessment checklist is invaluable for needed, ongoing assessments.

PARATHYROID DISORDERS

Hypoparathyroidism

History

- Surgery of the thyroid or neck (as the most common cause is accidental removal of the parathyroid glands during surgery)
- Numbness and tingling in fingertips, lips, toes
- Fatigue
- Dry skin
- Muscle aches

Physical Examination

- Paresthesia in fingertips, lips, toes
- Muscle spasms

Consideration

- Signs and symptoms are related to the hypocalcemia that results from the decreased secretion or activity of PTH

Hyperparathyroidism

History

- History of kidney stones, osteoporosis
- Abdominal pain, joint or bone pain
- Fatigue, depression symptoms

Physical Examination

- Elevated blood pressure
- Positive depression screening
- Abnormal labs and imaging

Consideration

- Enlargement of one of more of the parathyroid glands causing excess production of PTH results in hypercalcemia

THYROID DISORDERS

Hypothyroidism

History

- Fatigue, weakness, dyspnea on exertion
- Intolerance of cold temperatures
- Weight gain
- Constipation
- Decreased hearing
- Hoarseness
- Coarse, brittle hair; dry skin
- Myalgia, arthralgia
- Difficulty concentrating
- Heavy menstrual bleeding (women)

Physical Examination

- Cognitive dysfunction, slow movement, or slow speech
- Bradycardia, diastolic hypertension
- Delayed relaxation of tendon reflexes
- Signs of carpal tunnel syndrome, paresthesia
- Periorbital edema and enlargement of the tongue
- Nonpitting edema (myxedoma)
- Pleural effusion, ascites

Considerations

- Key assessments indicating hypothyroidism are related to metabolic changes that result from lack of thyroid hormone.

- A goiter is visible, diffuse or nodular enlargement of the thyroid gland; resultant thyroid activity may result in hypothyroidism *or* hyperthyroidism (**Figure 7.6**).

Hyperthyroidism

History

- Increased perspiration and heat intolerance
- Itching, thinning of hair
- Dysphagia due to goiter, weight loss
- Urinary frequency and nocturia
- Amenorrhea or oligomenorrhea (women)
- Anxiety, emotional lability

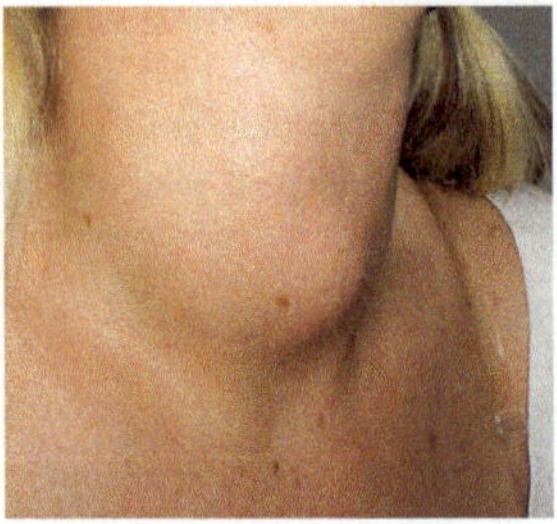

FIGURE 7.6 Goiter.
Source: Image Courtesy of Drahreg01.

Physical Examination

- Hyperpigmentation
- Stare and lid lag, impairment of eye muscle function
- Proptosis or exophthalmos, periorbital edema
- Tachycardia, systolic hypertension, atrial fibrillation
- Weakness, tremor, and palpitations

Considerations

- Older adults often have isolated symptoms that warrant evaluation, including unexplained weight loss, decreased appetite, weakness, and new onset of atrial fibrillation.
- Graves' disease, an autoimmune disease that causes hyperthyroidism, can precipitate thyroid eye disease, which causes upper eyelid retraction, lid lag, conjunctivitis, and bulging eyes (exophthalmos).

Thyroid Cancer

History

- Dysphagia
- Hoarseness
- History of childhood head or neck irradiation
- Family history of thyroid cancer

Physical Examination

- Palpable fixed, hard thyroid mass
- Lymphadenopathy

- Vocal cord paralysis

Considerations

- Thyroid nodules can be incidental findings during routine exams or imaging tests
- History and physical exam have low accuracy for predicting malignancy

PEDIATRIC CRANIOFACIAL DISORDERS

- *Cleft lip and palate* abnormalities result when the lip and/or palate do not completely form; degree varies from mild notch to severe large opening extending to the nasal cavity.
- *Craniosynostosis,* early fusion of the bones of the skull, results in increased intracranial pressure and/or skull abnormalities; differs from plagiocephaly, which is a flat area on the head or side of the infant's head resulting from positioning.
- *Down syndrome, trisomy 21*, is associated with craniofacial abnormalities that include flattened nasal bridge, shortened neck, small low-set ears, and slanted epicanthal folds.
- *Fetal alcohol syndrome* is associated with facial abnormalities, including smooth philtrum, thin upper lip, flat nasal bridge, short or upturned nose, and wide set eyes.
- *Hemangioma,* an abnormal collection of blood vessels in the skin that is faint at birth, but then appears larger and darker in the first few months after birth; also known as *port wine stain, salmon patch,* or *strawberry hemangioma*.
- *Treacher Collins syndrome,* a genetic disorder that causes maxillary hypoplasia and auricular deformities, in addition to a smaller skull or microcephaly
- *Turner syndrome,* a genetic disorder that affects development in females; appearance can include thickened neck, low hairline, prominent earlobes, and crowding of teeth.

PHYSICAL EXAMINATION DOCUMENTATION

Documentation should include results of inspection and palpation.

EXAMPLE OF NORMAL FINDINGS

Appears stated age, in no distress. Awake, alert, and oriented to person, place, and time. Articulates clearly, ambulates without difficulty. Skin warm, dry, intact without obvious lesions or edema; turgor with quick response. Hair with even distribution and pattern.

Normocephalic, no lesions, lumps, scaling, or tenderness of head or scalp. Face symmetric, no weakness or involuntary movements. Extraocular muscle function intact, no nystagmus. No ptosis or lid lag. Neck supple with full ROM, symmetric, no masses, tenderness, or lymphadenopathy. Trachea midline. Thyroid nonpalpable, nontender.

EXAMPLE OF ABNORMAL FINDINGS

Appears stated age, in no distress. Awake, alert, and oriented to person, place, and time. Articulates clearly, ambulates without difficulty. Blood pressure 140/90; heart rate, temperature, and respiratory rate within normal limits. BMI 40. Skin is dry without obvious lesions, generalized nonpitting edema of upper and lower extremities. Coarse, brittle, thinning hair. Normocephalic, no scaling, or tenderness of head or scalp. Face symmetric, no weakness or involuntary movements. Extraocular muscle function intact, no nystagmus. No ptosis or lid lag. Generalized periorbital puffiness noted. Neck supple with full ROM, symmetric, no tenderness or lymphadenopathy. Trachea midline. Diffuse, nodular thyroid enlargement noted.

REFERENCES

References for this chapter draw from Chapter 11, "Evidence-Based Assessment of Head and Neck," of the textbook *Evidence-Based Physical Examination: Best Practices for Health and Well-Being Assessment*. The references may be accessed in the digital version of the handbook at https://connect.springerpub.com/content/book/97808-0-8261-6466-7/chapter/ch07

8

Evidence-Based Assessment of the Eye

CLINICAL CONSIDERATIONS

- Changes in vision and/or eye pain may indicate systemic as well as ocular disease. Early detection and prompt referral can prevent long-term disabling effects.
- Patients who are at high risk for retinopathy benefit from vision screening with a dilated eye exam. Consider deferring an undilated eye exam; often, patients who have had an undilated eye exam believe that they have had the exam as recommended and forgo the specialist evaluation by dilated eye exam. The consequences of failing to have recommended dilated eye exams for these populations can be significant vision loss.
- The fundoscopic exam (direct ophthalmoscopy) in the undilated eye yields assessment findings that are limited. Because the pupils are neurologically designed to close significantly when light is shown in the eye, using an ophthalmoscope to view the posterior retina is restricted. Inform patients that any exam of an undilated eye is limited by the small field of view, despite the high magnification.
- Dilating a patient's pupils in the primary care setting has risks and challenges. Those with cataracts or small pupils or who are unable to cooperate will not benefit from a dilated eye exam. Dilated exams are unsafe for small children, infants, anyone who is hyperopic, and anyone who has had previous acute angle-closure glaucoma. There is a risk of precipitating acute angle-closure glaucoma when dilating a patient's pupils.

SUBJECTIVE HISTORY

COMMON REASONS FOR SEEKING CARE

- Eye pain
- Eye swelling and/or itching
- Eye redness and/or drainage
- Decreased visual acuity or vision loss
- Blurry vision or floaters, cloudy vision, diplopia (double vision)
- Photophobia (painful spasm on exposure to bright light)

HISTORY OF PRESENT ILLNESS

- **Onset:** When did symptoms start? Are symptoms recent? Recurring? Chronic?
- **Location:** Are symptoms unilateral or bilateral? Which part of the eye is being affected?
- **Duration:** Are symptoms persistent or transitory? Increasing or unchanged?
- **Characteristics:** How would you describe the symptoms? Is there itching, tearing, burning, foreign body sensation, photophobia, deep pain, pain on eye movement, tenderness to touch, flashing lights in vision, or floaters? Any vision changes—for example, loss in vision, decease in visual acuity, double vision, or blurry vision?
- **Aggravating factors:** Any recent eye injury, foreign body or chemical substance in eye, recent illness, stressors, sleep problems, and/or overuse of digital devices/screens?
- **Relieving factors:** What actions or activities decrease the symptoms, including flushing of the eye or application of heat or cold? If relieved, how long does the relief last?
- **Treatment:** What medications has the individual taken to help with the symptoms? Clarify dosage and frequency of OTC and prescribed medications.
- **Severity:** How severe are the symptoms on a scale of 0 to 10?

HEALTH HISTORY

Past Medical History

- Recent injury, trauma, or infection
- Past history of eye problems, disorders, diseases, injury, surgery
- Prescription eyewear, glasses, contacts; myopia, astigmatism
- If contact wearer, current practices, including daily cleaning, sleeping/napping in contacts, change contacts as prescribed

- History of systemic disease/disorder with ocular signs and symptoms:
  - **Metabolic endocrine**: Diabetes, thyroid disorders
  - **Vascular**: Hypertension, stroke, migraines, clotting disorders, sickle cell anemia
  - **Autoimmune**: SLE, sarcoidosis, temporal (giant cell) arteritis, RA, Sjogren's syndrome, myasthenia gravis
  - **Inflammatory bowel disease**: Crohn's, ulcerative colitis
  - **Idiopathic disorders**: MS
  - **Infective disorders**: CMV, HIV
  - **Neoplastic disorders**: Melanoma, pituitary adenoma, metastatic carcinoma, lymphoma
  - **Congenital disorders**: Marfan syndrome, Down syndrome, neurofibromatosis

Medications

- Prescribed and OTC medications or supplements, including dose and frequency
- Use of any eye drops, contact lens solutions, or solutions to flush or dilate the eyes

Allergies

- Allergies to medications; seasonal, environmental, and/or food allergies
- Reaction to allergens, including ocular symptoms, anaphylaxis

Preventive Care Considerations

- Diet includes fruits, vegetables high in vitamin A, antioxidants
- Use of sunglasses to limit sun exposure/damage
- Regular handwashing and avoidance of touching the eye
- Health behaviors, including sleep and rest, strategies to avoid eye strain, limit screen time

FAMILY HISTORY

- **Ocular history**: Glaucoma, cataracts, retinal detachment, blindness
- **Visual history**: Poor visual acuity, macular degeneration
- **History of diseases impacting vision**: Diabetes, hypertension, stroke, migraines, genetic disorders, clotting disorders, sickle cell anemia, ulcerative colitis, Marfan syndrome

SOCIAL HISTORY

- Use of tobacco, including cigarettes, smokeless tobacco, e-cigarettes or vaping, cigars
- Environmental exposures at work or at home
- Occupational, educational, or recreational vision requirements, use of protective eyewear
- Risk factors for HIV exposure
- Typical use of alcohol, episodes of binge drinking, alcohol misuse
- Use of prescription medications, OTC drugs, or illicit substances for nonmedical purposes

REVIEW OF SYSTEMS

- **General:** Weight loss or gain, fatigue, fever, pain
- **Head/neck**: Acute or recurrent headache, neck pain, lymphadenopathy
- **Ear, nose, and throat:** Ear pain, nasal congestion, rhinorrhea, sinus pain, sore throat, and itchy ears, nose, or throat
- **Eyes:** Additional symptoms of redness, discharge, blurry vision, eye pain, vision loss
- **CV/Respiratory:** Shortness of breath at rest or with exertion, cough, chest pain, orthopnea
- **GI/GU:** Nausea, vomiting; likelihood of pregnancy
- **MSK**: Inflamed joints, arthritis, weakness, gait or posture defects, need for assistive devices
- **Neurologic**: Numbness, dizziness, light sensitivity, asymmetric facial movements
- **Endocrine**: Polyuria, polydipsia, polyphagia
- **Integumentary**: Itching; rashes; lesions changing shape, size, or color; nonhealing sores/wounds
- **Mental health**: Depression, sadness, worry, insomnia; changes in memory, concentration

RED FLAGS IN SUBJECTIVE HISTORY

- Acute angle-closure glaucoma is uncommon and should be treated as a medical emergency. See **Box 8.1** for a list of symptoms.

BOX 8.1 Red Flags in Subjective History That Indicate Possible Acute Angle-Closure Glaucoma

- Sudden onset of severe eye pain
- Acute change in visual acuity, loss of vision
- Halos around lights, double vision, photophobia
- Eye redness
- Severe headache
- Nausea and vomiting

PHYSICAL EXAMINATION

Examination of the eye by the generalist clinician involves inspection in conjunction with various clinical techniques that incorporate careful observation.

INSPECTION

Inspect eyelids, eyelashes, conjunctivae, sclera, corneas, and irises for abnormal lesions, rashes, redness, swelling, or drainage.

ASSESSMENT OF CORNEAL LIGHT REFLEX

- **Hirschberg test**: Shine a light directly in front of the patient who is focusing on an object across the room (**Figure 8.1**). Observe where the light reflects back within the pupil of both eyes simultaneously.
- Corneal light reflex and observation are the primary methods for assessing eye alignment in infants. In young cooperative children, the cover test can also be used. To perform the cover test, have the child focus on an object straight ahead. Check for deviation in either

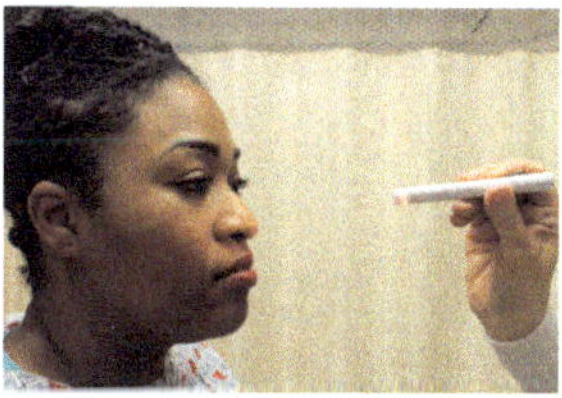

FIGURE 8.1 Hirschberg test to assess corneal light reflex.

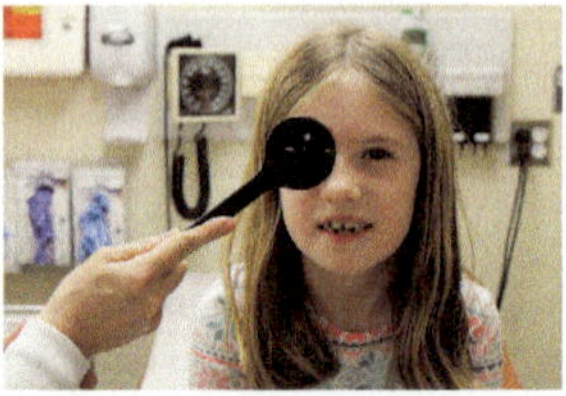

FIGURE 8.2 Pediatric binocular assessment with cover test.

eye. Cover one eye for 3 seconds (**Figure 8.2**). The tested, uncovered eye is observed for movement out of (or back into) its original position. The untested eye is uncovered, while the tested eye is again observed for any deviation out of (or into) alignment. Repeat for the other eye.

- Asymmetric corneal light reflex indicates misalignment of the eyes (strabismus; **Figure 8.3A**); inward deviation of the eye (esotropia) resolves when the opposite eye is covered (**Figure 8.3B**).

PUPILLARY ASSESSMENT

Pupillary Light Reflex

- If possible, perform the pupillary exam in a dimly lit room. Have the patient focus on an object across the room. Shine a light in each pupil, and note the size, position, shape, equality of the pupils, and their response to bright light (**Figure 8.4**). Note that each pupil should constrict with direct illumination and will also

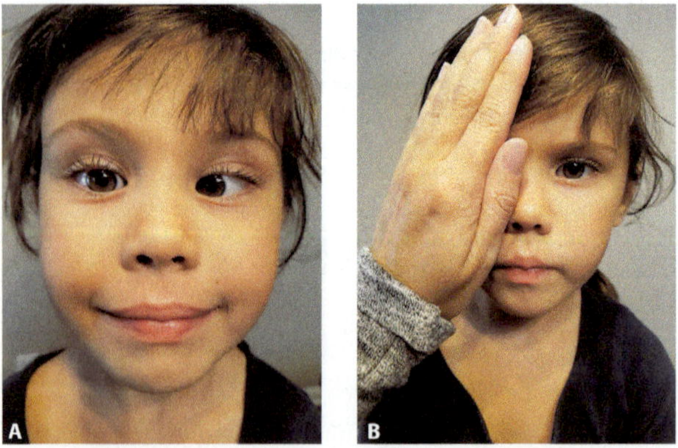

FIGURE 8.3 Esotropia. (**A**) Uncorrected. (**B**) Corrected during exam.

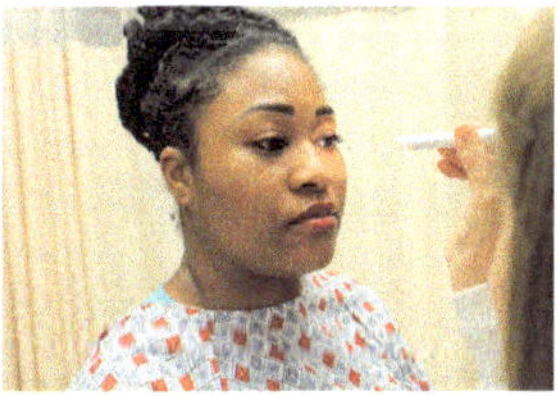

FIGURE 8.4 Assessing direct response to light.

constrict when a light is directed at the opposite pupil. Pupils should be equal in size, round, and react briskly with both direct and consensual response to light. Appropriate pupillary response requires an intact optic nerve, or CN II, and reflects the integrity of CN III, IV, and VI.

Accommodation Reflex

- Pupils should change in size when the eyes change focus on near and far objects. To assess this accommodation reflex, have the patient focus on a distant object, then focus on a penlight and slowly move the penlight toward the patient's nose. Both eyes should turn inward (convergence), and both pupils should constrict (accommodation). These functions are necessary for near and far vision.

VISUAL FIELD TESTING

- Confrontation visual field testing is used as a screening for integrity of CN II, visual field defects, scotomas (blind spots), and serious ocular disorders. Steps to test visual fields by confrontation:
    - Clinician should sit (or stand) approximately 2 feet away from the patient.
    - Clinician and patient should face one another.
    - Both cover one eye (as a mirror image) and maintain eye contact.
    - Clinician should extend an arm and raise a finger. Starting from the periphery, slowly advance the finger into the patient's field of vision. Ask the patient to say "now" when the finger becomes visible.
    - Assuming the clinician has normal peripheral vision, the patient should be able to see the finger at the same time the clinician does.
    - This should be repeated through all fields of vision. (Note that novice clinicians may incorrectly test only the right visual fields when testing the right eye, and the left visual fields when testing the left eye. Because the visual fields of both eyes overlap, each eye should be tested independently through temporal, upper, nasal, and lower visual fields.)

- Alternatively, the clinician can hold up a certain number of fingers peripherally, equidistant between themselves and the patient. The patient is asked to correctly identify the number of fingers. All quadrants (upper and lower, temporal, and nasal) should be tested.
- Confrontation visual field testing is highly specific but has limited sensitivity. To improve identification of any defects in central processing, the clinician may perform additional testing with both eyes open, presenting stimuli in the right and left visual fields simultaneously (**Figure 8.5**).

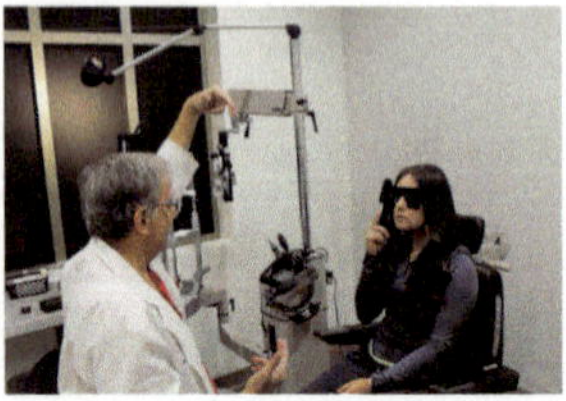

FIGURE 8.5 Simultaneous visual field testing by confrontation.

TESTING MOVEMENT OF THE EXTRAOCULAR MUSCLES

- Smooth and coordinated eye movement requires the use of the EOMs of each eye that are innervated by CN III, IV, and VI. Eye movement occurs in six cardinal fields of gaze.
- To assess EOMs, the clinician stands in front of the patient and asks the patient to follow the clinician's finger with their eyes while keeping the head still and steady in a neutral position. If the clinician uses their finger to trace an "H" or rectangular shape in front of the patient, all EOMs will be required by the patient to follow their finger smoothly (**Figure 8.6**). Note the importance of moving the finger far enough out laterally and vertically to elicit

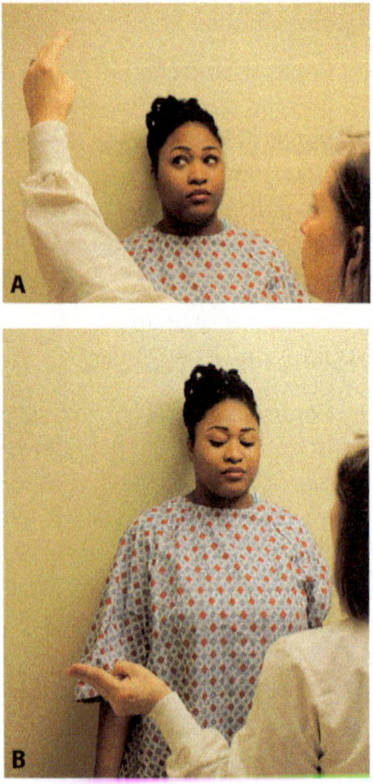

FIGURE 8.6 Assessment of extraocular muscles. (**A**) Assess upward gaze (top of the "H" on patient's right side). (**B**) Assess downward gaze (bottom of the "H" on patient's right side).

the full range of eye movements, and remember to assess movement across the entire "H" to assess the six cardinal fields of gaze: lateral and upward, lateral and downward, lateral, medial, medial and upward, medial and downward.

DIRECT OPHTHALMOSCOPY

- Direct ophthalmoscopy, or fundoscopy, is used to assess concerns related to the retina, macula, optic nerve, or vasculature of the eye. Signs, symptoms, and/or history that are concerning for serious eye disease or increased intracranial or IOP should be urgently referred. A dilated fundoscopic exam (facilitated by mydriatic drops) should be performed by an ophthalmologist or optometrist for diagnostic purposes.
- Inspection of the peripheral retina, optic nerve, macula, and vasculature of the eye using direct ophthalmoscopy is a particularly difficult technique because of the small field of view and magnification adjustments required for the individual who has poor visual acuity. It is even more challenging when the pupils are not dilated. To perform the exam as effectively as possible:
  - Darken the room; ask the patient to focus on an object far away to help dilate the pupil.
  - Clinician should place the ophthalmoscope firmly against their own cheek. The clinician and ophthalmoscope should move as one unit.
  - Use the right hand/eye to assess the patient's right eye and vice versa.
  - Look through the ophthalmoscope to determine whether it is in focus and adjust the diopter setting if needed.
  - Direct the light of the ophthalmoscope into the pupil at a medial angle and watch for the red reflex, the red or reddish-orange reflection of light from the fundus.
  - Slowly move toward the patient while following the red reflex. If the red reflex is lost, start over. Follow the red reflex all the way in until the vasculature is seen. Follow the direction of the blood vessels in until the optic disc is visualized.
- At this point, the clinician is approximately nose-to-nose with the patient (**Figure 8.7**) and can pivot the ophthalmoscope to view the remainder of the retina, macula/fovea, and blood vessels (**Figure 8.8**).

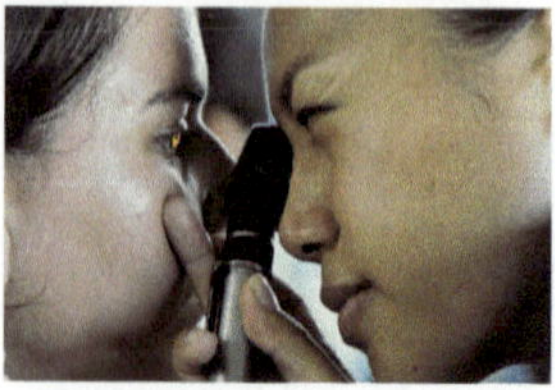

FIGURE 8.7 Ophthalmoscopy.

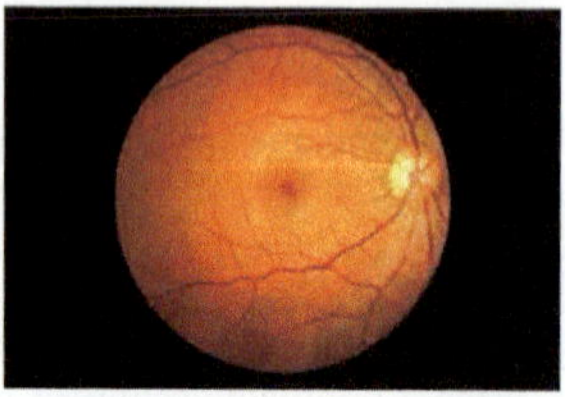

FIGURE 8.8 Normal fundal exam.

Assessment of the Red Reflex

- Assessment of the red reflex bilaterally is a priority for infants and young children who are unable to verbalize visual disturbances. Any asymmetry in red reflex, dark spots, or leukocoria (white reflex) is abnormal and may be indicative of cataracts, retinal disease, retinoblastoma, or ocular tumor (**Figure 8.9**).

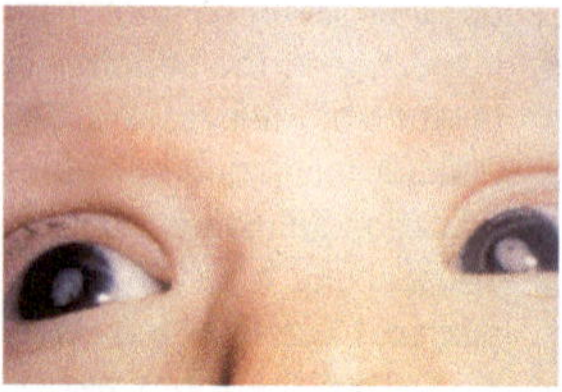

FIGURE 8.9 Infant with cataracts from congenital rubella syndrome. *Source:* Centers for Disease Control and Prevention.

- These abnormalities have been identified through lack of "red eye" in photographs. To best assess the red reflex in clinical practice, use an ophthalmoscope to visualize the pupil. Look through the ophthalmoscope while shining the light into the pupil. This technique works best in a dimly lit room with a calm, awake infant or young child. The clinician may need to view at different angles to elicit the reflex.

MEASUREMENT OF VISUAL ACUITY

- Visual acuity is not assessed on a routine basis as a component of physical exams in most cases, except for children; however, assessing visual acuity can provide useful data when patients present with clinical concerns as acute change in visual acuity may be a worrisome sign.
- Snellen visual acuity charts are widely used. They have been modified over the years for different languages and include numbers and pictures for children and others who cannot read the letters.

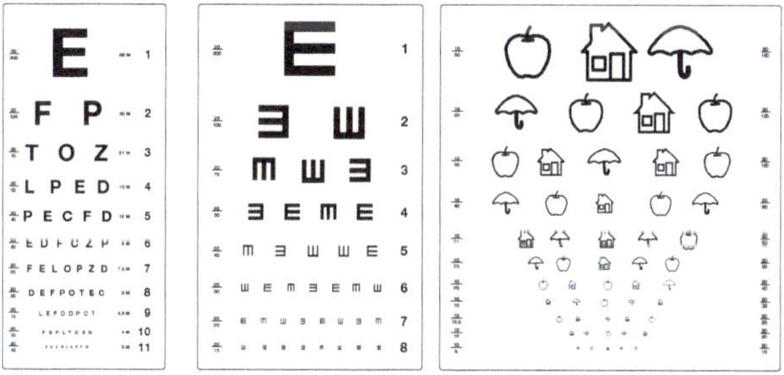

FIGURE 8.10 Snellen visual acuity chart.

- When testing visual acuity with a Snellen chart (**Figure 8.10**), the patient should stand at a 20-foot distance fro the chart. Each eye is tested independently—one eye is covered, while the other is used to read. The patient should be allowed to wear glasses; document results as "best corrected vision." Ask patient to read the line with the smallest characters that they can see. The numbers at the end of the line provide an indication of the patient's acuity compared with those who have normal vision. The larger the denominator, the worse the acuity. For example, 20/200 indicates that the patient can see at 20 feet what an individual with normal vision can see at 200 feet. If the patient is unable to read any of the lines on the chart, an estimate of what they are capable of seeing should be assessed (e.g., ability to count fingers, detect motion, or perceive light).

PEDIATRIC CONSIDERATIONS

- At each routine wellness visit, these assessments should be performed on all children aged newborn to 3 years:
  - Vision assessment, including visual fixation, tracking, visual interest, and attentiveness
  - Inspection of eyes, including lids, eyelashes, conjunctiva, corneas, sclera, irises, pupils
  - Assessment of corneal light reflex and movement of the eyes (EOMs)
  - Pupillary function, including reaction to light, accommodation, convergence
  - Red reflex (may appear gray or cream colored in infants with darker-pigmented skin)

- For children aged 3 years and older, age-appropriate visual acuity screening and fundoscopy should be included as components of the pediatric eye exam. Clinicians should complete these screening exams when children are able to be cooperative, and not when children are experiencing illness or fatigue.

PREGNANCY CONSIDERATIONS

Numerous physiologic effects occur within the body during pregnancy, and the eye is no exception. Normal physiologic changes include:

- Decrease in corneal sensitivity
- Slight increase in corneal thickness
- Changes in corneal curvature
- Contact lens intolerance as a result of a change in corneal curvature, increased corneal thickness/edema, or an altered tear film
- Decreased or transient loss of accommodation

CONSIDERATIONS FOR THE OLDER ADULT

Age-related changes include:

- Eyelid laxity and deepening of the lines of expression
- Changes in corneal curvature and decreased corneal luster
- Increased resistance to the outflow of aqueous humor in the trabecular network
- Hardening (nuclear sclerosis) of the lens
- Less collagen, which causes liquefaction of vitreous humor
- Decline in visual function, including function of the lens, resulting in presbyopia (far-sightedness)
- Decreased contrast sensitivity resulting in reduced depth perception
- Increased susceptibility to age-related diseases (e.g., macular degeneration)

RED FLAGS IN OBJECTIVE EXAM

- Timing is everything. Do not hesitate to refer patients to ophthalmology for abnormal findings associated with ocular assessment and vision.
- Red flags indicating serious neurologic or ocular disorders are listed in **Box 8.2**.

BOX 8.2 Red Flags in Objective Exam That Are Indications of Serious Neurologic or Ocular Disorders

- Intense eye redness of conjunctiva, sclera, lens, cornea
- Severe, purulent discharge from eye(s)
- Lens opacities, hazy cornea
- Loss of vision, visual field defects, change in visual acuity
- Pupil dilation or pupils unequal in size or shape
- Slow or absent pupil reaction to light
- Papilledema
- Periorbital or orbital erythema, edema, and tenderness
- Ptosis, painful or limited extraocular movements

EVIDENCE-BASED RESOURCES

- **American Academy of Ophthalmology:** www.aao.org
- **American Association for Pediatric Ophthalmology and Strabismus:** https://aapos.org
- **American Diabetes Association:** www.diabetes.org
- **American Optometric Association:** www.aoa.org
- **Choosing Wisely Campaign:** www.choosingwisely.org
- **U.S. Preventive Services Task Force:** www.uspreventiveservicestaskforce.org

ABNORMAL FINDINGS

The abnormal findings and differential diagnoses listed in this section are in alphabetical order, not in order of prevalence. The list is not exhaustive.

CATARACTS

History

- Cloudy, blurry vision
- Poor night vision; halos around lights

- Typically symptoms have progressed slowly, over years
- Risk factors: Diabetes, smoking, alcohol use, prolonged exposure to ultraviolet sunlight

Physical Examination

- Cloudy changes to the lens of the eye
- Missing or irregular red reflex (often leads to the discovery of cataracts in children)

Considerations

- Incidence increases with age
- Pediatric cataracts are either present at birth (congenital) or develop in early childhood

CONJUNCTIVITIS

History

- Burning, itching, foreign-body sensation, and/or eye drainage
- Contact lens wearers have increased risk

Physical Examination

- Common signs: Injection or redness and swelling of the conjunctiva, eye drainage

Considerations

- The etiology of conjunctivitis needs to be differentiated to ensure appropriate treatment.
    - Chemical irritants and fungal organisms can infect the eye and lead to conjunctivitis.
    - The incidence of conjunctivitis in patients with COVID-19 is being studied to determine exposure and transmission risks
    - The three most common causes or types of conjunctivitis are viral, bacterial, and allergic.

Allergic Conjunctivitis

History

- Itchy eyes; intense itching of eyelids
- Watery or clear mucoid drainage
- Co-occurring extraocular allergy symptoms, rhinorrhea

Physical Examination

- Reddened sclera from injected conjunctivae
- May have edema and erythema of eyelids, loss of lashes (**Figure 8.11**)
- May have hypertrophy of conjunctiva resembling "cobblestones"
- Associated signs of allergies, including rhinitis, allergic shiners

Considerations

- Caused by reaction to allergens such as pollen, ragweed, dust mites, molds, pet dander, medicines, or cosmetics
- Not contagious, occurs more commonly in people with other allergic conditions like asthma or eczema

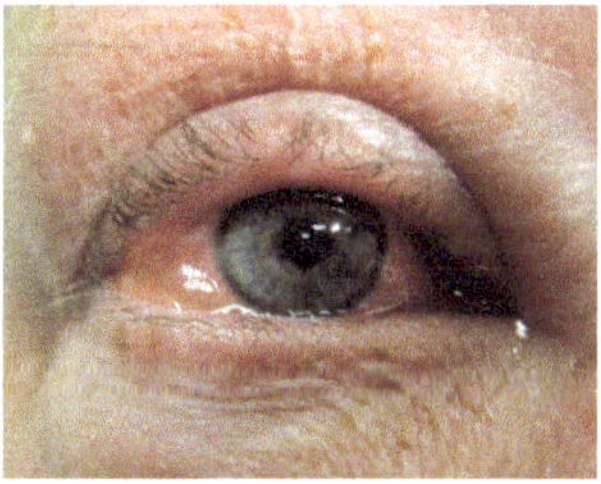

FIGURE 8.11 Allergic conjunctivitis.
Source: Image courtesy of James Heilman, MD.

Bacterial Conjunctivitis

History

- Significant crusting and matting of eyelashes from mucopurulent drainage, especially after waking
- May be unilateral, although commonly spreads to both eyes
- In children, comorbid otitis media is common

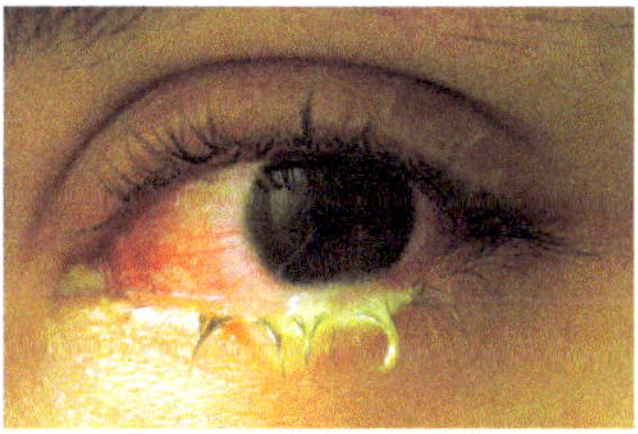

FIGURE 8.12 Bacterial conjunctivitis.
Source: Image courtesy of Tanalai.

Physical Examination

- Scleral erythema, injected conjunctivae
- Purulent eye discharge (**Figure 8.12**); may have lid swelling

Considerations

- Referred to as *pink eye,* highly contagious
- More common in children than adults
- If present in newborn, gonorrhea or chlamydia may be causal agent; treatment needed to prevent sepsis and vision loss

Viral Conjunctivitis

History

- Usually occurs concomitantly with symptoms of upper respiratory infection
- Symptoms often begin in one eye, but can be in both

Physical Examination

- Reddened sclera and watery drainage (**Figure 8.13**)

Considerations

- Most common viral cause: Adenoviruses

- Conjunctivitis caused by viruses like measles or herpes simplex virus present with additional extraocular, cutaneous lesions consistent with the causative agent

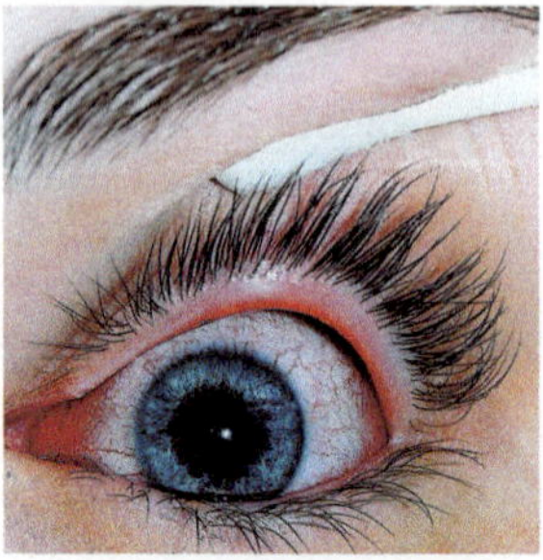

FIGURE 8.13 Viral conjunctivitis.
Source: Image courtesy of Joyhill09.

CORNEAL ABRASION

History

- Injury to the eye caused by foreign body, contact lens, trauma
- Excruciating eye pain that precludes normal daily activities
- Inability to open the affected eye due to foreign body sensation

Physical Examination

- Fluorescein-staining reveals abrasion on surface of the cornea.
- If a foreign body is suspected, the clinician may perform a lid eversion, "flipping" the lid inside out to inspect for a retained foreign body.

Consideration

- Penetrating trauma (ruptured globe) should be ruled out with a penlight exam by evaluating eye structures and pupil function; assess for clear drainage of aqueous humor.

DACRYOSTENOSIS

History

- Newborn with excess tearing
- Dacryostenosis is a congenital lacrimal duct obstruction that typically resolves spontaneously by 6 to 12 months of age; gentle massage may help relieve the blockage

Physical Examination

- Persistent clear eye discharge without reddened sclera

Considerations

- Can be acquired in other age groups after injury or surgery
- Dacryocystitis, an infection of the nasolacrimal duct system, is a rare complication of dacryostenosis; key signs and symptoms

include erythema, swelling, warmth, and tenderness of the nasolacrimal sac, and/or purulent eye drainage

DIPLOPIA

- Causes of diplopia (double vision) depend primarily on whether the diplopia is monocular or binocular. Binocular diplopia is present when both eyes are open and absent when one eye is closed. Monocular diplopia persists even when one eye is closed.
- Monocular diplopia is suggestive of local unilateral eye disease or refractive error. Causes of monocular diplopia include cataracts; high astigmatism error; keratoconus, a collagen vascular condition causing a very steep cornea; displacement or subluxation of the lens, highly associated with Marfan syndrome.
- Binocular diplopia results from ocular misalignment. Sudden development should be evaluated urgently to rule out neurologic disorders, vascular pathologies, or mass/lesion etiologies. Common causes include strabismus; palsy of CN III, IV, or VI; myasthenia gravis or Graves' disease; trauma to the eye muscles.

GLAUCOMA

Acute Angle-Closure Glaucoma

Optic neuropathy characterized by unequal or elevated IOP from insufficient drainage or excessive production of aqueous humor. It can lead to vision loss if untreated.

History

- Dramatic onset of symptoms (see Box 8.1 for red flags).

Physical Examination

- Severely elevated and/or asymmetric IOPs
- Conjunctival injection
- Fixed or sluggish, dilated pupil (**Figure 8.14**)

Considerations

- Causes sudden and severe damage to the optic nerve
- Should be treated as a medical emergency!

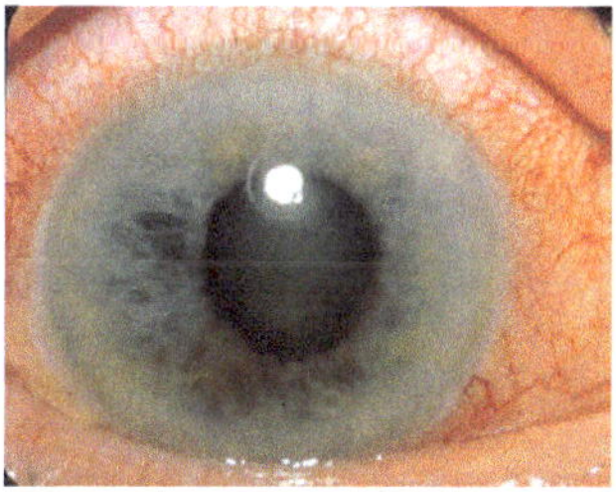

FIGURE 8.14 Acute angle-closure glaucoma.
Source: Image courtesy of Jonathan Trobe, M.D.

Open-Angle Glaucoma

Glaucoma is optic neuropathy characterized by unequal or elevated IOP from insufficient drainage or excessive production of aqueous humor. It can lead to vision loss if untreated.

History

- Patchy blind spots in the peripheral or central vision
- Tunnel vision in advanced stages
- Risk factors: Family history, ethnicity, age over 65

Physical Examination

- Asymmetric IOPs
- May have retinal hemorrhages

Considerations

- Known as the *silent blinder* because it is often asymptomatic

MACULAR DEGENERATION

History

- Patients over 50 years of age most at risk
- Increased difficulty adapting to low light levels; increased blurriness of printed words
- Difficulty recognizing faces

Physical Examination

- Reduced central vision in one or both eyes
- Fundoscopic exam may reveal focal areas of retinal pigment loss, lesions

Consideration

- An Amsler grid can be used to detect vision changes associated with macular degenerations (**Figure 8.15**).

OPTIC NEURITIS AND RETROBULBAR NEURITIS

This is an inflammatory condition of the optic nerve.

History

- Sudden onset of unilateral visual loss, unilateral orbital pain
- Occurs most often in ages 18 to 45 years
- Loss of color vision in the affected eye

Physical Examination

- Absent or diminished pupillary response
- Visual field defects (central or peripheral)
- Fundoscopy may reveal papilledema, flame-shaped hemorrhages, and vitreous cells

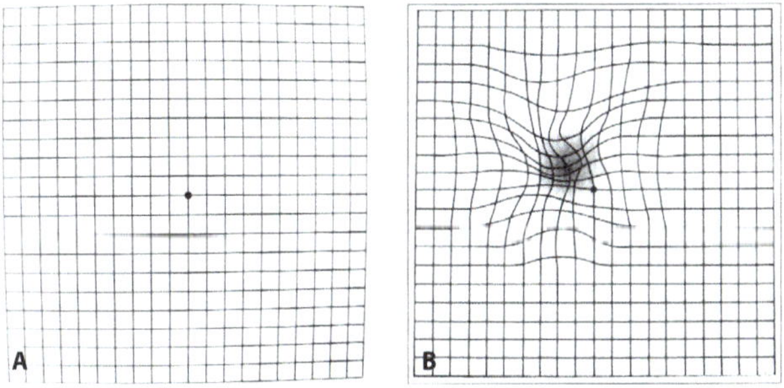

FIGURE 8.15 Amsler grid. (**A**) Amsler grid used to detect changes in vision. (**B**) Distorted Amsler grid.
Source: Image A courtesy of Rosmarie Voegtli. Image B courtesy of National Institutes of Health and National Eye Institute.

Consideration

- Causes include multiple sclerosis, infective organisms (including viruses), granulomatous inflammatory conditions, tuberculosis, syphilis, sarcoidosis, and autoimmune disorders

ORBITAL AND PERIORBITAL CELLULITIS

Periorbital cellulitis is an infection of the anterior portion of the upper and/or lower eyelid(s). Orbital cellulitis is an infection of the tissue in the orbit (eye socket).

History

- With either type of cellulitis, history includes eye pain with eyelid swelling and erythema.
- Orbital cellulitis generally presents with more severe clinical features: pain with eye movements, impaired eye movement, and proptosis (forward displacement of the globe).

Physical Examination

- Both conditions cause eyelid swelling and erythema surrounding the eye (**Figure 8.16**)

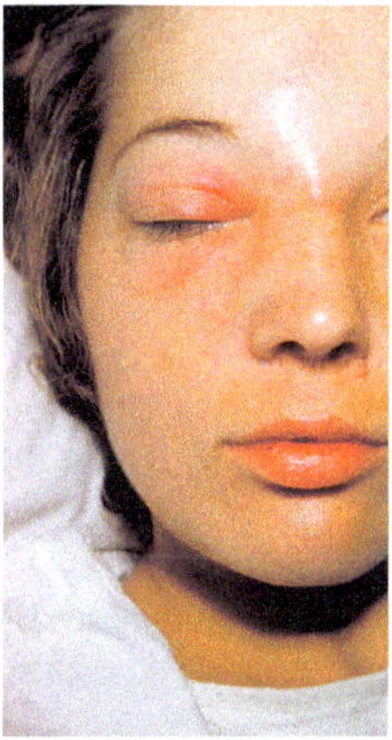

FIGURE 8.16 Orbital cellulitis.
Source: Centers for Disease Control and Prevention /Dr. Thomas F. Sellers, Emory University.

Considerations

- Most common cause of periorbital cellulitis: Infection secondary to local skin trauma.
- Most common causes of orbital cellulitis: Acute sinusitis, ophthalmic surgery, orbital trauma.

PINGUECULUM

Benign growth of the conjunctiva.

History

- Chronic dry eyes
- Recurrent exposure to wind, dust, and ultraviolet light or sunlight

Physical Examination

- Growth appears as a yellow bump on the inner canthus of the conjunctiva (**Figure 8.17**).

Consideration

- Can progress to pterygium.

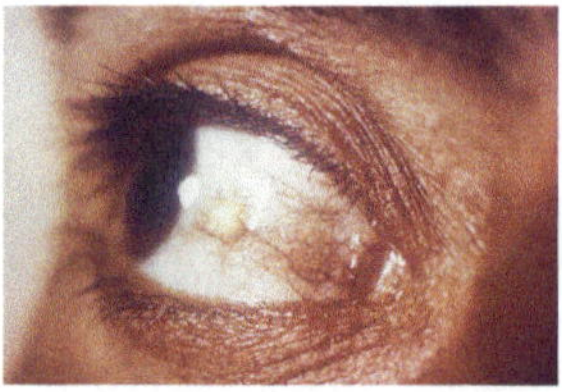

FIGURE 8.17 Pinguecula.
Source: Centers for Disease Control and Prevention.

PTERYGIUM

Benign growth of the conjunctiva.

History

- Chronic dry eyes
- Recurrent exposure to wind, dust, and ultraviolet light or sunlight

Physical Examination

- Growth of fleshy tissue that often arises from the pinguecula (**Figure 8.18**)

Consideration

- Can potentially obstruct vision by causing an astigmatic distortion of the cornea

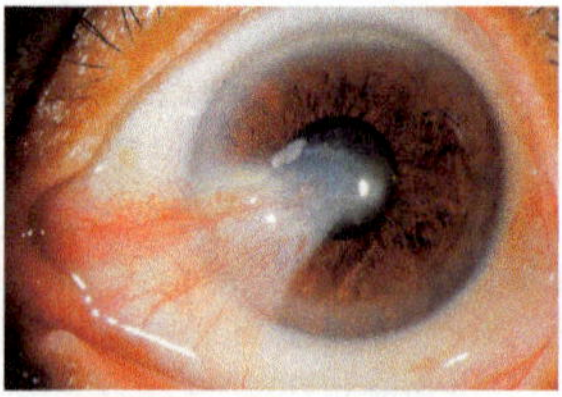

FIGURE 8.18 Pterygium.
Source: Image courtesy of Jmvaras.

RETINAL ABNORMALITIES

Retinal Floaters

A condition in which specks, black spots, or threads "float about" in a person's vision. These floaters move as the eyes move and are most noticeable to people when looking at a plain, bright background. Common causes are age-related. However, more serious conditions like posterior vitreous detachment can be an underlying cause.

Retinal Tears

In some cases of posterior vitreous detachment, the vitreous can pull away hard enough to tear the retina. A torn retina may result in a torn retinal vessel, which results in blood leaking into the vitreous (vitreous hemorrhage). Any case of floaters should be evaluated for retinal tear by a specialist.

Retinal Detachment

Occurs when the retinal cells separate from the layer of blood vessels that supply the retina. Signs and symptoms include acute onset of floaters, flashes of light (photopsia), blurred vision, and impaired peripheral vision. Any acute visual changes are concerning for a serious condition and should be evaluated urgently by an ophthalmologist. Infants and young children who present with suspicion of abusive head trauma should be evaluated emergently for retinal tears, hemorrhage, or detachment.

RETINOPATHY

Diabetic Retinopathy

Condition in which damage to the retina causes visual impairment.

History

- Floaters, blurry vision, poor night vision, impaired color vision, and blank/dark areas in the field of vision.
- Both eyes are typically affected
- Occurs more often in patients with chronic diabetes (>5 years) and history of uncontrolled blood sugar (HbA1c significantly above 7.0).

Physical Examination

- Defects in visual acuity, visual fields
- Chronically elevated blood-sugar levels
- Fundoscopic exam may reveal micro-aneurysms, retinal hemorrhages, cotton-wool spots, and macular edema (**Figure 8.19**)

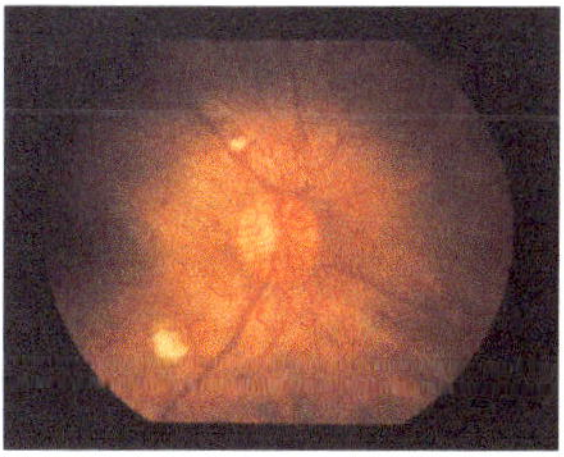

FIGURE 8.19 Proliferative diabetic retinopathy.
Source: National Institutes of Health and National Eye Institute.

Considerations

- Diabetic retinopathy occurs primarily in two forms: proliferative and nonproliferative, which refer to whether there is growth of abnormal blood vessels on the retina.
- Causes vision loss, glaucoma, retinal detachment, and blindness

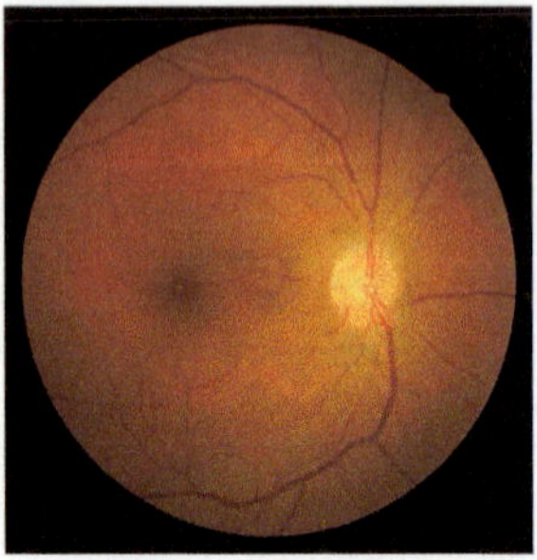

FIGURE 8.20 Hypertensive retinopathy.
Source: Image courtesy of Frank Wood.

Hypertensive Retinopathy

History

- Floaters, blurry vision
- Occurs more often in patients with chronically elevated blood pressure, those with a genetic predisposition, or younger patients with secondary hypertension

Physical Examination

- Chronic uncontrolled hypertension
- Fundoscopic exam can reveal arteriolar constriction, arteriovenous crossing or nicking, retinal hemorrhages, blurred disc margins (**Figure 8.20**)

Consideration

- Visual changes can occur with advanced disease; less common to cause blindness

Retinopathy of Prematurity

History

- Occurs in a small percentage of premature infants born less than 31 weeks' gestation.
- Infants at risk are those who require intensive respiratory support, such as oxygen therapy

Physical Examination

- Digital retinal imaging is a useful tool to screen and document retinal changes.

Consideration

- The condition is thought to be a result of disorganized growth of retinal blood vessels, which can cause retinal scarring and detachment. Oxygen toxicity and hypoxia may also contribute to the development of retinopathy of prematurity.

SCLERITIS AND EPISCLERITIS

Scleritis

Scleritis is the inflammation of the sclera or choroid of the eye.

History

- Severe "boring" or penetrating pain, watery discharge, extreme photophobia

Physical Examination

- Exquisite tenderness to palpation
- Severe inflammation, injection of sclera
- Decreased visual acuity

Considerations

- Associated with SLE, rheumatoid arthritis, ankylosing spondylitis, inflammatory bowel disease, and infectious diseases
- Scleritis can be anterior or posterior, diffuse, focal, nodular, or necrotizing

Episcleritis

Localized inflammation of the episcleral tissues (outer covering of the sclera). Unlike scleritis, this condition is self-limiting and benign with mild discomfort.

History

- Red eye without discharge of drainage

Physical Examination

- May note a discrete, elevated area of inflamed episcleral tissue (nodular type) or an area of diffuse, vascular congestion in the absence of an obvious nodule (simple type)

Considerations

- Typically involves only one sector or area of the episclera
- Resolves over a few weeks

STRABISMUS

Strabismus is a misalignment of the eyes that is often congenital and occurs with various degrees of severity. The misalignment occurs because of an imbalance in EOM function.

History

- More common in children than adults
- Particularly more common in children with neurologic disorders like cerebral palsy

Physical Examination

- Asymmetric corneal light reflex and abnormal cover test; the axis of misalignment can occur in one of several directions. As one eye fixates, the other eye may deviate inward (esotropia), outward (exotropia), upward (hypertropia), or downward (hypotropia).

Considerations

- Pseudostrabismus describes a condition in which the eyes appear to be misaligned when in fact they are not. If patients or young children have undeveloped facial features or a variation in the slant of palpebral fissures, symmetric corneal light reflex confirms pseudostrabismus not strabismus.
- Strabismus can lead to amblyopia (reduced vision) or blindness, as the child's developing brain prioritizes vision in the aligned eye and disregards the visual stimulus in the deviated eye, adversely affecting visual development. Persistent loss of visual stimulation in the affected eye eventually leads to the amblyopia. Early intervention and treatment are crucial.
- Acute onset of strabismus in an older adult can be indicative of a more serious condition, for example, a CN VI or CN III palsy, and should be considered a medical emergency.

STY (HORDEOLUM)

An acute pustular infection of the eyelid margin.

History

- Redness of the eyelid, tearing
- No changes in vision

Physical Examination

- Red, tender papule/pustule on the eyelid margin (**Figure 8.21**)
- The sty can present externally at the area of an eyelash follicle or tear gland, or internally just under the conjunctival side of the eyelid

Considerations

- A sty, or hordeolum, may evolve into a chronic inflammatory lesion (chalazion), which presents as a firm, rubbery nodule within the eyelid.
- When an individual presents with eyelid redness but not

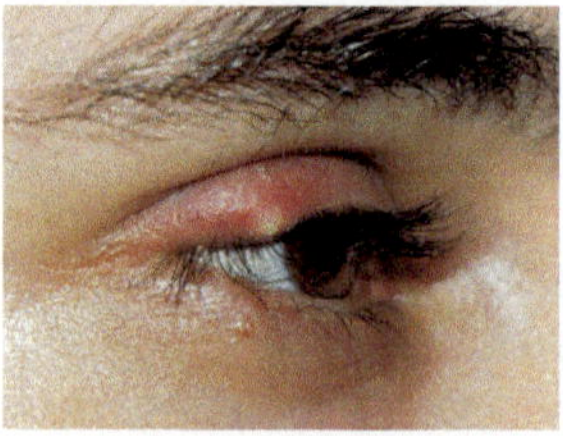

FIGURE 8.21 Sty of upper eyelid.

tearing, the condition is more likely blepharitis, inflammation of the eyelids, which can be caused by infection or systemic illnesses, such as seborrheic dermatitis, rosacea, or dry eye syndromes.

SUBCONJUNCTIVAL HEMORRHAGE

Demarcated area of ruptured blood vessels just beneath the surface of the eye.

History

- Asymptomatic; no itching, drainage, pain, or discomfort

Physical Examination

- Distinct collection of blood within the sclera (**Figure 8.22**)
- Differs from more generalized hyperemia associated with acute conjunctivitis

Considerations

- Can be caused by traumatic injury to the head or eye, but may also occur with Valsalva-associated coughing, straining, or vomiting; from anticoagulant therapy; or with contact lens insertions or removal
- Condition is diagnosed by clinical appearance. If the patient presents with a history of head trauma, further evaluation is needed.

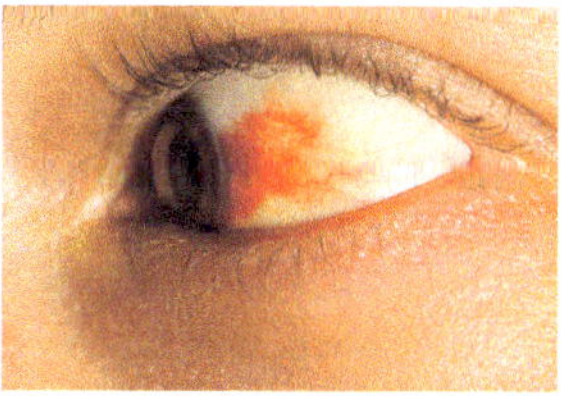

FIGURE 8.22 Subconjunctival hemorrhage.
Source: Image courtesy of Daniel Flather.

UVEITIS

An inflammatory condition of the uveal tract.

History

- Usually appears suddenly, with nonspecific symptoms of eye pain, redness, severe photophobia, diminished vision

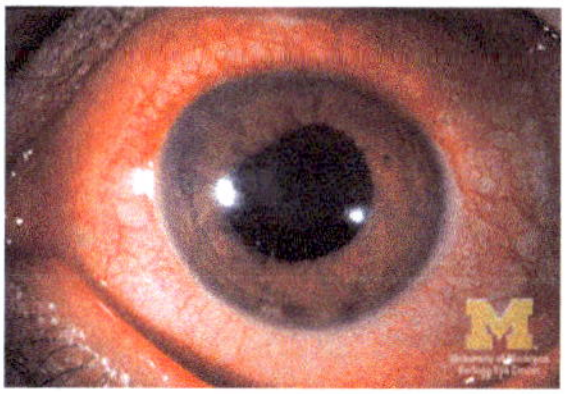

FIGURE 8.23 Uveitis.
Source: Image courtesy of Jonathan Trobe, M.D.

Physical Examination

- Reduced visual acuity
- Deep hyperemia extends beyond the conjunctiva (**Figure 8.23**)

- Physical findings vary depending on portion of the uveal tract affected—anterior chamber (iritis), ciliary body, posterior chamber (retinitis), or dissemination throughout

Consideration

- Cause varies depending on the etiology of the inflammation. Infectious causes include herpes; CMV; toxoplasmosis; syphilis; tuberculosis; and West Nile, Ebola, and Zika viruses. Systemic or immune conditions include spondyloarthritis, sarcoidosis, juvenile idiopathic arthritis, psoriatic arthritis, IBD, MS, Vogt–Koyanagi–Harada syndrome, Behçet syndrome, Sjögren's syndrome, and SLE.

PHYSICAL EXAMINATION DOCUMENTATION

Documentation should include results of inspection and special tests.

EXAMPLE OF NORMAL FINDINGS

Visual fields full by confrontation, EOMs intact, no nystagmus. No ptosis, lid lag, discharge, or crusting. Corneal light reflex symmetric, no strabismus. Conjunctiva clear, sclera white, no lesions or redness; PERRLA. Fundi: Optic discs with sharp margins, retinal background has even color without hemorrhages or exudate.

EXAMPLE OF NORMAL FINDINGS FOR PEDIATRIC WELLNESS EXAM

Visual acuity 20/20 with use of Snellen Tumbling E chart for each eye and both eyes. EOMs intact, smooth, with no nystagmus, ptosis, or lid lag. Corneal light reflex symmetric, cover test indicates no strabismus. Conjunctiva clear, sclera white, no lesions, redness, or discharge noted. PERRLA. Red reflex equal bilaterally.

REFERENCES

References for this chapter draw from Chapter 12, Evidence-Based Assessment of the Eye, of the textbook *Evidence-Based Physical Examination: Best Practices for Health and Well-Being Assessment*. The references may be accessed in the digital version of the handbook at https://connect.springerpub.com/content/book/97808-0-8261-6466-7/chapter/ch08

9

Evidence-Based Assessment of Ears, Nose, and Throat

CLINICAL CONSIDERATIONS

- When evaluating a patient with hearing loss, use tuning forks to confirm diagnosis.
- To visualize the tympanic membrane in an adult, pull the helix up and back. In children under the age of 3, the angle of the ear canal is less acute, so the clinician will need to pull back and down on the posterior helix to see the tympanic membrane.
- Pneumatic otoscopy is recommended to evaluate for effusion in the middle ear and can be very helpful when evaluating children.
- If a patient presents with otalgia with a normal exam, consider other pathology such as TMJ disorders, cervical pain, dental abscess, and cancer of the oropharynx and larynx.
- Rhinoscopy is a commonly overlooked part of the ear, nose, and throat exam. It should be completed in any patient who presents with an ear/nose/throat concern.
- When performing an oral exam, have the patient remove their dentures to ensure all of the oral mucosa is evaluated.
- If you cannot get a good view of the posterior pharynx because the patient is guarding, have the patient pant in and out or yawn. This will elevate the soft palate, while relaxing the tongue.

SUBJECTIVE HISTORY

COMMON REASONS FOR SEEKING CARE

Otalgia, nasal congestion/rhinitis, sore throat

HISTORY OF PRESENT ILLNESS

- **Onset:** When did the symptoms start? What was the individual doing when they became symptomatic? Did this occur suddenly, or has it been developing gradually?
- **Location:** Does the symptom have associated pain or discomfort? If so, where is the discomfort located? Which ear is affected? Is the nasal discharge one side or both?
- **Duration:** How long do symptom(s) last? Over what period of time has the ear/nose/throat symptom(s) developed? Have the symptoms been occurring for days/months/years?
- **Characteristics:** Is the pain aching, burning, sharp, dull, or throbbing? What color is the nasal/ear exudate?
- **Associated symptoms:** Have there been any fevers, chills, or night sweats? Any eye drainage or itching, ear drainage, hearing loss, tinnitus, anosmia, enlarged lymph nodes, coughing, postnasal drip, or sinus pain or pressure? Is there any pus on the back of the throat?
- **Aggravating factors:** What actions, activities, or body positions make the symptoms worse? Does it hurt to swallow? Does laying on the ear or swimming make the pain worse? Has exposure to smells, dust, pollen, smoking, or activities caused an increase in symptoms?
- **Relieving factors:** What actions, activities, or body positions decrease the symptoms? If relieved, how long does the relief last?
- **Treatment:** What medications has the individual taken to help with the symptoms? Have nasal corticosteroids or allergy medications or injections ever been tried? Clarify dosage and frequency of any medications. Are there any pain or cold/sinus medications being used for the symptoms?
- **Severity:** How severe are the symptoms on a scale of 0 to 10? Do the symptoms affect the patient's quality of life? Are the symptoms worsening?

HEALTH HISTORY

Past Medical History

- History of ENT illnesses throughout their life span
- Premature birth history, low birth weight, or birth complications such as severe asphyxia or low Apgar scores
- Previous diagnoses of asthma, sleep-disordered breathing, CF, migraine, stroke, ciliary dyskinesia, autoimmune disorders, anemia, hematologic disorders, GERD, Parkinson's

- Previous emergency room visits or hospital stays for ear/nose/throat or respiratory problems
- Previous head and neck procedure(s) or surgery, including myringotomy with tympanostomy tubal placement
- History of trauma to the nose
- Previous history of eczema or asthma
- Viral diseases such as EBV, meningitis, or recent viral upper respiratory infection
- History of frequent ear infections as child/adult, sudden hearing loss, eardrum rupture, deviated or perforated septum, recurrent sinus infections, nasal polyps, conjunctivitis, vitamin deficiencies, lichen plantus, frequent strep throat/ tonsillitis, tonsilliths, sexually transmitted infections
- Anatomic malformation of the head or neck, craniofacial abnormalities (e.g., cleft palate)
- History of allergy testing and results
- Exposure to radiation
- Frequency of routine dental exams and cleanings
- Comorbidities or risk factors related to ear/nose/throat disease
- Recent exposure to individual with flu, flu-like symptoms, or COVID-19 symptoms
- Known or suspected pulmonary, cardiac, liver, or renal disease
- History of malignancy
- Recent surgery, hospitalization, or immobility
- Pregnancy status, note likelihood of pregnancy or if currently or recently pregnant

Medications

Prescribed or OTC medications or supplements, including dose and frequency: NSAIDs, antibiotic use (aminoglycosides), oxymetazoline, anticoagulants (prescribed and OTC), chemotherapy, HPV vaccination, steroids (including oral steroid inhalers), bisphosphonates, hormones, OTC saline rinses or saline irrigations, recent antibiotic use

Allergies

- Allergies to medications or seasonal, environmental, and/or food allergies
- If yes to being allergic to any substance or environmental trigger, clarify reaction:
  - Swelling of tongue, lips, face?
  - Dyspnea, wheezing, dizziness?

Immunizations

Risks for vaccine-preventable illnesses; vaccine status; date of last influenza, HPV, and tetanus vaccinations

Pediatric Considerations

- Sniffing or tripod position (may indicate epiglottis in children)
- Number of ear infections in the past 6 months
- Family members or school contacts with illness
- Concern for a possible foreign body (in ear, nose, or throat)

FAMILY HISTORY

- Hearing loss, especially in childhood
- Head and neck cancers
- Allergic rhinitis
- Asthma
- Eczema
- Sinus disease
- Bleeding disorders
- Ciliary dyskinesia
- Autoimmune disorders
- Genetic malformations
- HIV
- Laryngeal disorders
- Thyroid disorders
- Perinatal viral infections such as CMV, HPV, rubella, herpes, toxoplasmosis, or syphilis

SOCIAL HISTORY

- Tobacco use, including chewing tobacco, snuff, e-cigarettes, cigarettes, and cigars: Pack-years (or equivalent), secondary exposure, quitting history and attempts, current desire to quit
- Alcohol use: Frequency, quantity, type
- Illicit drug use, especially intranasal use
- Use of headphones, gun use, attendance at loud music concerts; playing in a band
- Occupation:
    - Operation of heavy machinery, exposure to loud noises
    - Exposure to wood dust, chemicals, asbestos, nickel
    - Teachers, speakers, singers, or professionals who use their voice often
- Recreation: Frequent swimming

- Use of paan (betel quid)
- High-risk sexual behavior or exposure to HPV

REVIEW OF SYSTEMS

- **General:** Fatigue, fevers, unintended weight loss, weakness
- **Eyes:** Eye pain, double vision, blurry vision
- **ENT:** Dental pain or caries, trismus, change in voice, hoarseness, odynophagia
- **Lymphatics:** Lymphadenopathy
- **CV:** Chest pain, palpitations
- **Respiratory**: Shortness of breath, cough, wheezing
- **GI:** Abdominal pain, gastroesophageal reflux, diarrhea, constipation, blood in stool
- **Neurologic:** Headaches, facial palsies, dizziness, numbness
- **Skin:** Rashes, ulcers, sores, lumps

RED FLAGS IN SUBJECTIVE HISTORY

- Suspected foreign body in the ear or nose
- History of sudden or rapidly progressive hearing loss
- Unilateral hearing loss of sudden or recent onset
- ENT symptoms associated with unintentional weight loss or other systemic symptoms
- History of pain, active drainage, or bleeding from an ear
- Acute, chronic, or recurrent episodes of dizziness
- Evidence of congenital or traumatic deformity of the ear
- Unilateral or pulsatile tinnitus
- Head or neck mass

PHYSICAL EXAMINATION

GENERAL SURVEY

- **Vital signs:** Temperature, pulse rate, respiratory rate, blood pressure
- Rate, rhythm, depth, and effort of breathing
- Posture and position

INSPECTION OF THE EAR

- Inspect the outer ear. Look for erythema, edema, tissue deformity, lesions, or masses.
- Use an otoscope to see the ear canal and tympanic membrane. Clinician should place the otoscope in their dominant hand and

place the nondominant hand on the helix, then pull up and back (**Figures 9.1 and 9.2**).

- The otoscope can be held several different ways based on the preference and comfort of the clinician. One way is to put the handle between the thumb and fingers, wrapping the hand around the handle, with the handle pointing toward the floor. This works well when examining adult patients and you do not expect much movement of the head.
- Pneumatic otoscopy is recommended for evaluation of effusion in the middle ear. Pneumatic otoscopy is a method of examining the middle ear by using an otoscope with an attached rubber bulb to change the pressure in the ear canal (**Figure 9.3**). Changing the pressure in the ear helps the clinician to determine whether the tympanic membrane moves. If the middle ear is well aerated, the tympanic membrane will move from the pressure exerted with the rubber bulb. In an ear has an effusion, the tympanic membrane cannot move because fluid is pushing against it.

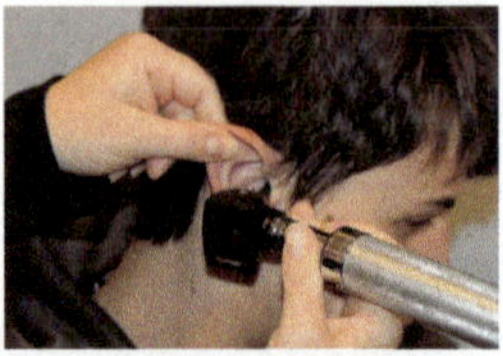

FIGURE 9.1 Adult ear exam technique.

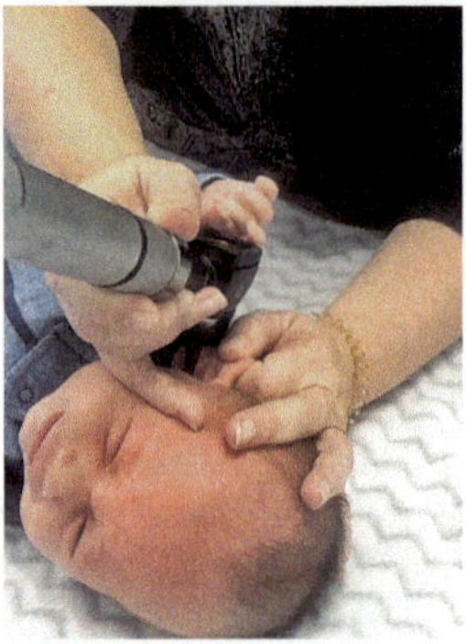

FIGURE 9.2 Infant ear exam technique.

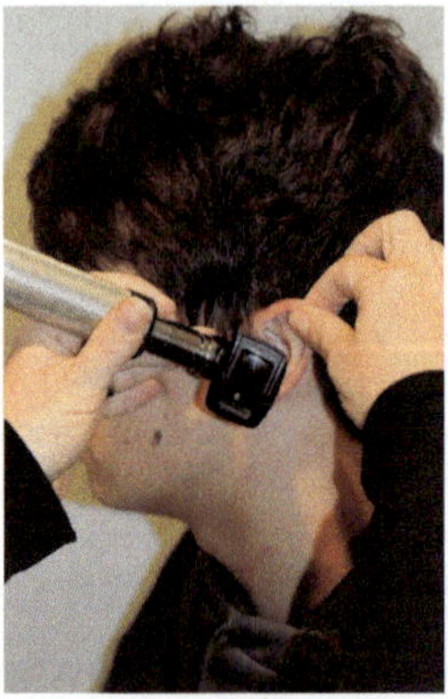

FIGURE 9.3 Pneumatic otoscopy.

PALPATION OF THE EAR

Palpating the tragus and mastoid, or pulling up on the pinna, can provide information as to if there is an ongoing, infective process as these maneuvers will generally produce pain if inflamed.

ASSESSING AUDITORY ACUITY

- The patient will be asked to occlude one ear canal. If the patient cannot do this, the clinician can press on the tragus, occluding the ear canal. The clinician should stand behind the patient or cover their mouth to ensure that the patient does not read the clinician's lips.
- Standing about 1 to 2 feet away, the clinician should exhale fully and whisper softly three words or numbers toward the unoccluded ear. The words or numbers should be equally accented syllables like "baseball" or "99." If the patient repeats them back correctly, the hearing is considered normal. If the patient does not respond correctly, repeat using three different words or numbers. The patient is considered to pass if they repeat three out of six answers correctly.

Finger Rub Test

- Standing in front of the patient, the clinician should hold their hands to the side of the patient's head. Gently rub the fingers on one side together, asking whether the patient hears the sound. Repeat on the other side.
- Wait for the patient's response. Repeat again with both hands asking whether the patient hears them equally on both sides.

ASSESSING AIR AND BONE CONDUCTION

The tuning fork exam should be used in addition to the physical exam when evaluating hearing. This provides valuable information and can assist in distinguishing diagnoses that are consistent with a conductive or sensorineural hearing loss. The following are screening tests and do not replace formal audiometry.

Weber Screening Test

- In a quiet room, lightly hit the fork to start a light vibration. The clinician can do this by hitting the tuning fork on their knuckles/elbow or stroking the forks between their fingers. Once vibration is felt, lightly place the 512-Hz tuning fork on the patient's scalp at midline (**Figure 9.4**). Ask the patient whether they hear the tone louder in the left ear, the right ear, or if it is equally loud in both ears. The exam is considered normal if the sound is heard equally in each ear.
- In unilateral conductive hearing loss, the sound lateralizes to the affected ear (it will be heard louder in the affected ear). In unilateral sensorineural hearing loss, the sound lateralizes away from

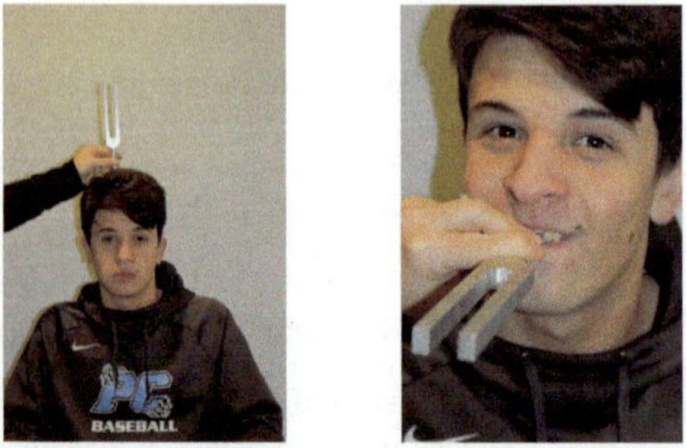

FIGURE 9.4 Weber exam techniques.

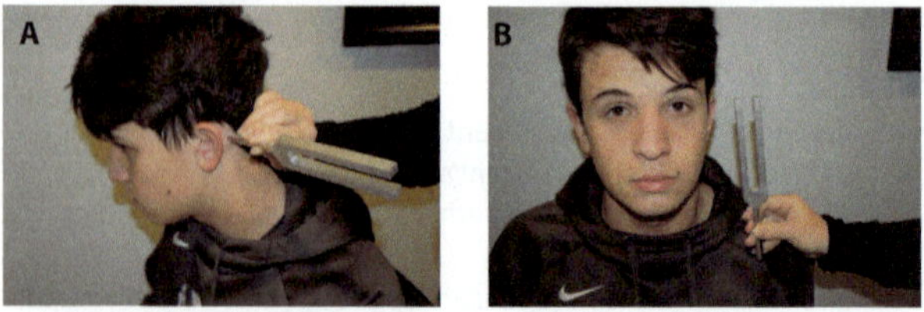

FIGURE 9.5 Conducting the Rinne test. (**A**) Assessing bone conduction. (**B**) Assessing air conduction.

the affected ear (it will be heard louder in the normal ear). If nothing is heard, try again or move the turning fork onto the upper front teeth. This cannot be done if the patient is edentulous or has false teeth.

Rinne Test

- Place a lightly vibrating 512-Hz tuning fork on the mastoid bone behind the ear (**Figure 9.5A**). Ask the patient to cover the opposite ear with their hand. When the patient can no longer hear the sound, move the vibrating tuning fork in front of the same ear canal. Avoid touching the ear. The "U" portion of the tuning fork should face forward in order to maximize the sound for the patient. The patient should report when they can no longer hear the vibratory sound.
- A normal test is when the patient continues to hear the vibratory sound for twice the amount of time when the tuning fork is held next to their ear (**Figure 9.5B**) than when it was placed on their

mastoid bone. This indicates that AC is greater than BC, signifying a normal test.

- The Rinne test would detect unilateral conductive hearing loss if the vibratory sound is heard through the bone as long or longer than through the air (AC < BC or AC = BC).

AUDIOMETRY

Testing Recommendations

- Tympanometry should be done in a patient with suspected otitis media. This can be available in some medical offices or performed by a licensed audiologist.
- In patients with a complaint of hearing loss, an audiogram by a licensed audiologist is recommended.
- Any abnormal tuning fork exam findings should prompt a referral for an audiologic evaluation.

PEDIATRIC CONSIDERATIONS

- In children under the age of 3, the angle of the ear canal is less acute, so the clinician will need to pull back and down on the posterior helix. This allows for proper placement of the speculum into the external ear canal. A parent or assistant can help stabilize the head for you.
- It may be difficult to see the posterior pharynx in an infant. It is best visualized when the infant is crying. If you cannot get good visualization, listen to the quality of the infant crying, as this can indicate if there is any obstruction or restriction of the airway.

INSPECTION OF THE NOSE AND SINUSES

- Inspect the outside of the nose. Look for shape, deformity, lesions, asymmetry, and deviation. Assess the nares as the patient breathes in and out of the nostrils. To assess for nasal obstruction, press on one naris at a time, asking the patient to breathe in and out, assessing airflow through the nasal vestibules.
- Palpate the sinuses to evaluate for tenderness. Palpate the frontal sinuses, which are located under the eyebrows, without pressing on the eyes. Palpate the maxillary sinuses, which are located approximately 1 cm lateral to the nasal bridge bilaterally.
- Inspect the inside of the nose with an otoscope and the largest ear speculum available. Have the patient tilt the head back and press the nasal tip up to open the nasal vestibule. Grabbing the otoscope between the thumb and index finger, brace the

otoscope using your fifth digit against the patient's cheek (**Figure 9.6**). This will stabilize the scope and prevent sudden jerking movements in the nose.

- Look posteriorly and superiorly to visualize the anterior septum, anterior inferior turbinate, and possibly the middle turbinate. Evaluate the septum for deviation, lesions, perforation, bleeding, and/or crusting. Assess the nasal cavity and mucosa for color, lesions, drainage, ulcerations, and polyps. Assess the turbinates for color, size, polyps, lesions, and ulcerations.

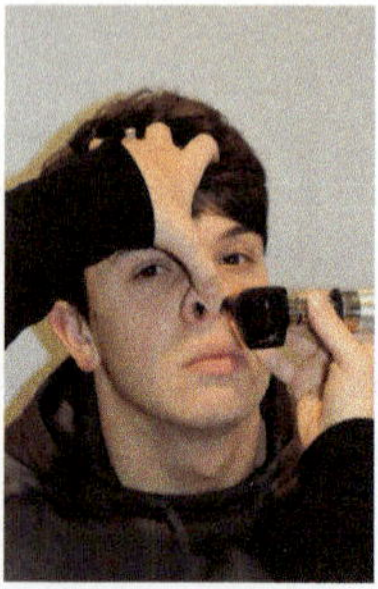

FIGURE 9.6 Otoscope technique for anterior rhinoscopy.

INSPECTION OF THE MOUTH AND POSTERIOR PHARYNX

Lips

- Inspect the oral cavity, starting with the lips. Ensure the lips are symmetrical at the oral commissure. Asymmetry can indicate stroke or facial nerve palsies.
- Assess the lips for color, lesions, and closure. Nonhealing lesions on the lip can indicate cancer.

Mouth

- Inspect the mouth with a light source and tongue depressor.
- Inspect the gingiva and dentition for caries, abscesses, periodontal disease, and lesions. Note the condition of the teeth and provide education on oral hygiene if poorly maintained.
- Look at the floor of the mouth under the tongue for pooling of saliva or ulcerations, which could indicate cancer.

Tongue

- Inspect the buccal mucosa, dorsal tongue, ventral tongue, floor of the mouth, retromolar trigone, hard palate, and soft palate. Use the tongue blade to help pull back the buccal mucosa, lift the tongue, or depress the tongue to get good visualization of the posterior tongue, lateral sides of the tongue, ventral tongue, and floor of mouth. Check for masses, ulcerations, and discolorations (red or white patches).

- Ask the patient to stick out the tongue and move it from side to side, assessing for fasciculation, symmetry, and function of CN XII. In infants and young children, have the patient sit on a parent's or adult's lap. The parent/adult should hold the head stable while the clinician examines the mouth with a tongue blade and light source. Inspect the frenulum of the tongue.

Posterior Pharynx

- Inspect the posterior pharynx by asking the patient to say "ahh" (**Figure 9.7**). Watch the soft palate elevate. This examines the function of CN X.
- Assess the uvula for deviation. Deviation can indicate peritonsillar abscess or CN X paralysis.
- Inspect the posterior pharynx, tonsillar pillars, retromolar trigone, soft palate, and uvula.
- Inspect the tonsils for symmetry, size, crypts, exudates, white spots (tonsilliths), and/or masses.

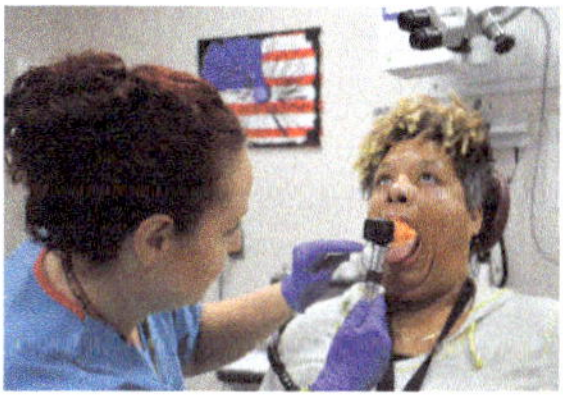

FIGURE 9.7 Inspection of oral cavity and posterior pharynx.

PALPATION OF THE MOUTH AND JAW

- With gloved hands, ask the patient to stick out their tongue. Move it side to side assessing for color, lesions, asymmetries, rough texture/smooth texture, and/or white/red patches (**Figure 9.8**).
- Next palpate the entire tongue—lateral surfaces, dorsal surface, ventral surface, and floor of mouth (**Figure 9.9**). If there is asymmetry of the tonsils or a concern of a sore throat in a patient who is a tobacco user, palpate the tonsils and base of tongue. Oral or tonsillar lesions can cause referred pain to the ear.

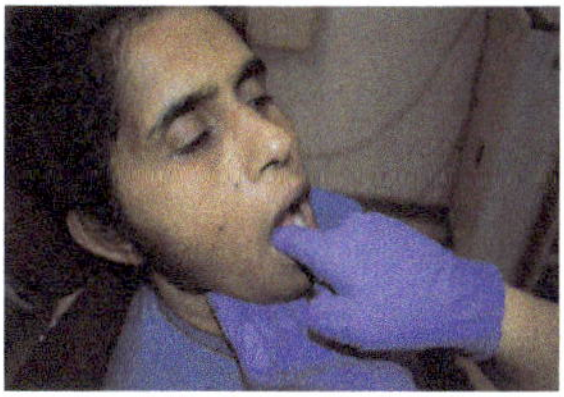

FIGURE 9.8 Palpation during the oral examination.

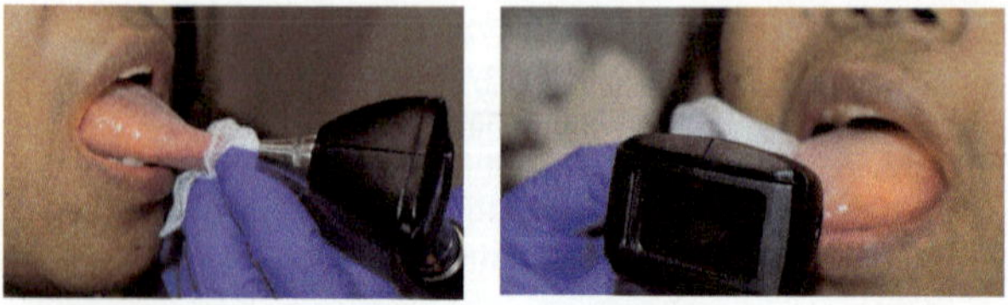

FIGURE 9.9 Inspection and palpation of the tongue.

TEMPORAL MANDIBULAR JOINT

- Palpate and examine the TMJ. Assess the patient opening and closing the mouth and palpate the TMJ joint with adduction and abduction of the jaw (**Figure 9.10**). Patients with TMJ arthritis may have pain that radiates to the ear, causing ear pain.
- The clinician can also feel for crepitus or shifting of the joint when affected patients open their mouth.

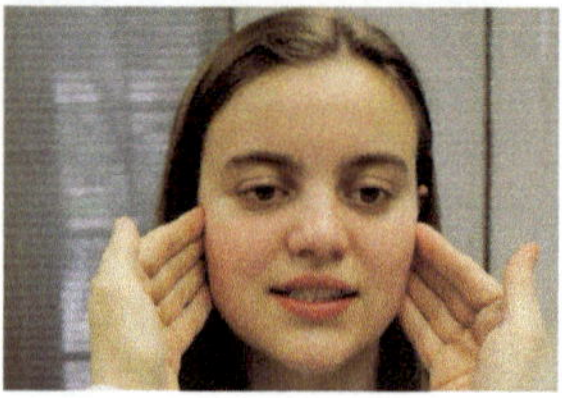

FIGURE 9.10 Assessing the temporal mandibular joint.

PEDIATRIC CONSIDERATIONS

- OME can cause significant hearing problems in children, resulting in speech and learning delays. Clinicians should assess children between the ages of 2 and 12 who exhibit speech or learning problems.
- Subtle symptoms of poor balance, behavioral problems, school performance issues, or speech delay may also point to an underlying hearing problem. It is important to rule out otitis media with effusion in these children as management can improve hearing outcomes.
- An additional consideration in the pediatric population is the heightened activity of the tonsil and adenoid tissue from the ages of 4 to 10. The most common bacterial infection that affects this area is GABHS, which causes tonsillitis.
- The Paradise criteria for tonsil infection include a sore throat plus at least one of the following features: temperature over 38.3 °C (100.9 °F), adenopathy, tonsil exudate, or a positive culture for GABHS.

EVIDENCE-BASED RESOURCES

Ears

Rosenfeld, R., Shin, J., Schwartz, S., Coggins, R., Gagnon, L., Hackell, J. M., Hoelting, D., Hunter, L. L., Kummer, A. W., Payne, S. C., Poe, D. S., Veling, M., Vila, P. M., Walsh, S. A., & Corrigan, M. D. (2016). Clinical practice guideline: Otitis media with effusion (update). *Otolaryngology—Head and Neck Surgery, 154*(Suppl. 1), S1–S41. https://doi.org/10.177/0194599815623467

Stachler, R., Chandrasekhar, S., Arcer, S., Rosenfeld, R., Schwartz, S., Bontempo, L. J., Faucett, E. A., Finestone, S. A., Hollingsworth, D. B., Kelley, D. M., Kmucha, S. T., Moonis, G., Poling, G. L., Roberts, J. K., Stachler, R. J., Zeitler, D. M., Corrigan, M. D., Nnacheta, L. C., & Satterfield, L. (2012). Clinical practice guideline: Sudden hearing loss. *Otolaryngology—Head and Neck Surgery, 146*(Suppl. 1), S1–S35. https://doi.org/10:1177/0194599812436449

Tunkle, D., Bauer, C., Sun, G., Rosenfeld, R., Chandrasekhar, S., Cunningham, E. R., Jr., Archer, S. M., Blakley, B. W., Carter, J. M., Granieri, E. C., Henry, J. A., Hollingsworth, D., Khan, F. A., Mitchell, S., Monfared, A., Newman, C. W., Omole, F. S., Phillips, C. D., & Robinson, S. K., … Whamond E. J. (2014). Clinical practice guideline: Tinnitus. *Otolaryngology—Head and Neck Surgery, 151*(Suppl. 2), S1–S40. https://doi.org/10.1177/0194599814545325

U.S. Preventative Services Task Force. (2018). *Draft research plan: Hearing loss in older adults: Screening*. https://www.uspreventiveservicestaskforce.org/uspstf/document/draft-research-plan/hearing-loss-in-older-adults-screening-2021

Nose

Rosenfeld, R., Piccirillo, J., Chandrasekhar, S., Brook, I., Kumar, K., Kramper, M., Kramper, M., Orlandi, R. R., Palmer, J. N., Patel, Z. M., Peters, A., Walsh, S. A., & Corrigan, M. D. (2015). Clinical practice guideline (update) adult sinusitis. *Otolaryngology—Head and Neck Surgery, 152*(Suppl. 2), S1–S39. https://doi.org/10.1177/0194599815572097

Seidman, M., Gurgel, R., Lin, S., Schwartz, S., Baroody, F., Bonner, J., Dawson, D. E., Dykewicz, M. S., Hackell, J. M., Han, J. K., Ishman, S. L., Krouse, H. J., Malekzadeh, S., Mims, J. W. W., Omole, F. S., Reddy, W. D., Wallace, D. V., Walsh, S. A., Warren,

(continued)

EVIDENCE-BASED RESOURCES (*CONTINUED*)

B. E., ... Nnacheta, L. C. (2015). Clinical practice guideline: Allergic rhinitis. *Otolaryngology—Head and Neck Surgery, 152*(1 Suppl.), S1–S43. https://doi.org/10.1177/0194599814561600

Throat

National Institute for Health and Center Excellence. (2017). *Head and Neck Cancers* (NICE Quality Standard No. 146). Retrieved on January 19, 2019 from https://www.nice.org.uk/guidance/qs146

Pynnonen, M., Gillespie, B., Roman, B., Rosenfeld, R., Tunkel, D., Bontempo, L., Brook, I., Chick, D., Colandrea, M., Finestone, S., Fowler, J., Griffith, C., Hensen, Z., Levine, C., Mehta, V., Salama, A., Scharpf, J., Shatzkes, D., Stern, W., ... Corrigan, M. (2017). Clinical practice guidelines: Evaluation of the neck mass in adults. *Otolaryngology—Head and Neck Surgery, 157*(Suppl. 2), S1–S30. https://doi.org/10.1177/0194599817722550

Stachler, R., Francis, D., Schwartz, S., Damask, C., Digoy, G., Krouse, H., McCoy, S., Ouellette, D., Patel, R., Reavis, C., Smith, L., Smith, M., Strode, S., Woo, P., & Nnacheta, L. (2018). Clinical practice guideline: Hoarseness. *Otolaryngology—Head and Neck Surgery, 158*(Suppl. 1). https://doi.org/10.1177/0194599817751030

ABNORMAL FINDINGS

EAR

Otitis Media

An infection or inflammation that involves the middle ear.

History

- Otalgia (typically unilateral)
- Reported fever, may have additional symptoms of upper respiratory infection concurrent or prior to symptoms
- Difficulty hearing typically described as muffled hearing

Physical Examination

- Bulging, erythematous TM (**Figure 9.11**); posterior to TM, purulent fluid noted inside middle ear

- Weber lateralization to the affected ear
- No movement of TM with pneumatic otoscopy or autoinsufflation

Consideration

- Otitis media can be purulent and symptomatic with otalgia and fever, or there can be serous or mucoid fluid behind the TM that may or may not cause hearing impairment and rarely other associated symptoms.

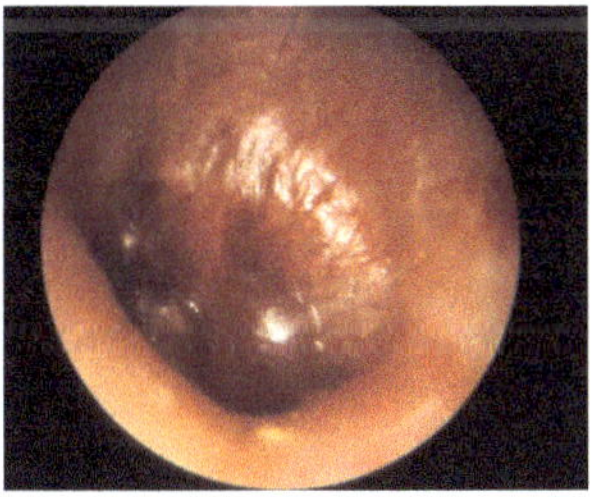

FIGURE 9.11 Otitis media.
Source: Image courtesy of B. Welleschik.

Otitis Media With Effusion

Fluid accumulates behind an intact TM.

History

- Hearing loss often described as muffled hearing
- Aural fullness/pressure
- May report vertigo or tinnitus
- Often following an upper respiratory infection or with seasonal allergies

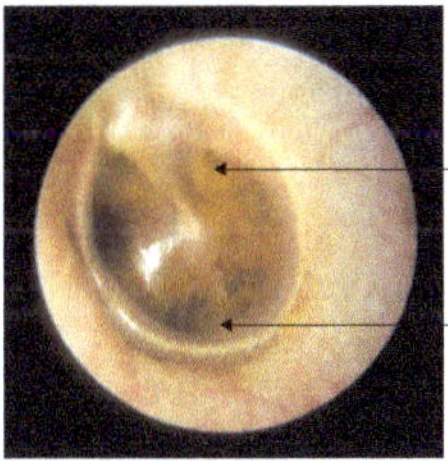

FIGURE 9.12 Otitis media with effusion.
Source: Image courtesy of Michael Hawke, MD.

Physical Examination

- Amber fluid behind the TM (**Figure 9.12**); bubbles behind the TM
- Weber lateralizes to the affected ear
- Audiogram will reveal conductive or mixed hearing loss of affected ear

Considerations

- OME may occur spontaneously because of poor eustachian tube function or as an inflammatory response following an AOM.
- Between 60% and 70% of OME will resolve spontaneously within 3 months.

Cholesteatoma

A condition in which squamous epithelium becomes entrapped either behind the ossicles or within the crevices of the temporal bone and causes bony erosion, hearing loss, and TM perforations.

History

- Difficulty hearing
- History of chronic ear infections and/or eustachian tube dysfunction
- Chronic otorrhea
- May experience vertigo and tinnitus

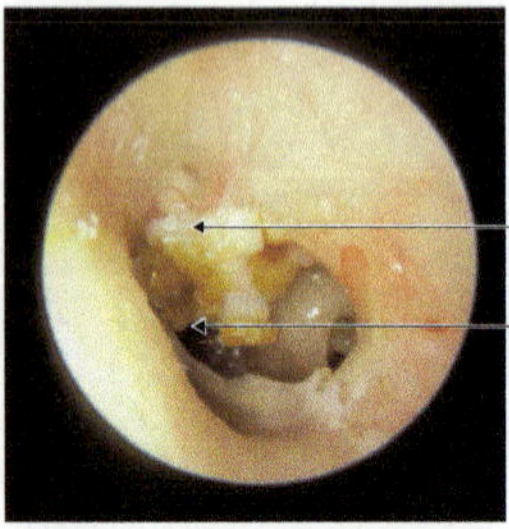

FIGURE 9.13 Cholesteatoma with upper canal erosion.
Source: Image courtesy of Michael Hawke, MD.

Physical Examination

- Accumulation of debris most often in the upper ear above the malleus (pars flaccida); debris can resemble white skin and/or may be mixed with cerumen
- Bony erosion of the upper ear canal (scutum erosion; **Figure 9.13**)

Considerations

- Cholesteatoma is due to long-term eustachian tube dysfunction and/or repeated middle ear infections, resulting in severe retraction of the tympanic membrane around these osseous structures.
- If cholesteatomas are left untreated, they can cause hearing loss, infections, dizziness, and injury to the facial nerves.

Eustachian Tube Dysfunction

An ear condition that occurs when there is negative pressure in the middle ear and the TM is pulled into the middle ear cavity.

History

- Difficulty hearing usually described as muffled hearing
- Difficulty popping or equalizing pressure in ear
- Otalgia, tinnitus
- Aural fullness in affected ear
- History of frequent ear infections

Physical Examination

- TM is sucked into the middle ear space, creating a pocket
- Weber lateralizes to affected ear

Consideration

- Blockage of the Eustachian tube isolates the middle ear space from the outside environment, creating a negative pressure that pulls the TM inward, causing pressure, pain, and accumulation of fluid.

Hearing Loss

Hearing loss can have multiple causes and presentations. See **Table 9.1** and **Figure 9.14**.

TABLE 9.1 Causes of Hearing Loss With Expected Exam Findings

Causes of Hearing Loss	Assessment Noted on Exam
Conductive Hearing Loss	
Cerumen	Yellow, orange, brown waxy substance in the ear canal blocking visualization of the TM
Otitis media with effusion (most common in children)	Usually painless with amber fluid behind the TM; usually can see air bubbles
Acute otitis media	On inspection, bulging TM with purulent material behind TM
Tympanic membrane perforation	Hole in the TM with view into the middle ear
Otosclerosis	Not visible on exam but will demonstrate conductive hearing loss
Otitis externa	Erythema, edema, exudate within the ear canal; can have white, yellow debris or purulent drainage
Ear canal mass/middle ear mass (glomus tumor, osteomas)	White, hard round masses within the ear canal (osteomas) or red pulsating mass within the middle ear that may extend through the TM
Tympanosclerosis	Scarring on the TM; usually white in color
Cholesteatoma	White skin debris or hard cerumen that usually occurs in the pars flaccida
Causes of Sensorineural Hearing Loss*	
Presbycusis	Gradual, symmetric, high frequency, permanent hearing loss that occurs over the age of 60

(*continued*)

TABLE 9.1 Causes of Hearing Loss With Expected Exam Findings (*continued*)

Causes of Hearing Loss	Assessment Noted on Exam
Noise exposure	Exposure to loud noise, typically over 85 decibels; the louder the sound, the shorter amount of time it takes to cause hearing loss
Hereditary	In infants, this can affect between one and three children per 1,000; newborn hearing screening can detect this hearing loss
Ototoxicity	Certain drugs are known to cause ototoxic effects in the cochlea: aminoglycoside antibiotics, platinum-based chemotherapeutic medications, loop diuretics, salicylates/nonsteroidal anti-inflammatory drugs NSAIDs
Sudden idiopathic hearing loss	Considered a medical emergency and needs to be identified early in order to preserve hearing; physical exam reveals normal ear exam and Weber lateralizes away from affected ear; immediate referral to otolaryngologist is indicated
Autoimmune hearing loss	Very rare; symptoms include fluctuating hearing loss and possibly vertigo
Ménierès disease	Inner-ear disorder believed to be caused by too much endolymph inside the cochlea
Vestibular Schwannoma	Rare, affects one to two per 100,000 people, slow growing, benign tumor; physical exam findings reveal normal otoscopy; if tumor is large, patient may have facial paresis due to compression of CN VII (facial nerve)
Infections (meningitis, viral labyrinthitis)	In meningitis, patient may have severe headache, fevers, cranial nerve palsies, and decreased hearing; in viral labyrinthitis, some patients may have precipitating viral upper respiratory infection causing vertigo, as well as decreased or sudden hearing loss

CN, cranial nerve; NSAIDS, nonsteroidal anti-inflammatory drugs; TM, tympanic membrane.

*In all of these situations, otoscopy is normal. Weber would lateralize away from the affected ear. Air conduction should be louder than bone conduction.

Tinnitus

Typically described as ringing in the ears but can be any type of sound one hears that is not external.

History

- Subjective sound reported as hissing, ringing, buzzing, humming, or chirping in one or both ears; can be reported as pulsatile (sound like heartbeat is in the ear); heard constantly or intermittently
- Can occur in one or both ears
- Causes interference with concentration and hearing
- Can lead to decreased quality of life

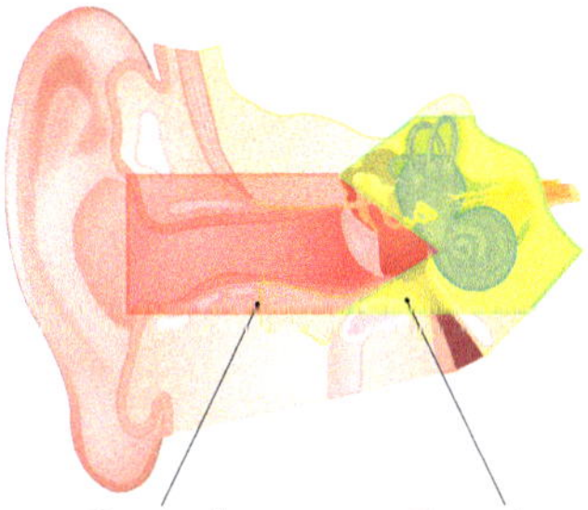

FIGURE 9.14 Conductive and sensorineural hearing loss. Conductive hearing loss occurs when sound waves do not reach the inner ear. Sensorineural hearing loss occurs when sound waves are not processed correctly.

Physical Examination

- Otoscopic exam is typically normal.
- Audiogram typically shows hearing loss.

Consideration

- Tinnitus is a subjective perception of sound that originates in the brain and not an outside source.

Malignant Otitis Externa

The sequela of a severe outer ear infection, mostly from *Pseudomonas aeruginosa* or *Staphylococcus aureus.*

History

- Otalgia, otorrhea
- Change in hearing
- Immunocompromised status or uncontrolled diabetes
- Granulation at the bony cartilaginous junction of the ear canal

Physical Examination

- Pain with manipulation of the auricle
- Culture from otorrhea is positive for *Pseudomonas aeruginosa*
- Facial weakness in severe cases
- Osteomyelitis noted on CT temporal bone or gallium scan

Consideration

- The infection begins as an external otitis media and progresses into an osteomyelitis of the temporal bone.

NOSE

Allergic Rhinitis

An inflammatory IgE-mediated disease triggered by exposure to allergens.

History

- Sneezing, nasal congestion
- Itchy eyes, nose, or throat
- Nasal congestion

Physical Examination

- Postnasal drip
- Clear, watery, bilateral rhinorrhea
- Pale, boggy nasal mucosa
- Swelling of turbinates
- Puffiness/darkening around eyes or "allergic shiners"
- Posterior pharynx cobble stoning
- Nasal polyps (occasional)

Consideration

- AR can also be associated with other conditions such as atopic dermatitis, eczema, asthma, sleep-disordered breathing, conjunctivitis, rhinosinusitis, and otitis media.

Nonallergic Rhinitis

An inflammation of the nasal tissues with an etiology that is not immune related and most often due to a virus or irritant. It results in nasal congestion, rhinitis, and sneezing.

History

- Environmental triggers (e.g., pollen, grass)
- Postnasal drip
- Congestion, sneezing
- Lack of nasal itching is the *key difference between this and AR*

Physical Examination

- Edematous turbinates
- Rhinorrhea (clear)
- Allergy testing is negative for IgE

Consideration

- Usually viruses or environmental irritants will trigger it, but it can be triggered by medications or pregnancy.

Sinusitis

An inflammation of paranasal sinus cavities (**Figure 9.15**) due to a virus, bacteria, fungus, or an allergic reaction.

History

- Bacterial sinusitis: Symptoms persist over 10 days or worsen after an initial improvement
- Viral sinusitis: Symptoms peak at day 3 and gradually decline within 10 to 14 days
- Acute sinusitis: Duration of symptoms last <4 weeks
- Chronic sinusitis: Symptoms persist >12 weeks
- Three core symptoms: Purulent nasal drainage, facial pain/pressure, nasal obstruction/congestion
- Additional symptoms: Cough, headache, maxillary dental pain, aural fullness, sinus tenderness, anosmia

Physical Examination

- Purulent nasal drainage
- Edematous, erythematous nasal mucosa
- Injected throat, with purulent mucus in posterior pharynx
- Possible head and neck lymphadenopathy
- Occasional anatomic findings such as deviated septum, turbinate hypertrophy, nasal mass, and/or nasal polyps (more likely found in chronic sinusitis)

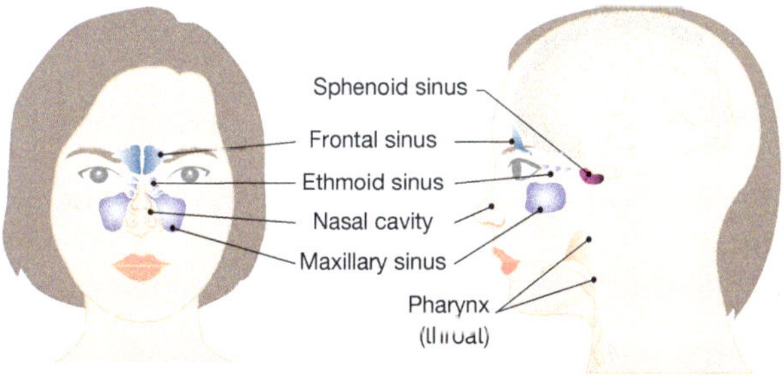

FIGURE 9.15 Paranasal sinuses.

Consideration

- Sinusitis can be acute or chronic in nature. With chronic sinusitis, there can be a history of allergic rhinitis and allergies.

Epistaxis

Bleeding from the nose caused by a ruptured blood vessel.

History

- Reported digital trauma
- Use of certain medications (e.g., warfarin)
- Dry environment
- History of elevated blood pressure, hypertension, vascular malformations, or coagulopathies
- History of or current upper respiratory infection and/or allergic rhinitis
- Reported trauma to the nose or face
- Use of inhaled illicit drugs (cocaine)
- Alcoholism
- History of nasal cannula use

Physical Examination

- Septal deviation
- Active bleeding of nose either anteriorly or posteriorly
- Nasal obstruction
- Blood clots inside the nose
- Prominent vasculature on anterior septum

Consideration

- Anterior epistaxis is most common (90%–95%) in the Kiesselbach's plexus. It is common among children aged 2 to 10 years and adults aged 50 to 80 years.

Nasal Polyp

Mucus-filled lobular lesion that occurs within the nose and paranasal sinuses (**Figure 9.16**).

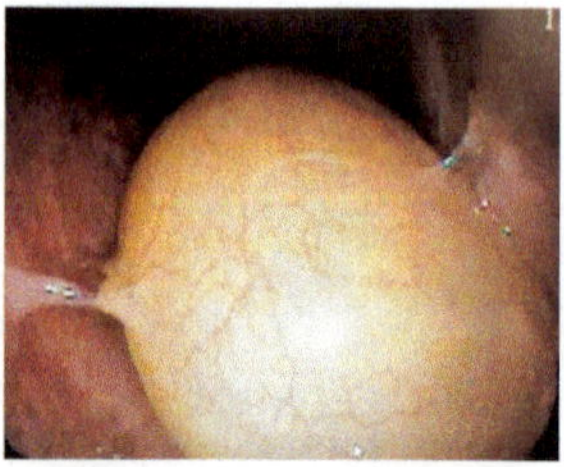

FIGURE 9.16 Nasal polyp left nares between inferior turbinate and septum.

History

- Nasal congestion, postnasal drip, rhinorrhea
- Will likely have allergy symptoms such as itchy watery eyes, itchy nose, sneezing

- May have a history of chronic sinus infections because of the obstruction
- History of CF, allergic fungal sinusitis, aspirin allergy

Physical Examination

- Nasal obstruction
- Boggy pale, enlarged turbinate(s)
- Round symmetric pale grape-like mass

Consideration

- Nasal polyps can occur in response to a foreign body in the nose.

Septal Perforation

Refers to a hole within the septum of the nose.

History

- History of cocaine use
- Epistaxis
- Crusting

Physical Examination

- May be entirely asymptomatic
- A whistling noise occurs when breathing through the nose
- Malodorous smell in nose
- Hole in the septum (It can be tiny or involve the majority of the septum.)
- Saddle nose deformity

Consideration

- Septal perforation can be a result of trauma to the nose, post-surgical trauma or due to an iatrogenic cause.

THROAT

Acute Pharyngitis

Edema, odynophagia, and/or scratchiness in the pharynx typically due to a viral or bacterial infection.

History

- Sudden onset sore throat; often accompanied by rhinorrhea, cough, fever, fatigue, malaise, and/or myalgia
- Odynophagia
- Absence of a cough (typical of streptococcal pharyngitis)
- History of exposure to strep throat

Physical Examination

- Anterior and posterior cervical lymphadenopathy
- Fever
- Tonsillar hypertrophy
- White exudate on tonsils
- Palatal petechiae (**Figure 9.17**)
- Erythematous rash that blanches with a sandpaper quality (scarlet fever or scarlatina)

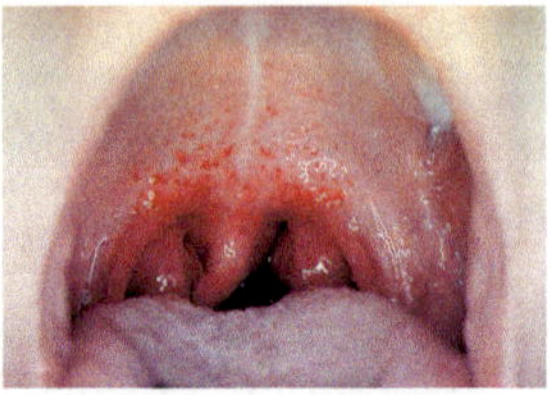

FIGURE 9.17 Strep pharyngitis.
Source: Centers for Disease Control and Prevention/Heinz F. Eichenwald, MD.

Consideration

- Bacterial (or streptococcal) pharyngitis needs to be treated with antibiotics to prevent complications including rheumatic fever and glomerulonephritis.

Angioedema

Swelling of the deeper layers of skin in response to an allergen, commonly affecting the eyes, cheeks, and lips.

History

- History of medications known to cause reactions (e.g., ACE inhibitors, antibiotics)
- History of allergies (e.g., certain foods, latex, insect venom)
- Can be a hereditary disorder

Physical Examination

- Sudden swelling of the face, lips, and/or tongue, but can occur in any part of the body
- Swelling of the airway
- Sudden, severe shortness of breath or trouble breathing
- Voice changes
- Stridor
- May have other allergic reaction symptoms such as pruritus or rash
- Edema of lips, around the eyes; may cause edema of oral mucosa and tongue

Consideration

- If not treated, severe cases can be life threatening due to risk of airway compromise.

Aphthous Ulcer

Small, painful lesions that occur inside the lips or on the tongue, buccal or palatal mucosa, and floor of mouth and are frequently referred to as cold sores.

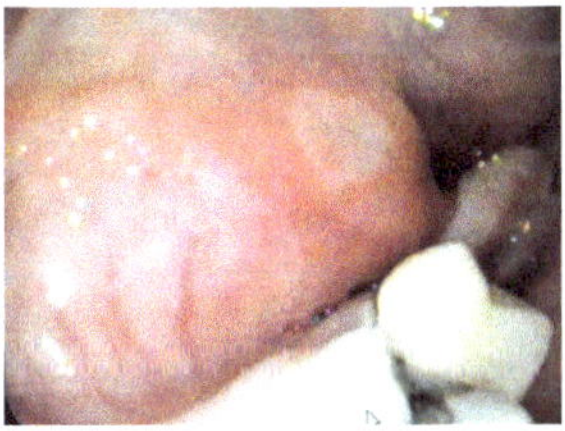
FIGURE 9.18 Aphthous ulcer.

History

- Painful, burning, or tingling sensation at the site of the ulcer
- More common during an immunocompromised state
- May report a fever
- Lasts about 1 to 2 weeks

Physical Examination

- Shallow ulcer with white or yellow center surrounded by erythema (**Figure 9.18**)
- Can occur on ventral tongue, gingiva, or buccal mucosa

Consideration

- They typically self-resolve without treatment.

Herpangina

A contagious illness most often caused by Coxsackie group A viruses.

History

- Typically found in young children (ages 3–10)
- More frequent in the summer and fall months
- Reported high fever
- Reported fussiness or refusing to eat in young children
- Headache, anorexia, sore throat
- Odynophagia

Physical Examination

- High fever
- Ulcerative lesions in the mouth and throat; similar lesions on feet, hands, buttocks
- Vomiting

Consideration

- Herpangina is most commonly spread through contact with respiratory secretions or via the fecal–oral route. It is similar to HFMD; see Chapter 5, "Evidence-Based Assessment of Skin, Hair, and Nails."

Leukoplakia

Thin white lesion on the mucosal surface anywhere within the oral cavity. It is usually not painful and does not brush or rub off.

History

- History of heavy smoking or chewing tobacco, heavy alcohol use
- Often asymptomatic
- Nonpainful, nontender

Physical Examination

- White, thick patches on mucosa and/or tongue
- Can be thickened or hardened patches
- Can be seen along with raised, red lesions
- Does not rub off

Consideration

- It can be a premalignant lesion in some cases. They are diagnosed with a biopsy.

Oral Candidiasis

A white lesion due to a fungal infection involving the mucosal surfaces, commonly referred to as thrush.

History

- Often seen in infants and the elderly
- Immunocompromised status
- Use of an inhaled steroid
- Wears dentures
- History of diabetes, HIV, or cancer
- Reports soreness or pain around area; difficulty eating or swallowing
- Reduced feeding (infants)
- Loss of taste

Physical Examination

- White lesion that will leave an erythematous base when scraped off
- Generally has a flaky type appearance involving several areas
- Patches are typically found on tongue or inner cheek
- Can spread to roof of mouth, gingiva, tonsils, or posterior pharynx (**Figure 9.19**)

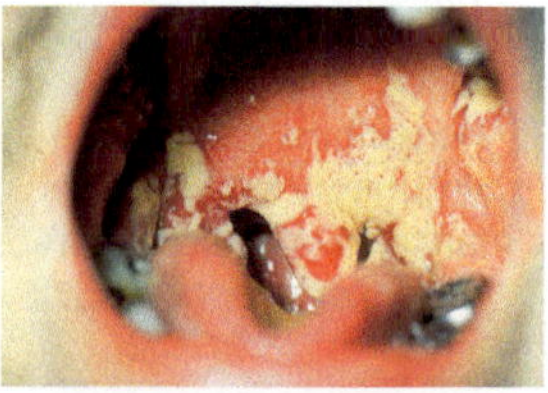

FIGURE 9.19 Oral candidiasis. *Source:* Centers for Disease Control and Prevention.

Consideration

- It can be spread from the infant to the mother during breastfeeding.

Nasal/Oral Cancers

Malignancy in the nasal/oral cavities, typically due to a squamous cell carcinoma.

History

- History of HPV
- History of smoking or chewing tobacco, heavy alcohol use
- Poor oral hygiene
- Pain
- Dysphagia
- Odynophagia
- Hoarseness
- Unilateral otalgia, nasal obstruction, rhinorrhea, sinus infections, epistaxis, or orbital symptoms

Physical Examination

- Unintentional weight loss
- Neck mass
- Red or white patch or ulcer on the lips, tongue, cheeks, floor of the mouth, hard and soft palate, sinuses, and pharynx (throat) that does not resolve
- Tender to palpation
- May be firm and/or fixed on palpation
- Loose teeth
- Adenopathy

Consideration

- There are many kinds of head and neck cancers but many of them have the same risk factors, specifically, tobacco and heavy alcohol use.

PHYSICAL EXAMINATION DOCUMENTATION

Documentation should include results of inspection and palpation.

EXAMPLE OF NORMAL FINDINGS

Conjunctiva clear without erythema or drainage bilaterally. Pupils are equal, round, and reactive to light and accommodation. Vision 20/20 on Snellen chart. No frontal or maxillary sinus tenderness on palpation. No tragus or pinna tenderness bilaterally. Tympanic membranes are pearly grey and translucent with no bulging or retraction. Cone of light visible at 5 o'clock in right ear and 7 o'clock in left ear. Nasal turbinates are nonedematous and nonerythematous bilaterally without drainage. Dentition is intact with no caries. Oral membranes are moist and pink. The posterior pharynx is nonerythematous. Tonsils are 1+ without exudate. No occipital, preauricular, postauricular, posterior cervical, anterior cervical, submandibular, submental, or supraclavicular lymphadenopathy.

EXAMPLE OF ABNORMAL FINDINGS

No tragus or pinna tenderness bilaterally. Right TM is pearly grey and translucent with no bulging or retraction. Left TM with clear fluid, no movement of TM with insufflation. Nasal turbinates edematous with clear drainage bilaterally. Posterior pharynx erythematous with cobblestoning and clear drainage. Tonsils 1+ without exudate. No occipital, preauricular, postauricular, posterior cervical, submandibular, submental, or supraclavicular lymphadenopathy. Several shotty anterior cervical lymph nodes palpated.

REFERENCES

References for this chapter draw from Chapter 13, "Evidence-Based Assessment of Ears, Nose, and Throat," of the textbook *Evidence-Based Physical Examination: Best Practices for Health and Well-Being Assessment*. The references may be accessed in the digital version of the handbook at https://connect.springerpub.com/content/book/97808-0-8261-6466-7/chapter/ch09

10

Evidence-Based Assessment of Nervous System

CLINICAL CONSIDERATIONS

- Develop a routine for the neurological examination. Perform the examination the same way each time to ensure no portion of the examination is missed or forgotten.
- Several neurological conditions do not present with neurological deficits.
- Older adults may present with altered levels of cognition, not associated with or occurring as part of neurological disease.
- Depression screening is important in older adults to determine whether changes in cognition are related to depression or as part of a neurological disorder.

SUBJECTIVE HISTORY

COMMON REASONS FOR SEEKING CARE

Headaches, dizziness/vertigo, weakness

HISTORY OF PRESENT ILLNESS

- **Onset:** When did the symptoms start? What was the individual doing when they became symptomatic? Did this occur suddenly, or has it been developing gradually?
- **Location:** Does the symptom have associated pain or discomfort? If so, where is the discomfort located? Is the headache on one side or both? Is the weakness localized to one area of the body or is it generalized?

- **Duration:** How long do symptom(s) last? Over what period of time has the neurological symptom(s) developed? Do the symptoms come and go or are they always present?
- **Characteristics:** Is the headache aching, pulsating, sharp, shooting? Would you describe the headache as the thunderclap, abrupt onset headache? Did the headache wake you from sleep? Would you describe the dizziness as lightheadedness, disequilibrium, or like the room is spinning?
- **Associated symptoms:** Do you experience any nausea, vomiting, vision changes, confusion, weakness, or aura with the headache? Does the weakness worsen with effort? Does the weakness include sensory loss?
- **Aggravating factors:** What actions, activities, or body positions make the symptoms worse? Is the headache exacerbated by light, sound, noise, or smell? Can you identify any triggers (e.g., dehydration, certain foods, alcohol, fatigue, stress) for the headache? Is the dizziness worse with movement or going from sitting to standing? Is the weakness worse with movement or when completing certain activities? If so, what activities?
- **Relieving factors:** What actions, activities, or body positions decrease the symptoms? If relieved, how long does the relief last? Does the headache improve with sleep or going into a dark room? Does the weakness improve with rest?
- **Treatment:** What medications has the individual taken currently or in the past to help with the symptoms? Clarify dosage and frequency of any medications.
- **Temporal:** Are the symptoms worse at a certain time of day? Do you wake up in the morning with a headache?
- **Severity:** How severe are the symptoms on a scale of 0 to 10? Do the symptoms limit participation in activities or daily activities? Are the symptoms worsening?

HEALTH HISTORY

Past Medical History

- **History of trauma**: Concussion/brain injury, spinal cord injury or localized injury, central nervous system insult, seizures, birth trauma, stroke
- Premature birth history or neurological disease diagnosed during childhood
- Previous diagnoses of meningitis, encephalitis, lead poisoning, poliomyelitis

- Previous emergency room visits or hospital stays for neurological problems
- Previous or current history of neurological disorders, neuro/brain surgeries, or any residual effects
- History of migraines or headaches
- History of deformities, congenital anomalies, genetic syndromes, developmental delays in children
- Hand, eye, foot dominance
- Recent illness or tick bite

Comorbidities or Risk Factors Related to Neurological Diseases

- History of CV or circulatory problems: Hypertension, aneurysm, peripheral vascular disease, stroke
- History of diabetes or endocrine disorders
- Known or suspected respiratory, cardiac, or renal disease
- History of malignancy
- History of autoimmune disorders
- Recent surgery, hospitalization, or immobility
- Pregnancy status: note likelihood of pregnancy or if currently or recently pregnant
- Recent infection with *Campylobacter jejuni*, EBV, cytomegalovirus

Medications

- **Prescribed medications:** Dose, frequency, last time blood levels were checked (if applicable)
- OTC medications or supplements, including dose and frequency
- Any new medications that have been recently started or had the dosage adjusted
- Any medication-induced tardive dyskinesia

Allergies

- Allergies to medications; seasonal, environmental, and/or food allergies
- If yes to being allergic to any substance or environmental trigger, clarify reaction

Immunizations

- Risks for vaccine-preventable illnesses
- Vaccine status; date of last influenza, meningococcal, *Haemophilus influenza* type B, pneumococcal, tetanus, polio
- History of Guillain-Barre syndrome following vaccine

Pediatric Considerations

- **Gestation**: Mother's health during pregnancy? Exposures or illnesses during pregnancy? Fetal abnormalities identified during the prenatal stage? Substance use during pregnancy?
- **Birth history**: Delivery eventful or uneventful, vaginal or C-section, prolonged or abrupt? Prolapsed cord, malpositioned placenta, premature rupture of membranes, or abruptio placentae? Any respiratory distress after birth? Any apneic episodes? Did the child require oxygen, pulse oximetry monitoring, or support for breathing as an infant? Apgar scores at birth?
- **Growth and development history**: Meeting developmental milestones (motor, adaptive, language, and personal–social behavior)? Has there been any regression of developmental milestones? Suboptimal growth or poor weight gain (based on pediatric growth charts)? Academic performance?
- **Eating and nutritional history**: How has the child been eating? Is the infant breast or bottle fed? Has the child's eating patterns changed?

FAMILY HISTORY

- **Neurological disorders**: ALS, AVMs, brain tumors, headaches (migraine, cluster), Alzheimer's, Creutzfeldt-Jakob, Huntington's, Parkinson's, MS, stroke, cerebral palsy, epilepsy, trigeminal neuralgia, dementia, neurofibromatosis, muscular dystrophy
- Metabolic disorder, thyroid disease, hypertension, diabetes
- Developmental delays, learning disorders, intellectual disability, ADHD
- Addiction (and/or use of alcohol or drugs during pregnancy)
- Family patterns of dexterity and dominance

SOCIAL HISTORY

Environmental Exposures

- Current and past occupations
- Exposure to pollutants, neurotoxins, insecticides, herbicides, fungicides, other harmful chemicals and/or irritants in the work environment
- Low-level chronic exposure to hazardous substances at work or at home

Lifestyle Behaviors (Including Substance Use)

- Typical use, type, amount of alcohol consumed
- Use of prescription medications or illicit substances for nonmedical purposes

- Use of OTC drugs for reasons other than health-related
- Use of tobacco, including cigarettes, smokeless tobacco, e-cigarettes or vaping, cigars
- Caffeine use (amount, frequency of intake)
- Hygiene, ADL, finances, communication, shopping, ability to fulfill work expectations
- Social support system
- Use of cane or assistive device

REVIEW OF SYSTEMS

- **General**: Fever, chills, sleeplessness, fatigue, dizziness, unintentional weight loss
- **HEENT**: Visual disturbances/visual difficulty, tearing or redness of eyes
- **CV/respiratory**: Respiratory irregularities, bruits, thrills
- **GI/GU**: Nausea, vomiting, urinary frequency, hesitancy, urgency, incontinence
- **Neurological**: Weakness, numbness/tingling, change in sensation, loss of consciousness, headaches, falls, dizziness, tremor, sensory disturbances, changes in balance or coordination, confusion
- **MSK**: Headache, backache, nuchal rigidity, unsteadiness when standing/walking, myalgias, arthralgias
- **Mental health**: Depression; anxiety; changes in mentation, memory, or mood

PHYSICAL EXAMINATION

GENERAL SURVEY

- Assess/compare vital signs to past measurements to identify possible disease/pre-disease markers.
- Height, weight, and BMI calculation should be completed and compared to previous visits to identify signs of chronic disease or weight loss.
- Note patient's demeanor, speech, presence of a resting tremor, affect, ability to articulate and communicate.

INSPECTION

- Observe patient's gait, balance, and coordination. Listen to the patient's response to questions, which provides information regarding the patient's ability to follow directions. Important to note for older adults as depression is more common in elders and those with chronic diseases, including neurological disorders such as dementia, MS, and Parkinson's.

- Inspection of the face includes attention to symmetry, shape, features, facial expression, symmetry of eyebrows, eyes, ears, nose, mouth; and position of nasolabial fold and inspecting for facial muscle atrophy and tremors (see Chapter 7, "Evidence-Based Assessment of Head and Neck").
- **Neurological physical assessment**: Mental status, cranial nerves, proprioception/cerebellar function, sensory function, reflexes.

MENTAL STATUS EXAMINATION

Refer to the mental status exam in Chapter 16, "Evidence-Based Assessment of Mental Health and Substance Use."

CRANIAL NERVES

Olfactory (I)

- Tested when the patient is unable to discriminate odors. Ensure patient's nares are clear. Ask the patient to occlude one naris at a time and close their eyes while you hold an open vial under their nose. Ask the patient to breathe deeply. Use a different aroma to test the other side. Repeat two to three times with two to three different odors. Patients are expected to perceive an odor on each side and identify it.

Optic (II)

- Testing of distant and near vison, ophthalmoscopic examination of optic fundi, with special attention to the optic disc, and testing visual fields by confrontation and extinction.
- Test each eye separately and both eyes together. In patients with partial vision loss, testing of both eyes can reveal a visual field deficit, whereas testing with one eye will miss this finding. See Chapter 8, "Evidence-Based Assessment of the Eye."

Oculomotor, Trochlear, and Abducens (III, IV, VI)

- Tested with movement of the eyes through the six cardinal points of gaze.
- Visualizations of pupil size, shape, response to light, accommodation, and opening of the upper eyelids are described in Chapter 8, "Evidence-Based Assessment of the Eye."

Trigeminal (V)

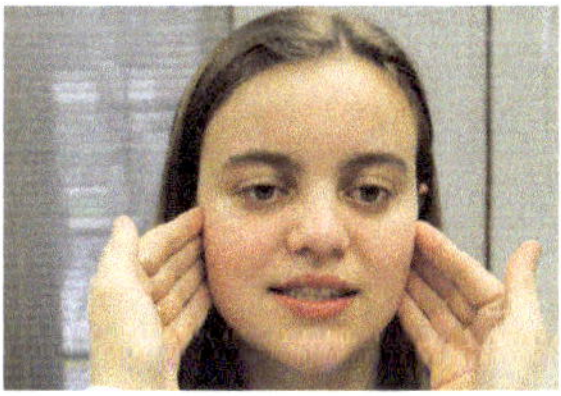

FIGURE 10.1 Motor function assessment of the trigeminal nerve.

- Primary function is to provide sensory and motor innervation to the face.
- **Motor function**: Observe face for muscle atrophy, deviation of the jaw to one side, and muscle twitching. Ask patient to clench teeth tightly as the muscles over the jaw are palpated, evaluating tone (**Figure 10.1**). Facial tone should be symmetric, without tremor.
- **Sensory function**: The three trigeminal nerve divisions are evaluated for sharp, dull, and light touch sensations. Have the patient close their eyes, then touch each side of their face at the scalp, cheek, and chin alternately using the sharp and smooth edges of a broken tongue blade or paper clip. Ask the patient to report whether each sensation is sharp or dull. Stroke the face in the same six areas with a cotton wisp, asking the patient to report sensation. Discrimination of all stimuli is expected over all facial areas (**Figure 10.2**).

Facial (VII)

- The facial nerve has both sensory and motor functions. It controls facial movements, taste, and movement of the lacrimal, submaxillary, and submandibular glands.
- Ask the patient to form specific facial expressions to test for facial symmetry (**Figure 10.3**).

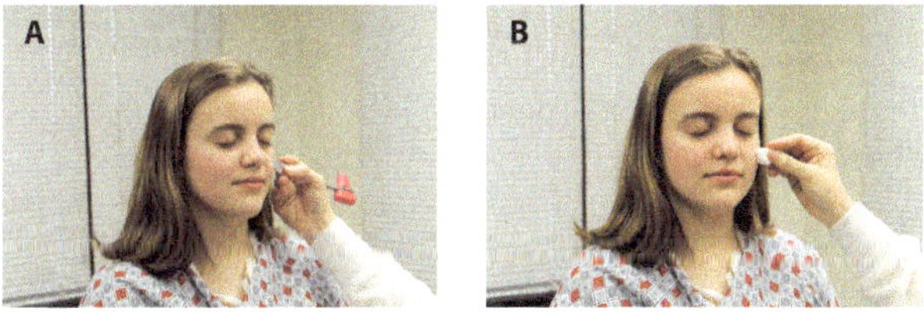

FIGURE 10.2 Evaluation of sensation in the trigeminal nerve divisions using **(A)** a dull edge and **(B)** a cotton ball.

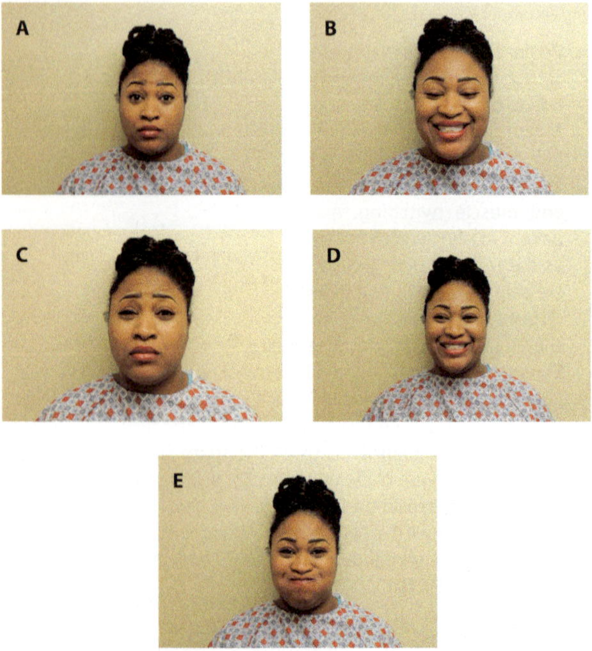

FIGURE 10.3 Facial nerve testing. Among other expressions, patient (**A**) raises eyebrows, (**B**) squeezes eyes shut, (**C**) frowns, (**D**) smiles, and (**E**) puffs out cheeks.

- Observe for tics, unusual facial movements, and asymmetry. Drooping of one side of the mouth, a flattened nasolabial fold, and/or sagging of the lower eyelid are signs of muscle weakness.

Vestibulocochlear (VIII)

- This cranial nerve is responsible for hearing and maintaining body balance.
- Assess hearing with the whispered voice test. Ask patient to repeat numbers whispered into one ear while blocking or rubbing your fingers next to the opposite ear. An audiometry examination can also be completed if a more thorough examination is necessary.
- Romberg test assesses vestibular function (position sense; **Figure 10.4**.)

Glossopharyngeal (IX) and Vagus (X)

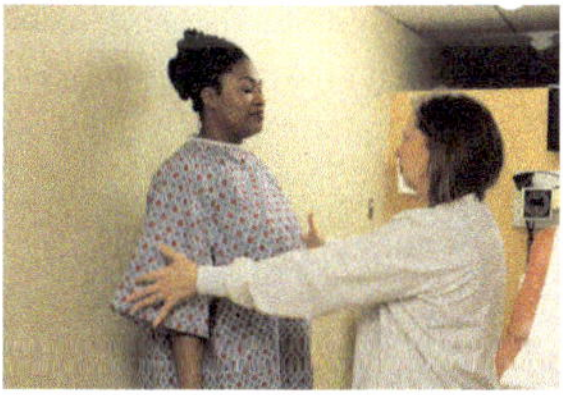

FIGURE 10.4 Romberg test.

- Tests the ability to identify sour and bitter tastes on the posterior third of each side of the tongue, gag reflex, ability to swallow, inspection of the palate and uvula, speech sounds.
- Observe for difficulty swallowing, assess for guttural speech or hoarse voice sounds.
- Sensory function of taste may be completed during the CN VII evaluation.
- Glossopharyngeal nerve function is simultaneously tested during the evaluation of the vagus nerve for nasopharyngeal sensation (gag reflex) and the motor function of swallowing.
- Gag reflex is initiated by touching the patient's posterior pharyngeal wall with an applicator while observing for upward movement of the palate and contraction of the pharyngeal muscles. Uvula should remain midline; drooping or absence of an arch on either side of the palate is abnormal.
- Motor function is evaluated with inspection of the soft palate for symmetry. Have the patient say "ah" and observe the movement of the soft palate. If there is damage to the vagus or glossopharyngeal nerve, the palate does not rise, and the uvula will deviate from midline. Have the patient sip and swallow water. Patient should be able to swallow easily.

Spinal Accessory (XI)

- Evaluation of the size, shape, and strength of the trapezius and SCM muscles.
- To test the trapezius muscle, stand behind patient and observe for atrophy or flickering movement of the skin (a symptom of disease of the nervous system). Place a hand on each shoulder and ask the patient to shrug upward; observe the strength and contraction of the muscles (**Figure 10.5**).

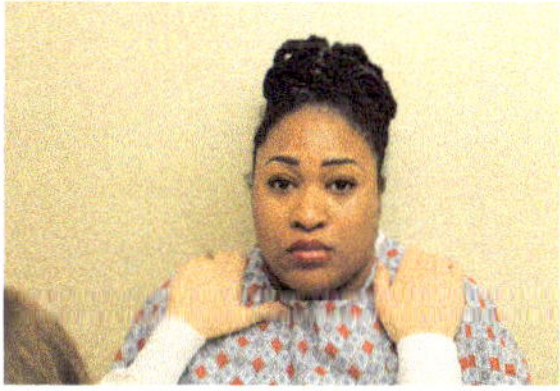

FIGURE 10.5 Testing the trapezius muscle.

- To test the SCM muscle, ask the patient to turn the head to each side against the clinician's hand, observing the contraction of the opposite SCM muscle and force of movement against the hand.

Hypoglossal (XII)

- This CN innervates all but one of the muscles of the tongue.
- Inspect the patient's tongue while at rest on the floor of the mouth and while protruded from the mouth, observing for size and shape. Have the patient move their tongue in and out of the mouth, side to side, and curled upward and downward.
- Test muscle strength by asking the patient to push the tongue against the cheek as the clinician applies resistance with an index finger or hand (**Figure 10.6**).
- Assess lingual speech sounds (l, t, d, n) by listening to the patient's speech (**Box 10.1**).

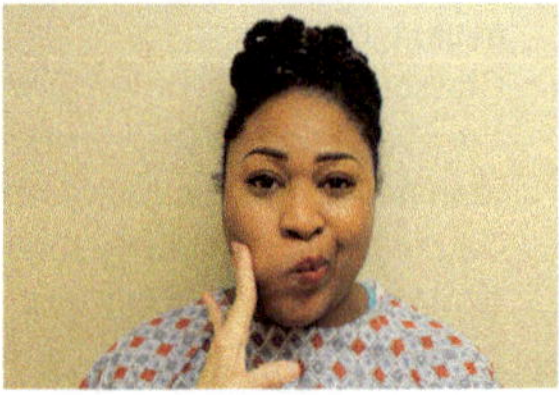

FIGURE 10.6 Testing muscle strength of the tongue.

BOX 10.1
MNEMONIC FOR CRANIAL NERVES

Olfactory	**O**n
Optic	**O**ld
Oculomotor	**O**lympus
Trochlear	**T**owering
Trigeminal	**T**ops
Abducens	**A**
Facial	**F**inn
Acoustic	**A**nd
Glossopharyngeal	**G**erman
Vagus nerve	**V**iewed
Spinal	**S**ome
Hypoglossal	**H**ops

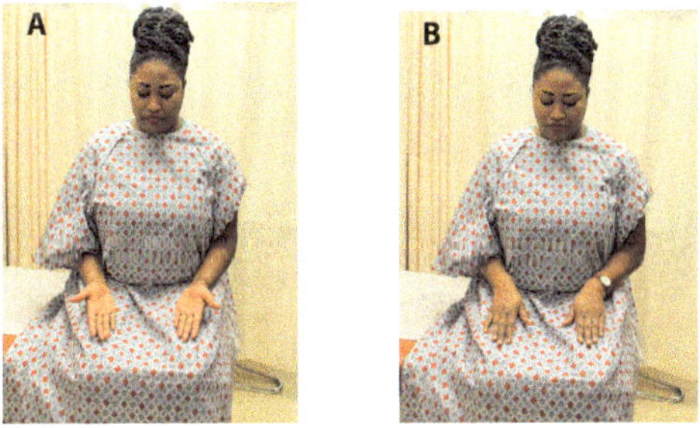

FIGURE 10.7 Testing rapid rhythmic alternative movements. Patient alternately places palms up (**A**) and down (**B**).

PROPRIOCEPTION AND CEREBELLAR FUNCTION

Coordination and Fine Motor Skills

Observe the patient's body position during movement and at rest. Look for involuntary movements (tics or tremors), muscle bulk, muscle strength, muscle tone, and the patient's coordination. Abnormal position may be due to mono- or hemiparesis from stroke.

Rapid Rhythmic Alternative Movements

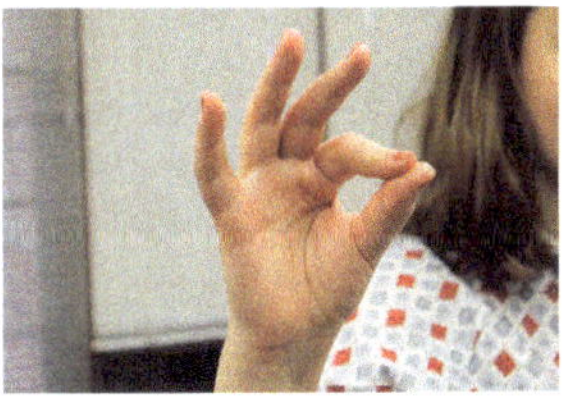

FIGURE 10.8 Testing rapid rhythmic alternating movements.

- Ask the seated patient to pat their knees with both hands, alternately turning the palms up and down and gradually increasing the speed of movements (**Figure 10.7**).
- Alternatively, ask the patient to touch the thumb to each finger on the same hand from the little finger and back. One hand is tested at a time, gradually increasing the speed (**Figure 10.8**). The clinician should model the movements for the patient before having the patient complete them. The patient should be able to accomplish these movements smoothly and rhythmically. Stiff, slow, or jerky clonic movements are abnormal.

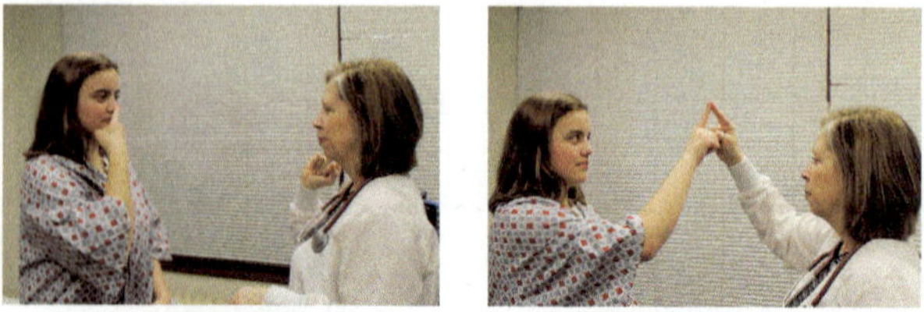

FIGURE 10.9 Finger-to-nose test.

Accuracy of Movements

- **Finger-to-nose test:** Tests accuracy of the patient's movements (**Figure 10.9**). The clinician moves their finger position several times during the test, which is then repeated on the other hand.
- **Heel-to-shin test**: An alternative method to test accuracy of movement. Test can be performed with the patient sitting or supine (**Figure 10.10**). The patient should be able to move the heel up and down the shin in a straight line without deviating to the side.

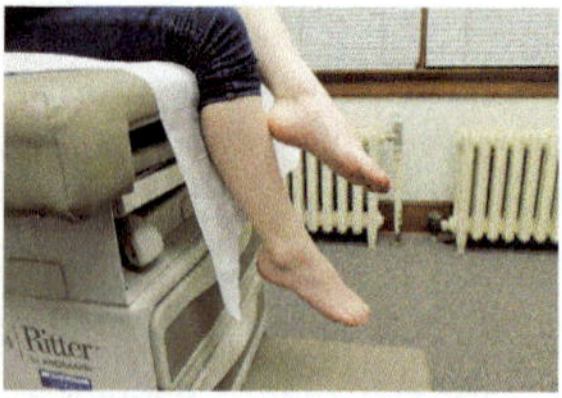

FIGURE 10.10 Heel-to-shin test.

Balance

- Complete the Romberg test (see "Vestibulocochlear [VIII]" section). Loss of balance is a positive sign, indicating cerebellar ataxia/dysfunction or sensory loss. If the patient staggers or loses balance, postpone other tests of cerebellar function that require balance. Other methods to evaluate balance:
  - Have patient stand with feet slightly apart and push the shoulders with enough effort to throw them off balance (be ready to catch patient if needed). Patient should be able to quickly recover balance.
  - Ask patient to close their eyes, hold their arms at the sides of the body, and stand on one foot, repeating the test on the opposite foot. Slight swaying is normal; patient should be able to maintain balance on each foot for 5 seconds.
  - With eyes open, have patient hop in place on one foot and then the other (tests proximal and distal muscle strength). Patient should be able to hop on one foot for 5 seconds without

loss of balance. Observe for instability or need to continually touch the floor with the opposite foot or a tendency to fall. Difficulty hopping may be related to weakness, lack of position sense, or cerebellar dysfunction.

Gait

- Have the patient walk across the room or down the hall and turn and come back, observing posture, balance, swinging of the arms, and intact movement.
- The patient should then walk heel to toe in a straight line (tandem walking), walk on their toes, and then on their heels (**Figure 10.11**). Last, have the patient do a knee bend.

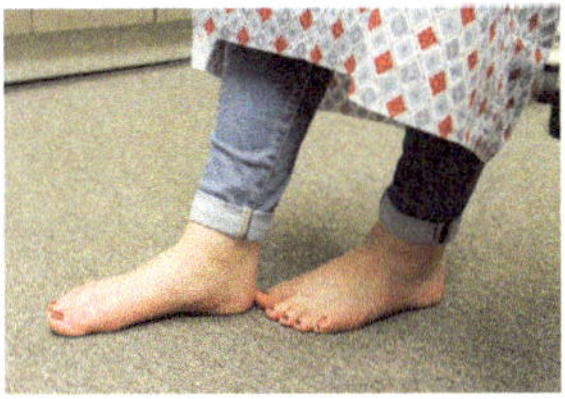

FIGURE 10.11 Assessment of gait using tandem walking.

- These tests assess for gait abnormalities that increase fall risk. An uncoordinated gait with reeling and instability is ataxic, which is seen in cerebellar disease, loss of position sense, and intoxication. Tandem walking may reveal ataxia, distal leg weakness, and is a sensitive test for corticospinal tract damage. See **Table 10.1** for abnormal gait pattern characteristics.

TABLE 10.1 Corticospinal, Basal Ganglia, and Cerebellar Motor Pathways

Pathway	Function
Corticospinal (pyramidal) tract	Mediation of voluntary movement; inhibition of muscle tone; coordination of complicated movements
Basal ganglia system	Controls muscle tone and body movements, including automatically performing a learned behavior
Cerebellar system	Coordinates muscle activity, sustains equilibrium, and maintains posture

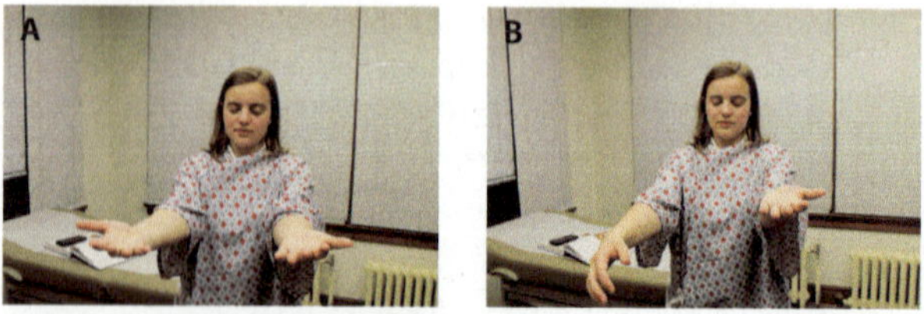

FIGURE 10.12 Testing for pronator drift. (**A**) Patient stands with eyes closed and arms straight forward with palms up. (**B**) Arms drifting sideward or upward after a brisk tap indicate a positive test.

- **Pronator drift testing**: Tests muscular strength, coordination, and good position sense (**Figure 10.12**).

Muscle Strength

- Normal muscle strength varies, so the normal standard should allow for age and gender. Patient's dominant side is usually stronger than nondominant side; differences may be hard to detect.
- Test muscle strength by asking patient to actively resist the clinician's movement:
  - **Biceps and brachioradialis at the elbow flexion and extension**: Patient pulls and pushes against clinician's hand.
  - **Extension at the wrist**: Patient makes a fist and resists as clinician presses down.
  - **Grip strength**: Clinician asks patient to squeeze two of their fingers as hard as possible and not let them go. Weak grip is seen in cervical radiculopathy, ulnar peripheral nerve disease, carpal tunnel syndrome, arthritis, and epicondylitis.
  - **Finger abduction**: Patient's hand is positioned down with fingers spread. Patient tries to prevent clinician from forcing fingers together (**Figure 10.13**). Weak finger abduction occurs in ulnar nerve disorders.
  - **Thumb opposition:** Patient touches the top of the little finger to the tip of the thumb. The clinician then attempts to break them apart.
  - **Muscle strength of the trunk:** Determined by flexion, extension, rotation, and lateral bending.

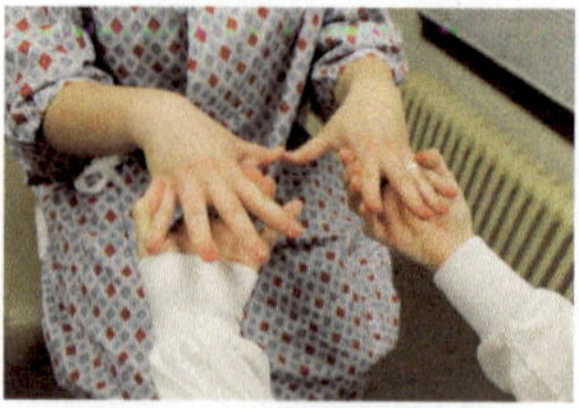

FIGURE 10.13 Finger abduction test.

- **Flexion at the hip:** Clinician places their hand on patient's midthigh and asks them to raise the leg against their hand
- **Adduction at the hips:** Clinician puts hands on the bed between the patient's knees and asks the patient to bring both legs together.
- **Abduction at the hips:** Clinician puts their hands on the outside of the patient's knees and asks patient to spread both legs against their hands.
- **Extension at the knee:** Clinician supports the knee in flexion and asks the patient to straighten the leg against their hand. Expect a forceful response as the quadriceps is the strongest muscle in the body.
- **Flexion at the knee:** Clinician positions the patient's leg so the knee is flexed with the foot resting on the bed. Clinician tells the patient to keep the foot down as they try to straighten the leg.
- **Foot dorsiflexion and plantar flexion at the ankle:** Clinician asks the patient to pull up and push down against their hand. Heel and toe walk assesses foot dorsiflexion/plantar flexion.

REFLEXES

Superficial Reflexes

- **Plantar reflex:** Using the end of a reflex hammer, stroke the lateral side of the foot from heel to ball, then across the foot to the medial side with the result of plantar flexion of the toes. This is a normal sign.
- **Abdominal reflex:** With the patient supine, stroke the four abdominal quadrants with the end of a reflex hammer. Stroking downward and away from the umbilicus elicits the lower abdominal reflexes, which respond with a slight movement of the umbilicus toward the area of stimulation. Reflex response should be equal and bilateral.

Deep Tendon Reflexes

- Biceps, brachioradialis, triceps, patellar, and Achilles reflexes are DTRs.
- Patient should be in a seated position. Test each reflex and compare it to the other side of the body. The reflex response should be symmetric, visible, and palpable. DTRs are obtained by positioning a limb with a slightly stretched tendon and quickly tapping the tendon to be tested with a percussion hammer.

TABLE 10.2 Deep Tendon Reflex Grading

Grade 0	No response
Grade 1+	Sluggish or diminished response
Grade 2+	Active or expected response (normal)
Grade 3+	Brisk/slightly hyperactive
Grade 4+	Brisk/hyperactive

The expected response is a sudden contraction of the muscle. If the tendon response is absent, consider a neuropathy. Consider upper motor neuron disorder with hyperactive reflexes. If deep tendon reflexes are symmetrically diminished or absent, use a technique of isometric contraction of other muscles which might increase reflex activity. Each reflex is scored as 0 to 4+ (**Table 10.2**).

- **Biceps reflex:** With the patient's arm bent at a 45-degree angle at the elbow, palpate the biceps tendon and place your thumb over the tendon and your fingers under the elbow. Strike your thumb with the reflex hammer to elicit contraction of the biceps muscle, causing flexion of the elbow (**Figure 10.14**).

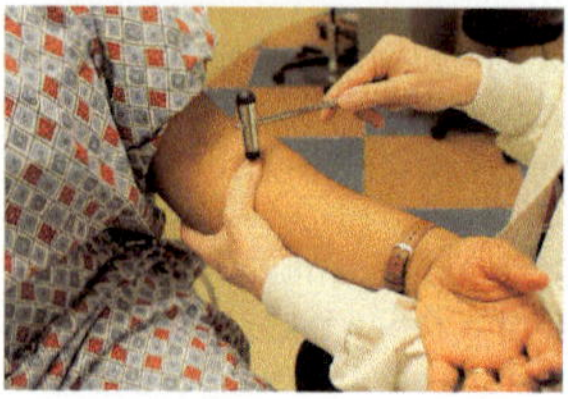

FIGURE 10.14 Biceps reflex test.

- **Brachioradialis reflex:** With the patient's arm bent at a 45-degree angle at the elbow, rest the patient's arm on yours. The patient's hand should be slightly pronated. Clinician directly strikes the brachioradial tendon 1 to 2 inches above the wrist with the reflex hammer (**Figure 10.15**). A normal response is forearm pronation and elbow flexion.

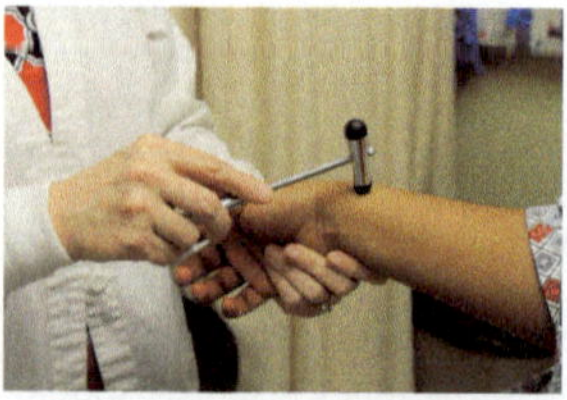

FIGURE 10.15 Brachioradialis test.

- **Triceps reflex:** With the patient's arm flexed at a 90-degree angle, support the patient's arm just above the antecubital fossa and palpate the antecubital fossa. Then directly strike the triceps tendon with a reflex hammer just above the elbow (**Figure 10.16**). A normal response is extension of the elbow.

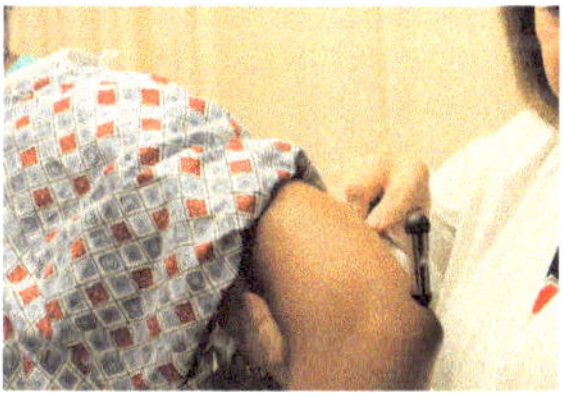

FIGURE 10.16 Triceps reflex test.

- **Patellar reflex:** With patient's knee flexed to a 90-degree angle, support the patient's upper leg with your hand to allow patient's lower leg to hang. Strike the patellar tendon just below the patella (**Figure 10.17**). A normal response is extension of the lower leg.

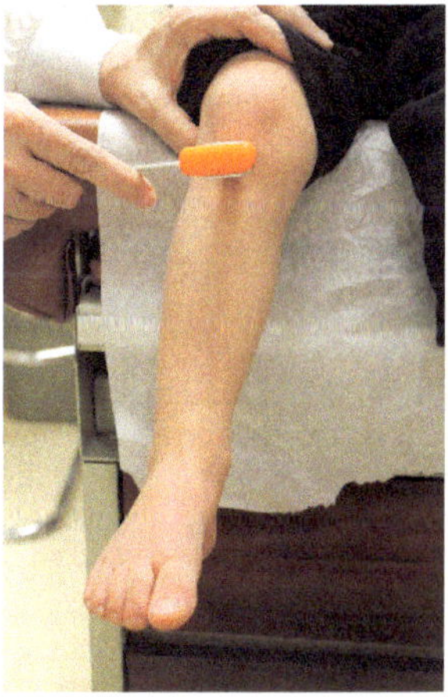

FIGURE 10.17 Patellar reflex test.

- **Achilles reflex:** With patient sitting and the knee flexed to a 90-degree angle, keeping the ankle in a neutral position, hold the patient's foot in your hand. Strike the Achilles tendon at the level of the ankle malleoli. A normal response is plantar flexion of the foot.

Primitive Reflex Testing in Infancy

- **Moro reflex:** Supporting the infant's head, body, and legs, the clinician suddenly lowers the body, causing the arms to abduct and extend, followed by relaxed flexion, during which the legs should flex.
- **Stepping reflex:** Clinician holds the infant under the arms, allowing one of the infant's feet to touch the surface of the examination table. The clinician observes for flexion of the hip and knee. The foot should touch the table while the other foot steps forward.

- **Palmar reflex grasp:** Clinician places a finger in the infant's hand, pressing against the palmar surface of the hand. The infant flexes all fingers to grasp the clinician's finger. A positive grasp reflex that lasts longer than 2 months indicates central nervous system damage.
- **Plantar reflex grasp:** Clinician touches the sole of the infant's foot at the base of the toes, causing the toes to curl.

SENSORY FUNCTION

- Evaluation requires testing of several kinds of sensations—for example, pain and temperature (spinothalamic tracts), position and vibration (posterior columns), light touch (spinothalamic tracts and posterior columns), and discriminative sensations that depend on pain, temperature, position, vibration, and light touch (the cortex).
- Evaluate sensation by asking the patient to identify stimuli on the hands, distal arms, abdomen, feet, and legs. Each sensation procedure is tested with the patient's eyes closed. Contralateral areas of the body are tested, and the patient is asked to compare sensations side to side. Normal findings: Minimal differences side to side, correct description of sensations (hot, cold, sharp, dull), recognition of the side of the body tested, location of sensation and recognition if proximal or distal to the site previously tested.
- When testing, the clinician focuses on the areas that have numbness, pain, motor, or reflex abnormalities. Compare symmetric areas on two sides of the body including arms, legs, and trunk. With pain, temperature, and touch sensation, compare distal to proximal areas of the extremities.
- Test fingers and toes first for vibration and sensation. If tests are normal, clinician can assume the more proximal areas are normal. Evaluation of light touch and superficial pain can be evaluated together.
- **Monofilament testing:** Testing with a 5.07 monofilament should be done on several sites of the foot for all patients with diabetic and peripheral neuropathy. With patient's eyes closed, the clinician places the monofilament on several sites of the plantar surface of each foot and one side of the dorsal surface of the foot in a random pattern (**Figure 10.18**). The clinician applies pressure for 1.5 seconds to each site without repeating a test site. The correct

amount of pressure is applied when the filament bends. Testing is positive if the patient cannot feel the monofilament.

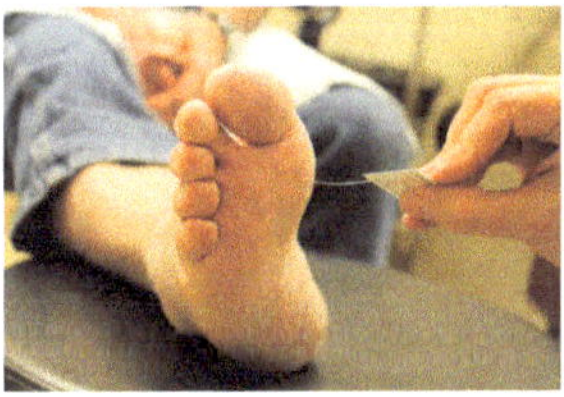

FIGURE 10.18 Monofilament test.

Primary Sensory Functions

- **Light touch:** Lightly touch the skin with a cotton wisp and ask the patient to respond when and where the sensation is felt.
- **Superficial pain:** Alternate the sharp and smooth edges of a broken tongue blade, Wartenberg wheel, or paper clip on the skin (**Figure 10.19**). Ask the patient to identify each sensation as sharp or dull and where the sensation is felt.

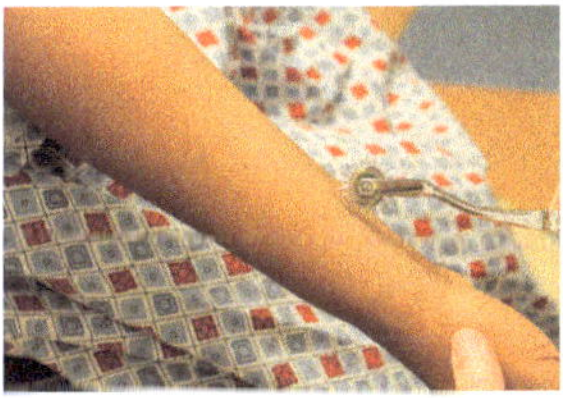

FIGURE 10.19 Testing superficial pain with a Wartenberg wheel.

- **Temperature:** Testing skin temperature is omitted if pain sensation is normal. If there are sensory deficits, use test tubes filled with hot and cold water. Ask the patient to identify whether the sensation is hot or cold and where the sensation is felt.

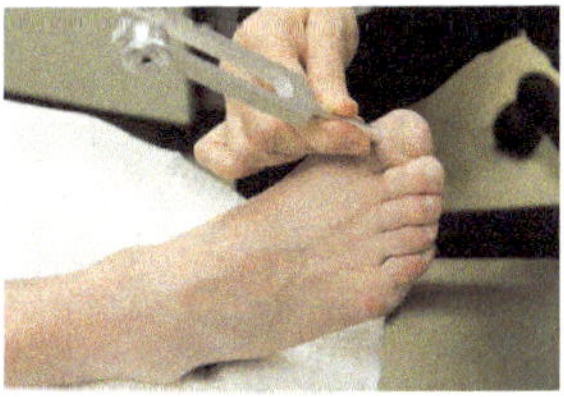

FIGURE 10.20 Testing vibration with a low-pitched tuning fork.

- **Vibration:** Place the stem of a low-pitched tuning fork (128 Hz) against a bony prominence at the toe or finger joint; ask patient to identify when/where the buzzing sensation is felt **Figure 10.20**).
- **Proprioception joint position sense:** Assess the patient's ability to sense the position of their joint. This should be completed on the great toe of each foot and a finger on each hand (**Figure 10.21**). Hold the joint by the lateral aspect in the neutral position. Move the finger/toe up and down; ask the patient

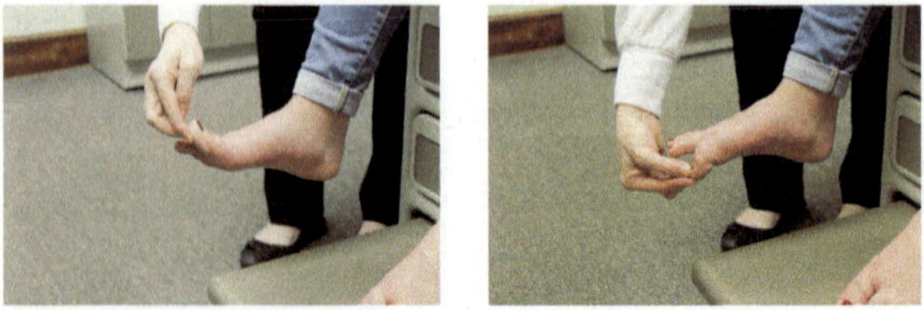

FIGURE 10.21 Testing proprioception joint position sense.

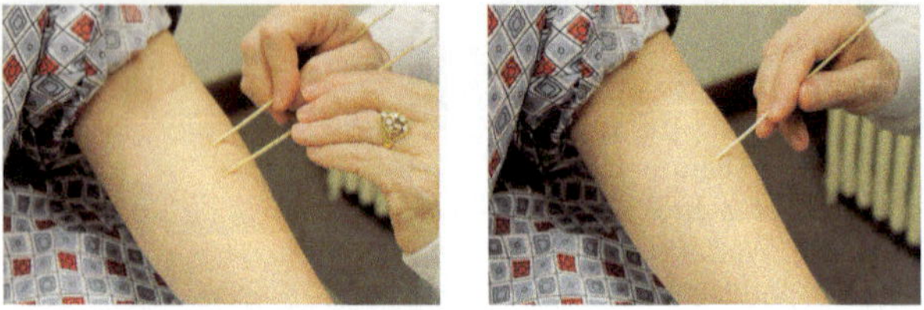

FIGURE 10.22 Two-point discrimination test.

to identify whether the joint is forward, backward, or in the neutral position. If they cannot, it is considered an abnormal finding.

SPECIAL TESTS

Cortical Sensory Function

- Discriminatory sensory function tests assess the patient's ability to interpret sensation. Patients with lesions in the sensory cortex or posterior spinal cord would be unable to complete these tests. The patient's eyes should be closed during testing.
- **Stereognosis:** Tests patient's ability to identify a familiar object by touch. Place a key or coin in the patient's hand; ability to identify the object is a normal response.
- **Two-point discrimination:** Using two ends of a paper clip, alternate touching the patient's skin at various locations with one or two points of the paper clip (**Figure 10.22**). Patient's ability to identify one- or two-point touch is a normal response.
- **Extinction phenomenon:** Simultaneously touch two areas on each side of the body (such as the cheek or hand) with the broken end of a tongue blade. The patient should be able to discriminate the number of touches and where they are felt bilaterally.

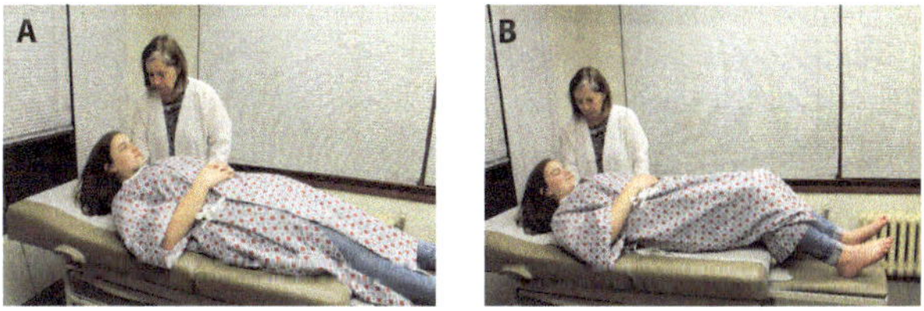

FIGURE 10.23 Brudzinski's sign test. (**A**) Clinician flexes the patient's neck forward. (**B**) Test is positive when the patient bends the hips and knees in response to neck flexion.

- **Graphesthesia:** With the blunt end of an applicator, draw a number or shape on the palm of the patient's hand. Repeat the test using a different figure on the other hand. Patient should be able to identify the shape or number.
- Other special tests are used when the clinician suspects meningeal irritation, which can occur with meningitis or subarachnoid hemorrhage:
    - **Brudzinski sign:** Clinician should not use this test if there is injury or fracture of the cervical vertebrae or cervical cord (**Figure 10.23**).
    - **Kernig's sign:** With patient lying flat, flex the patient's leg at the hip and knee, then slowly extend the leg and straighten the knee. Normally, the patient should feel some discomfort behind the knee with extension. A positive test reveals pain with knee extension.

RED FLAGS IN HISTORY AND PHYSICAL EXAM

- History of cancer or immunosuppression
- History of trauma, fall, or loss of consciousness
- History of previous stroke or TIA
- Family history of a progressive neurological disorder
- Reported progressive neurological dysfunction
- Face drooping
- Sudden numbness or weakness of the face, arm, or leg, especially unilateral
- Sudden confusion, trouble speaking, or issues understanding speech
- Sudden trouble seeing in one or both eyes, abrupt vision loss, or double vision
- Sudden trouble walking, dizziness, or loss of balance/coordination

- Sudden severe headache
- Abrupt onset of motor and sensory deficits
- Seizure; status epilepticus
- Paralysis
- Syncope
- Memory loss
- Loss of already attained cognitive or developmental abilities
- Meningitis triad (fever, headache, neck stiffness)

EVIDENCE-BASED RESOURCES

- **American Academy of Neurology:** www.aan.com/policy-and-guidelines/guidelines
- **European Academy of Neurology:** www.ean.org/research/ean-guidelines/guideline-reference-center
- **International Headache Society:** www.ihs-headache.org/ichd-guidelines

ABNORMAL FINDINGS

BELL'S PALSY

An inflammation of the facial nerve typically of unknown cause.

History

- History of herpes simplex type 1 or Lyme disease
- Symptoms that typically develop abruptly (within hours) with maximum characteristics in 3 days
- Reported facial pain; pain around the ear
- Abnormal taste

Physical Examination

- Unilateral facial weakness and drooping; drooling
- Unilateral eyelid weakness; absence of a corneal reflex; reduced tearing

Considerations

- Believed to be the result of swelling and inflammation of the facial nerve due to reactivation of an existing (dormant) viral infection. Impaired immunity from stress, sleep deprivation, physical trauma, minor illness, or autoimmune syndromes are most likely triggers.

- Other conditions that cause facial paralysis (e.g., brain tumor, stroke, myasthenia gravis, Lyme disease) should be ruled out first.
- Patient usually recovers within 3 weeks.

CEREBRAL PALSY

A nonprogressive motor disorder secondary to damage of the fetal or infant brain.

History

- History of preterm birth, low birth weight, low Apgar score, neonatal encephalopathy, neonatal sepsis, meningitis
- History of maternal conditions, infections, Rh incompatibility
- Poor nutrition
- Reported sleep disruption

Physical Examination

- In infancy: Abnormal muscle tone, abnormal motor development, and feeding difficulties
- Difficulty with speech, language, and communication
- Difficulty eating, drinking, swallowing
- Pain: Musculoskeletal disorders, including scoliosis, hip dislocation, nonspecific back pain, increased muscle tone (dystonia, spasticity), muscle fatigue, headache, nonspecific abdominal pain, dental pain, dysmenorrhea
- Mental health disorders, including depression, anxiety disorder, antisocial behavior, learning disabilities, ADHD
- Vision and hearing Impairment
- Vomiting, regurgitation, reflux
- Constipation
- Epilepsy

Considerations

- Symptoms of CP differ in type and severity from one person to the next and may even change in an individual over time.
- Symptoms depend on which parts of the brain have been affected.

EPILEPSY

A neurological condition that causes recurring seizures.

History

- Possible history of perinatal anoxia, congenital brain malformation, genetic disorders, infectious disease, traumatic brain injury
- Seizures often triggered by sleep deprivation, dehydration, stress, alcohol, and/or drug use

- Commonly interferes with school, work, driving
- Children may experience physical complications from seizures and are at greater risk for negative self-image, anxiety, depression, and learning disabilities

Physical Examination

- Jerking movement of one or more extremities
- Nystagmus
- Abrupt movement of head to one side or the other
- Moans or cries
- Fearful or sad emotions
- Humming or buzzing noises
- Intense or unpleasant smells or tastes
- Tingling in one area or side of the body
- Flashing lights in a portion of the visual fields

Consideration

- Status epilepticus is considered a medical emergency due to an increased chance of death.

HEMORRHAGIC STROKE

Bleeding directly into the brain tissue, caused by leakage from intracerebral arteries.

History

- Trauma history
- History of hypertension, previous stroke, coagulopathies, or anticoagulant therapy
- Reported nausea, vomiting, headache
- Advanced age
- History of alcohol abuse and/or cocaine use

Physical Examination

- Altered level of consciousness
- Seizures
- Weakness or paralysis of an extremity, half of the body, or all extremities
- Facial droop
- Monocular or binocular blindness; blurred vision
- Dysarthria and trouble understanding speech
- Vertigo or ataxia
- Aphasia
- Subarachnoid symptoms: Sudden onset of severe headache, signs of meningitis (nuchal rigidity), photophobia and eye pain, nausea and vomiting, syncope

Considerations

- Less common than ischemic stroke, associated with a higher mortality rate
- Patients may have neurological deficits similar to ischemic stroke, but are more likely to have headache, altered mental status, seizures, nausea and vomiting, and/or pronounced hypertension.

INTRACRANIAL TUMOR

An abnormal growth in the cranial cavity that may be benign or due to malignancy. Brain tumors include glioblastomas, meningioma, and pituitary tumors.

History

- Persistent headaches that wake patient from sleep
- Appetite loss
- Nausea and vomiting

Physical Examination

- Ringing and hearing loss in one ear
- Reduced visual acuity, loss of vision
- Changes in behavior and personality
- Children may exhibit irritability, lethargy, cranial nerve palsies, weight loss
- Seizures
- Confusion
- Papilledema
- Aphasia
- Nystagmus
- Ataxia
- Unilateral weakness

Consideration

- Brain CT scan or MRI needed to confirm diagnosis.

ISCHEMIC STROKE

An embolus from atrial fibrillation or atherosclerotic disease that causes a sudden loss of blood circulation to the brain.

History

- History of smoking or excessive alcohol use
- History of oral contraceptive use or pregnancy in young women
- History of atrial fibrillation
- History of high cholesterol, hypertension, atherosclerosis, cancer, blood clots, and/or diabetes

- History of hematological disorders (e.g., factor V Leiden, prothrombin gene mutation, sickle cell anemia)
- Hypercoagulable states
- History of TIAs
- Recent travel

Physical Examination

- Sudden severe headache with no known cause
- Abrupt onset of hemiparesis or monoparesis
- Visual field deficits
- Facial droop
- Ataxia
- Nystagmus
- Aphasia: expressive and receptive
- Sudden numbness or weakness of the face, arm, or leg
- Abrupt decrease in level of consciousness

Considerations

- If ischemic stroke is not treated promptly, it can lead to brain damage or death; signs and symptoms need to be identified immediately to prevent morbidity and mortality.
- Tissue plasminogen activator given within 4.5 hours of the start of symptoms is most effective at breaking up the clot.

MENINGITIS

Inflammation of the meninges of the brain or spinal cord caused by bacterial, viral, or fungal organism colonization in the upper respiratory tract.

History

- Symptoms develop over several hours or 1 to 2 days
- History of exposure to a patient with a similar illness
- Classic triad for bacterial meningitis is fever, headache, and neck stiffness; however, patients may present with only one or two of these symptoms

Physical Examination

- Neck stiffness
- Lethargy, sleepiness
- Nausea, vomiting
- Photophobia
- Confusion, irritability
- Delirium
- Seizures

- Coma
- Altered mental status
- Nuchal rigidity
- Increased blood pressure with bradycardia
- Positive Brudzinski and Kernig signs
- Petechial and purpura rash with meningococcal meningitis
- Infants: Bulging fontanelle, paradoxical irritability (quiet when lying flat, crying when held), high-pitch cry, hypotonia

Considerations

- It is important to identify the causative agent in cases of meningitis.
- Bacterial meningitis (a medical emergency) must be the first and foremost consideration in the differential diagnosis of patients with headache, neck stiffness, fever, and altered mental status.

MULTIPLE SCLEROSIS

An inflammatory demyelinating disease characterized by episodic neurological function in the brain, spinal cord, and optic nerves.

History

- Onset typically between 20 to 40 years of age; occurs more often in women
- Reports fatigue, heat intolerance, depression, localized weakness, and decreased attention span, concentration, and memory loss
- History of vision problems (double vision, loss of vision)
- Reports bowel, bladder, and sexual dysfunction
- Constipation

Physical Examination

- Localized weakness
- Paresthesia
- Muscle cramping due to spasticity
- Dysarthria, nystagmus, and intention tremor
- Lhermitte's sign (an electric shock-like sensation that occurs with flexion of the neck and goes down the spine, often going into the limbs)
- Trigeminal neuralgia
- Irregular twitching of the facial nerves
- Focal sensory disturbances (decreasing proprioception and vibration)
- Hyper-reactive reflexes
- Increased muscle tone or stiffness in the extremities
- Optic neuritis: Unilateral loss of visual acuity, pain

Considerations

- Signs and symptoms depend on where the nerves are demyelinated.
- Four types of MS: Relapsing-remitting, secondary-progressive, primary-progressive, and progressive-relapsing. The type of MS provides information about the general course of the disease and responsiveness of the disease to treatment.

MYASTHENIA GRAVIS

A common autoimmune disease that affects neuromuscular junction transmission.

History

- Personal or family history of autoimmune diseases
- Symptoms can worsen with stress, illness, and fatigue

Physical Examination

- Weakness that worsens with activity
- Difficulty swallowing or speaking
- Drooping eyelids
- Double vision; ocular symptoms are most common
- Fatigue or weakness; facial weakness when puffing out cheeks
- Difficulty walking
- Hypophonia
- Respiratory compromise or failure
- Skeletal muscle weakness
- Positive serum antibodies

Considerations

- Etiology of disease is unknown.
- Diagnosis is based on history and physical exam findings and confirmed by electrodiagnostic testing and positive serum antibodies directed at proteins in the neuromuscular junction.

PARKINSON'S DISEASE

A slowly progressive neurodegenerative disorder affecting movement, muscle control, and balance, caused by destruction and loss of dopaminergic neurons.

History

- Early signs and symptoms may be subtle and difficult to detect or missed secondary to slow disease progression
- Elderly (older than 60 years of age are at the greatest risk of acquiring)

- Affects men more than women
- Menopause in women
- History of head trauma
- Working with environmental toxins including pesticides and herbicides
- Carrying the alpha-synuclein gene
- Reports numbness, tingling, and muscle soreness; difficulty swallowing

Physical Examination

- Nonmotor symptoms can sometimes be seen prior to motor symptoms
- Constipation, depression, cognitive dysfunction, dementia, psychosis
- Motor symptoms considered cardinal signs of Parkinson's disease: Rest tremors; slowness of movement, freezing, or unable to continue movements; rigidity; postural instability
- Motor symptoms: Pill-rolling movement of fingers bilaterally; head tremors; drooling; stooped posture; short steps, shuffling gait, accelerating gait to maintain posture; slow slurred speech, softened voice

Consideration

- Diagnosis based on signs/symptoms, patient history, physical exam, and neurological assessment.

PERIPHERAL NEUROPATHY

The most common type of neuropathy, which is caused by nerve lesions or tissue nerve damage that produces hyper-excitability of primary sensory neurons and cells in the dorsal root ganglia.

History

- Reports numbness, tingling, shooting, burning, or electric-shock sensations; occurs in the feet or hands
- All sensation is painful
- Gradual onset of symptoms; symptoms worsen at night
- History of diabetes
- History of alcohol abuse
- History of nutritional disorders
- Neurotoxic chemotherapy

Physical Examination

- Reduced touch sensation
- Reduced sensation in feet with monofilament examination

- Diminished posterior tibial or dorsalis pedis pulses
- Distal muscle weakness; cannot stand on toes or heels
- Skin ulcerations that the patient is unable to feel (most often on the extremities)

Consideration

- Due to lack of feeling and pain, patients are at high risk for skin ulcerations. They should be advised to always wear shoes and do skin checks every day.

TRIGEMINAL NEURALGIA

Causes recurrent paroxysmal sharp pain radiating into one or more branches of the trigeminal nerve.

History

- More common in older adults (greater than age 50); affects women more often than men
- Reports unilateral burning, stabbing, electric shock, excruciating facial pain in the chin or cheek
- Pain episodes may occur several times a day to several times/month
- Increased pain with chewing, swallowing, talking, brushing teeth, cold exposure
- Intermittent pain-free periods
- Inflammation of the maxillofacial region
- Inflammation of the ear, nose, throat
- Recent dental work
- History of multiple sclerosis

Physical Examination

- May have normal neurological assessment
- Slight sensory impairment in painful regions
- Pain occurs in one or more divisions of the trigeminal nerve

Consideration

- Other causes of trigeminal neuralgia include pressure of a tumor on the nerve or MS. Development of trigeminal neuralgia in a young adult suggests the possibility of MS.

PHYSICAL EXAMINATION DOCUMENTATION

EXAMPLE OF NORMAL FINDINGS

Patient is alert and oriented ×3. Affect, behavior, speech, and communication are appropriate. Public Health Questionnaire-9 score: 6. Recent and remote memory is intact. Cranial nerves I to XII are intact.

Pain, light touch, and vibratory sense are intact. Two-point discrimination is intact. Biceps, brachioradialis, triceps, patellar, and Achilles DTRs 2+ bilateral. Good muscle tone. Strength 5/5 upper and lower extremities (deltoid, biceps, triceps, quadriceps. and hamstrings). Finger to nose and heal to shin testing is normal bilateral. Rapid alternating movements are even, equal, and coordinated. Romberg test is negative. Gait is smooth and coordinated with a steady base. Coordination is intact as measured by heel walk and toe walk.

EXAMPLE OF CRANIAL NERVE DOCUMENTATION

(I) Able to accurately identify three scents (II, III, IV, VI); visual acuity (uncorrected) left eye 20/20, right eye 20/20; visual fields intact; PERRLA; EOM* intact without ptosis; (V) facial sensation normal, equal bilateral to sharp, dull, and light touch stimuli; corneal reflex present; facial tone symmetrical, without tremor. (VII) Facial muscle strength is normal and equal bilaterally; (VIII) whisper test negative bilaterally; (IX, X) palate and uvula elevate symmetrically with intact gag reflex, uvula midline without deviation; voice is normal; (XI) shoulder shrug 5/5 bilateral; (XII) tongue protrudes midline and moves symmetrically.

REFERENCES

References for this chapter draw from Chapter 14, "Evidence-Based Assessment of Nervous System," of the textbook *Evidence-Based Physical Examination: Best Practices for Health and Well-Being Assessment*. The references may be accessed in the digital version of the handbook at https://connect.springerpub.com/content/book/97808-0-8261-6466-7/chapter/ch10

11

Evidence-Based Assessment of the Musculoskeletal System

CLINICAL CONSIDERATIONS

- History questions for the patient who presents with chronic MSK problems include assessing for fever, weakness, inability to bear weight, stiffness, and/or swelling.
- History questions for the patient who presents with acute MSK injury include asking about the mechanism of injury and subsequent limitation in movement.
- To be both systematic and thorough when completing a physical exam related to injury or pain in a joint, remember to begin with inspection, then palpate and assess strength; proceed to assess ROM and use special tests to note joint stability if there are no obvious deformities or point tenderness.
- In the MSK exam, a solid knowledge of the bony landmarks and underlying anatomy along with precise palpation is invaluable. Tenderness over a particular bony or soft-tissue landmark can help to determine potential differential diagnoses.

SUBJECTIVE HISTORY

COMMON REASONS FOR SEEKING CARE

- Joint pain (shoulder, elbow, wrist, hand, hip, knee, ankle, or foot pain)
- Spine pain (neck or back pain)

HISTORY OF PRESENT ILLNESS

- **Onset:** When did the symptoms start? What was the patient doing when they became symptomatic? Did this occur suddenly, or has it been developing gradually?
- **Location:** Does the symptom have associated pain or discomfort? If so, where is the discomfort located? Can you please point to the exact location of the pain or discomfort? Does the pain radiate anywhere? Are any other parts of the body affected?
- **Duration:** How long do symptom(s) last? Over what period of time has the pain or symptom developed? Does the pain come and go or is it constantly present?
- **Characteristics:** How would you describe the pain—aching, burning, sharp, shooting, or deep? Is there any obvious deformity?
- **Associated symptoms:** Is there ever a click or pop associated with movement? Do you experience any other symptoms with it like weakness, stiffness, numbness, or tingling? Is there ever any instability or inability to bear weight? Are there any systemic symptoms (e.g., fever, unintended weight loss)? Are there any urinary symptoms (loss of bowel or bladder)?
- **Aggravating factors:** Was there a known injury? If so, what happened? What actions, activities, or body positions make the symptoms worse? Clarify level of activity that causes symptom exacerbation. Is it worse at night or during the day? Is the back pain worse with bowel movements or the Valsalva maneuver?
- **Relieving factors:** What actions, activities or body positions decrease the symptoms? Have limb elevation, ice, or heat been tried? If relieved, how long does the relief last?
- **Treatment:** What medications has the patient taken to help with the symptoms? Clarify dosage and frequency of any medications. Have steroid injections been used in the past? Have any alternative treatments been tried like chiropractic care or acupuncture?
- **Severity:** How severe are the symptoms on a scale of 0 to 10? Do the symptoms limit participation in activities? Are there associated symptoms? Are the symptoms worsening?

HEALTH HISTORY

Past Medical History

- History of MSK conditions throughout the life span
- Chronic diseases (including cancers, diabetes, autoimmune disorders, osteoporosis, renal diseases, thyroid disorders)
- Osteoarthritis
- Anemia

- Surgeries
- Radiation therapy
- Recent or past injury, trauma, or car accidents
- History of physical or occupational therapy

Medications

- Prescribed medications (dose/frequency), including statins, steroids, antacids, antidepressants, Depo-provera, thyroid replacement therapy, cancer chemotherapy drugs, bisphosphonates, estrogen
- OTC medications or supplements (dose/frequency), including NSAIDs, acetaminophen, glucosamine, calcium, vitamin D
- Cortisone injections

Pediatric Considerations

- Birth history:
  - Delivery eventful or uneventful, vaginal or C-section, prolonged or abrupt? Any nerve or bony injuries? Any interventions required during delivery or after birth?
  - Fetal abnormalities identified during the prenatal stage?
- Growth and development history:
  - Meeting developmental milestones? Motor skills appropriate for age?
  - Suboptimal growth or poor weight gain (based on pediatric growth charts)?
- Eating and nutritional history:
  - How has the child been eating? Specifically for the infant: Is the infant breast or bottle fed? Have the child's eating patterns changed?
- Sports participation:
  - Is the injury affecting the child's ability to play and/or function at school?
  - Sports participation (what sport[s], training, frequency of participation, history of injuries)
  - History of concussions? Broken bones?

FAMILY HISTORY

- Congenital diseases (including myopathies)
- Autoimmune disease (including rheumatoid arthritis)
- Gout
- Paget's disease of the bone

- Osteogenesis imperfecta
- Osteopenia/osteoporosis
- Muscular dystrophy

SOCIAL HISTORY

- Level of physical activity; typical exercise routines, including type of activity, frequency, warm-up/cool down routines, stretching programs, recent changes, increases or decreases and reasoning for this change; sports participation (e.g., type, frequency of training, cross-training)
- **Occupation:** How much movement during a typical workday and any repetitive motions that could put the patient at risk
- **ADL:** Is the patient able to dress themselves independently, brush their hair, put on their own socks? Are they strong enough to walk stairs, carry loads, and reach overhead?
- Smoking status
- Alcohol consumption
- Diet, looking for possible nutritional deficiencies

REVIEW OF SYSTEMS

- **General**: Fever, weight loss, weight gain, fatigue, malaise
- **HEENT**: Conjunctivitis, vision changes
- **CV**: Chest pain
- **Respiratory**: Shortness of breath
- **GI/GU**: Dysuria, vaginal/penile discharge, erectile dysfunction
- **Neurologic**: Weakness, numbness, loss of sensation, balance concerns, cranial nerve deficits
- **MSK**: Recent falls, decreased ROM, dropping things, decreased grip strength, changes in handwriting or fine motor movements, difficulty with completing ADL, multiple or diffuse joint pain, early morning stiffness, past injury or medical evaluation to affected area
- **Hematologic**: Anemia, bone pain
- **Skin**: Color, rash, erythema

PHYSICAL EXAMINATION

Completing the physical exam of the MSK system includes having an appreciation for the techniques of the exam: (a) inspection; (b) palpation, which includes noting muscle strength; (c) assessment of ROM; and (d) use of special tests, as well as understanding of how these techniques are used to assess the integrity of the MSK system.

GENERAL SURVEY

- **Vital signs:** Temperature, pulse rate, respiratory rate, blood pressure
- Posture and position
- Gross deformities

INSPECTION

- Observe the patient throughout the exam. Observe their gait as they walk through the office, their posture, and their ability to do things like remove their shirt. Note whether they are able to get out of a chair using only their legs, or do they need their arms? If they need their arms, do they favor one arm versus the other?
- Observing their handwriting and asking about changes in handwriting can be an early clue to a number of MSK or neurologic disorders.
- Identify any deformity, asymmetry, hypertrophy, or atrophy along with any skin changes including bleeding, bruising, swelling, and previous scars.
- Observe the anterior, posterior, lateral, and medial aspects of the joint and compare the affected joint to the joint on the opposite side of the body for symmetry.

PALPATION

- The palpation portion of the exam should include ROM and strength testing, followed by joint-specific special tests. The exam may or may not need an evaluation of deep tendon reflexes.
- After completing this portion of the exam, imaging and interventions should be considered based on current, evidence-based guidelines.

MUSCLE STRENGTH

- See Chapter 10, "Evidence-Based Assessment of Nervous System," for information on completing this exam.
- See **Table 11.1** for the muscle strength scale.

RANGE OF MOTION AND SPECIAL TESTS

- *ROM* is the full movement potential of a joint; it should be completed during every MSK visit.
- Most joints will have a contralateral joint in which to compare motion and angles.
- See **Box 11.1** for a definition of different types of movements.

TABLE 11.1 Muscle Strength Scale

Grade	Level of Function
0	No movement
1	Trace movement
2	Full passive range of motion
3	Full range of motion against gravity, no resistance
4	Full range of motion with resistance, though weak
5	Full range of motion, full strength

BOX 11.1
TYPES OF MOVEMENTS

Flexion: Any joint movement that decreases the angle between two bones; bending

Extension: Any joint movement that increases the angle and straightens the joint; opposite of flexion

Rotation: Can occur within the vertebral column, at a pivot joint, or at a ball-and-socket joint

Abduction: Moving the limb or hand laterally away from the body, or spreading the fingers or toes

Adduction: Moving the limb or hand toward or across the midline of the body, or bringing the fingers or toes together

Inversion: Turning of the foot to angle the bottom of the foot toward the midline

Eversion: Turning the bottom of the foot away from the midline

Supination: Rotation of the radius that returns the bones to their parallel positions and moves the palm to the anterior-facing (supinated) position

Pronation: The body movement that moves the forearm from the supinated (anatomical) position to the pronated (palm backward) position

Circumduction: Moving of the limb, hand, or fingers in a circular pattern, using the sequential combination of flexion, adduction, extension, and abduction motions; movement of a body region in a circular manner

Source: Betts, J. G., Young, K. A., Wise, J. A., Johnson, E., Poe, B., Kruse, D. H., Korol, O., Johnson, J. E., Womble, M., & DeSaix, P. (Eds.). (2013). *Anatomy and physiology.* OpenStax. http://cnx.org/contents/14fb4ad7-39a1-4eee-ab6e-3ef2482e3e22@8.24

Head

- Have the patient open and close their mouth, move their jaw from side to side, and protract/ retract their jaw. Palpate the TMJ during these movements; inquire about tenderness. With the patient's mouth open, place fingers below the zygomatic bone, anterior to the condyle. When the patient closes their mouth, the tip of the finger should be placed anterior to the tragus. Feel for any clicking, popping, or catching.
- When the patient is opening and closing the mouth, movement should be smooth and the mandible should not have left- or right-sided deviation. When opened, there should be enough room for three fingers between the incisors.
- The jaw jerk reflex can be used to evaluate for pathology along the fifth cranial nerve. Allow the patient's mouth to relax in a slightly open position; place a finger over the mentum of the face and tap it with a reflex hammer. A normal response is to see the mouth briefly close; an abnormal response is an exaggerated closing or repeated closing (clonus). This could indicate an upper motor neuron lesion.

Cervical Spine

- When inspecting, look for deformities or asymmetries. Note the patient's posture; inspect for increased or decreased cervical lordosis or excessive thoracic kyphosis. Note their head position and whether they hold their head to one side or the other.
- Watch their movements. Do they have fluid, coordinated movements? Or do they appear stiff, slow, or uncontrolled?
- Palpate each spinal process. The spine has several landmarks that can assist in palpation, including the mastoid process, individual spinous processes (C7 is usually the most prominent), and facet joints, which lie approximately one-inch lateral to each spinous process (**Figure 11.1**). These joints are not always palpable. Tenderness over the midline of

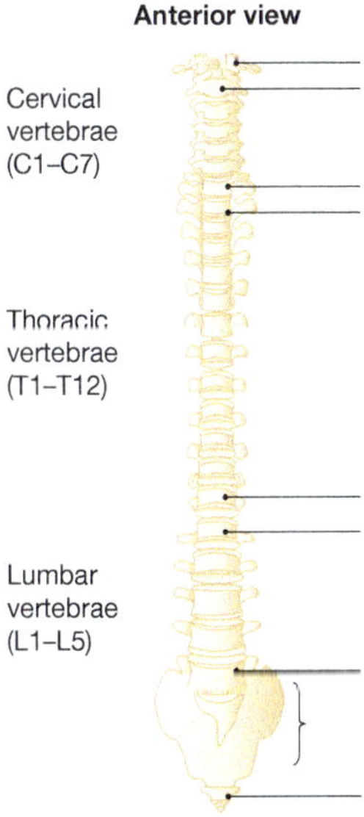

FIGURE 11.1 Spinal column.

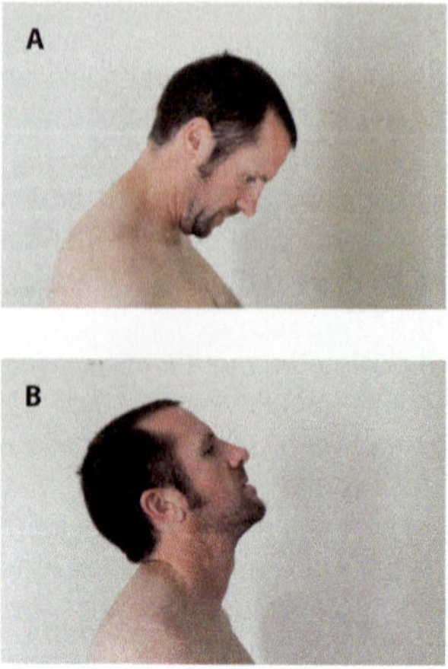

FIGURE 11.2 Range of motion of the cervical spine: (**A**) cervical flexion and (**B**) cervical extension.

the cervical spine when palpating the spinal processes could be indicative of a spinous process fracture.

- Palpate the soft tissue, including the paraspinal musculature, sternocleidomastoid muscle, and trapezius muscle.
- Do not test cervical ROM if unstable spine injury is suspected. Cervical ROM should include flexion, extension, lateral rotation to the left and right, and lateral bending to the left and right. The majority of flexion/extension occurs between the occiput and C1, with the majority of rotation occurring between C1 and C2.
- Cervical spine ROM normal values: flexion, 45 degrees; extension, 55 degrees; lateral rotation, 70 degrees; lateral bending, 40 degrees
- A proper cervical spine exam includes dermatome and myotome exams of the upper extremities, along with reflex testing of the biceps (C5), brachioradialis (C6), and triceps (C7; see **Figure 11.2** and **Table 11.2**).

TABLE 11.2 Dermatomes and Myotomes of the Upper Extremity

Nerve	Dermatome	Myotome	Associated Reflex
C5	Lateral upper arm	Deltoid	Biceps
C6	Radial side of forearm to thumb and index finger	Biceps, wrist extensors	Brachioradialis
C7	Middle finger	Triceps, wrist flexors, finger extensors	Triceps
C8	Ulnar forearm to fourth and fifth digits	Finger flexors and interossei muscles	None
T1	Ulnar side of elbow	Interossei muscles	None

Special Tests of the Cervical Spine

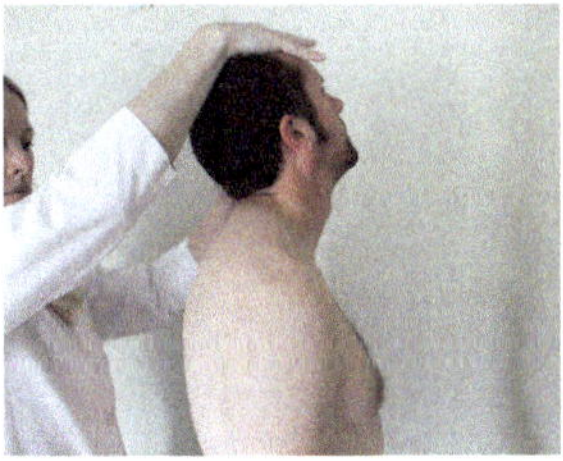

FIGURE 11.3 Spurling test.

- **Spurling test**: Identifies whethera nerve root is being compressed due to intervertebral disc pathology. Passively extend and rotate the patient's neck to the affected side. Slowly start applying axial pressure by pressing down on the top of the patient's head (**Figure 11.3**). Radicular pain extending down the arm on the same side as the test is considered a positive test. Be sure to rule out cervical instability, vertebral artery injury, and vertebral fracture before performing. It should not be performed in an acute trauma setting.
- **Extension–rotation test**: Used to eliminate facet joint etiology. Start by moving the patient into cervical extension, then laterally flex and rotate to the same side. Repeat with the contralateral side. Test is considered positive if the maneuver increases pain or causes numbness/tingling on the side of the neck being tested.

Thoracic/Lumbar Spine

- Inspect the spine, looking for increased lumbar lordosis, kyphosis, and side curvature of the spine (scoliosis).
- Spinal curvature is best examined by having the patient flex forward while observing the spinous processes, which should form a straight line. There are two natural lordoses; when viewed from the side, the spine should form a "S" shaped curve. The skin should be inspected for any abnormalities, including hairy patches, café-au-lait spots, or doughy lipomata. These findings could be indicative of underlying neurological pathology.
- Observe the iliac crests, gluteal folds, PSIS, and the ASIS while the patient is standing. Note any differences in height between the left and right sides.
- While the patient is supine, measure from the ASIS to the medial malleolus to check for true leg length discrepancies. Compare to apparent leg length discrepancies as measured from the umbilicus to the medial malleolus to evaluate for possible pelvic obliquity.

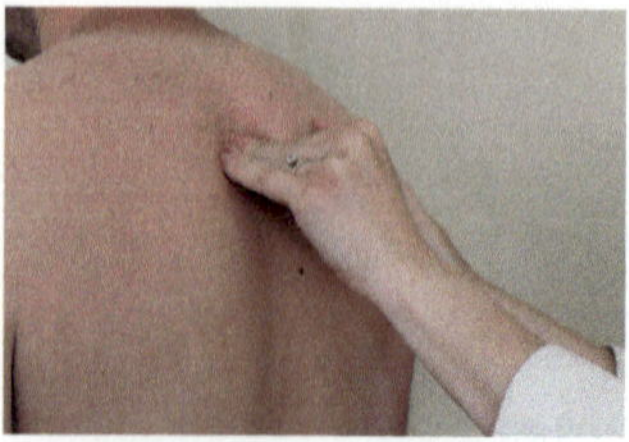

FIGURE 11.4 Palpation of spinal processes.

- Palpation of the lumbar and thoracic spines (**Figure 11.4**) should include patient spinous processes, iliac crests (approximately at L4 to L5 interspace), bilateral ASIS, greater trochanters, ischial tuberosities, and bilateral PSIS. The umbilicus often lies near the L3 to L4 interspace. Look for any step-off deformities. The transition from one spinous process to the neighboring ones should be smooth, with a slight divot between each.
- Normal values for the lumbar spine ROM are noted in **Figure 11.5**.

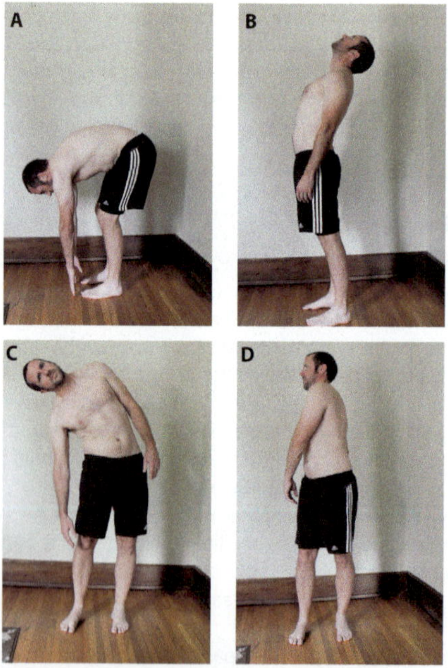

FIGURE 11.5 Range of motion of the spinal column. (**A**) Flexion: 40–60 degrees. (**B**) Extension: 20–35 degrees. (**C**) Lateral bending: 15–20 degrees. (**D**) Lateral rotation: 5–20 degrees.

TABLE 11.3 Dermatomes and Myotomes of the Lower Extremity

Nerve	Dermatome	Myotome	Associated Reflex
L4	Medial leg and medial foot	Anterior tibialis	Patella tendon
L5	Lateral leg and dorsum of foot	Extensor hallucis longus	None
S1	Lateral foot	Peroneus longus and brevis	Achilles tendon

- **Table 11.3** includes a listing of dermatomes originating from the spine that affect the lower extremities.

Special Tests of the Lumbar Spine

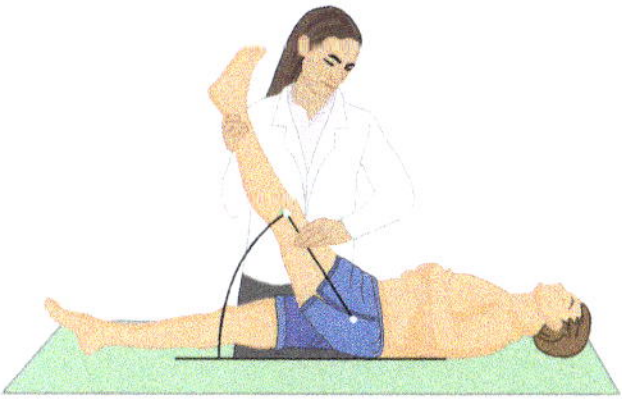

FIGURE 11.6 Straight leg raise.

- **Straight leg raise**: Identifies lumbar radiculopathy. Have the patient lie supine. Have patient lift one leg at a time to 90 degrees or as far as the patient can tolerate (**Figure 11.6**). Place your other hand on the knee to ensure full knee extension. Test is considered positive if there is pain between 30 and 70 degrees of hip flexion that radiates below the knee. To further confirm neurologic etiology, slightly lower the leg and dorsiflex the foot, which will also reproduce the radicular symptoms.
- **Valsalva maneuver**: Identifies whether pain is coming from the spinal canal. With the patient sitting, have them take a deep breath and bear down as if trying to have a bowel movement. Localized or radicular pain is considered a positive test.

Upper Extremities

Shoulder

- When inspecting the shoulder, evaluate the patient's arm swing. Does it appear equal or does the motion seem limited in one side? Movements should be smooth and coordinated. Use the contralateral side for comparison, not just during inspection but also when testing ROM, strength, and special tests.

- Look for any muscle atrophy (indicative of a nerve palsy or extreme deconditioning), deformity (fracture or dislocation), winging scapula, Popeye deformity, discoloration, or scars.
- Palpate the following bony landmarks (**Figure 11.7**): scapula (including the coracoid process, acromion process, spine of scapula, superior and inferior angles of the scapula, medial/lateral borders of the scapula); clavicle (including sternal end, acromial end, entire shaft); and humerus (including the deltoid tuberosity, the greater tuberosity [lateral], the bicipital groove, and the lesser tuberosity [medial]).
- Palpate the sternoclavicular joint, AC joint, sternoclavicular ligament, and the AC ligament.
- Palpate the following areas of soft tissue: insertion point of the rotator cuff muscles at greater tuberosity; axilla borders; serratus anterior muscles; pectoralis major muscles; upper, middle, and lower trapezius; deltoid (anterior, middle posterior bellies); sternocleidomastoid; biceps insertion and belly; and latissimus dorsi muscles.
- When palpating musculature, feel for tenderness and tone; compare muscles to contralateral side.
- **Apley's scratch test**: Ask patient to abduct and externally rotate their arms, then reach behind their back and touch the contralateral scapula. Have the patient abduct and internally rotate their

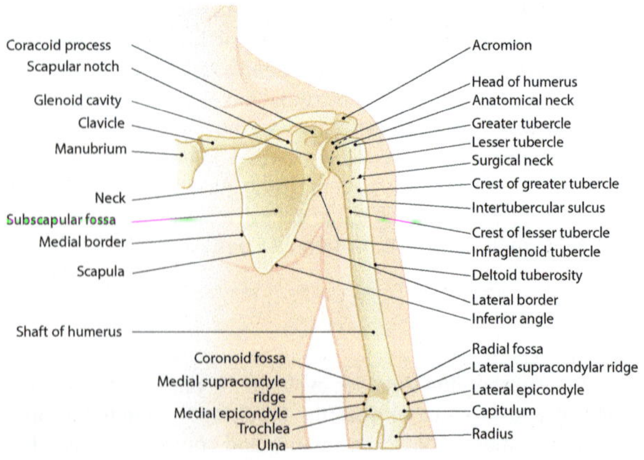

FIGURE 11.7 Bones of the shoulder.

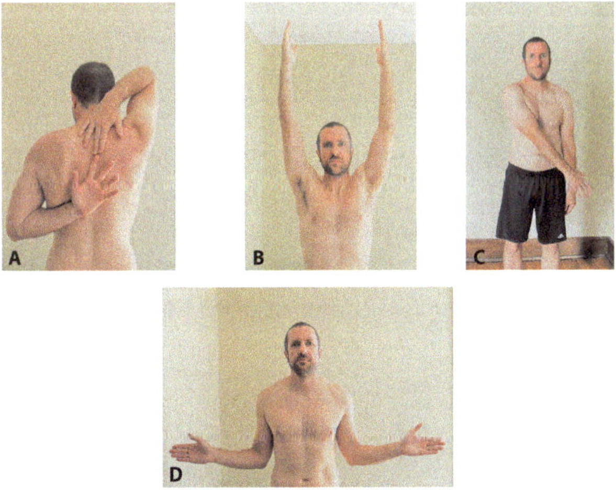

FIGURE 11.8 Shoulder range of motion. (**A**) Apley's scratch test. (**B**) Abduction: 180 degrees. (**C**) Adduction: 45 degrees. (**D**) External rotation: 90 degrees.

arm, then ask the patient to reach behind their back as if tucking in their shirt, and reach as far up their back as possible. Compare ROM bilaterally.

- To test active horizontal adduction, have the patient abduct their arms to 90 degrees, flex the elbow to 90 degrees, then reach across the front of their body and touch the contralateral AC joint.
- To test for full abduction ROM, have the patient externally rotate their arm to allow the humeral head to clear under the acromion.
- Passive ROM normal values are noted in **Figure 11.8**.
- Test all nine shoulder movements and compare bilaterally.

Special Tests of the Shoulder

- Shoulder tests should be completed in clusters, in contrast to completing a single test, to improve the reliability of results.
- **Hawkins–Kennedy test**: Helps to identify shoulder impingement, particularly of the supraspinatus. While holding the patient's elbow at 90 degrees with one hand, and their wrist with the other hand, flex the shoulder to 90 degrees, then internally rotate (**Figure 11.9**). Pain and apprehension are considered positive tests.
- **Neer Test**: Identifies supraspinatus impingement. While stabilizing the patient's scapula, passively forward flex the arm while the

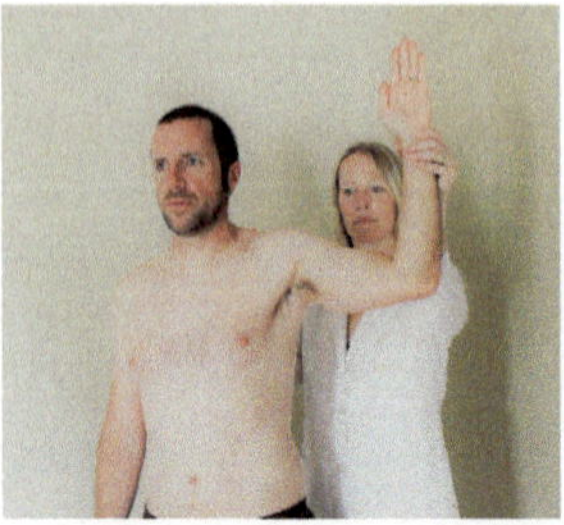

FIGURE 11.9 Hawkins–Kennedy test.

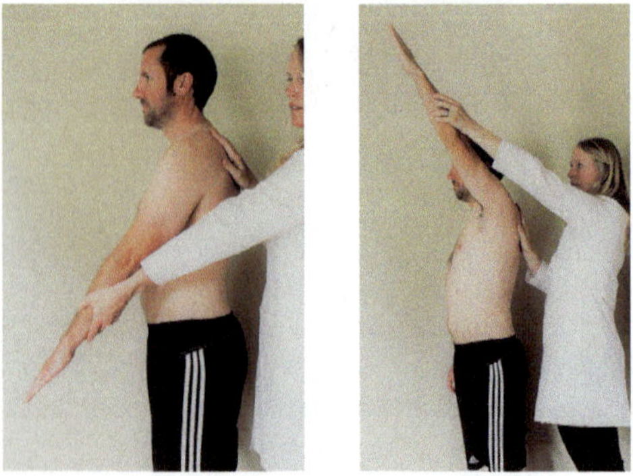

FIGURE 11.10 Neer test.

arm is in the pronated position (**Figure 11.10**). Pain and apprehension are considered positive tests.

- **Empty can test**: Identifies supraspinatus weakness, due to a tear, impingement, or a nerve injury. Have the patient abduct both of their arms to 90 degrees in the scapular plane (~30 deqrees of horizontal adduction; **Figure 11.11**). Next have them internally rotate the shoulder so their thumbs are pointing to the ground; ask the patient to try to actively resist adduction. A positive test is an inability to hold the arm in the testing position.
- **Painful arc test**: Ask the patient to forward flex the arm in 30 degrees of horizontal adduction. Ask them to slowly move their arms overhead to 180 degrees (**Figure 11.12**). Pain in the 60 to 120 degrees of flexion range is considered positive. Pain will often be worse with internal rotation and somewhat relieved with external rotation. A positive test indicates subacromial impingement.

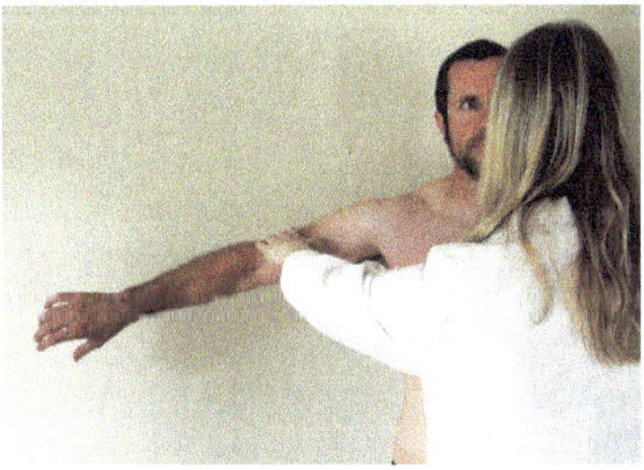

FIGURE 11.11 Empty can test.

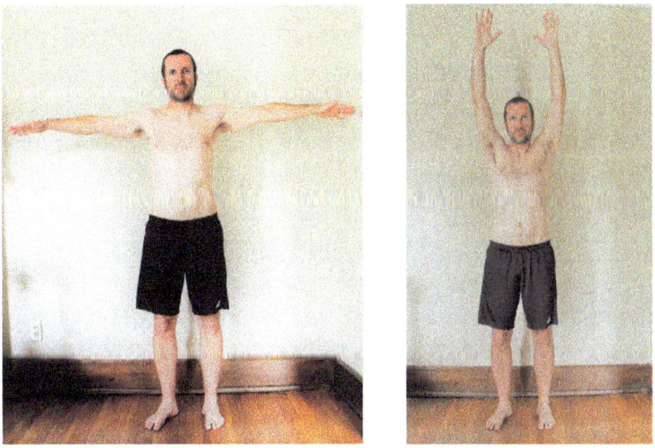

FIGURE 11.12 Painful arc test.

- **External rotation resistance test**: Identifies rotator cuff pathology, particularly of the infraspinatus and teres minor. While standing in front of the patient, have them flex their elbow to 90 degrees, then have them try to externally rotate the shoulder while providing resistance (**Figure 11.13**). Pain or weakness is considered a positive result. Repeat with arm abducted to 90 degrees.
- **Lag test**: Identifies rotator cuff pathology. With patient seated, have them flex their elbow to 90 degrees, then abduct to 90 degrees. Move them 5 degrees shy of full external rotation; ask them to hold the position. Inability to hold the position when support is removed is considered a positive test.

Elbow

- Examine the elbow in both flexion and extension. Identify the carrying angle with the elbow in extension. A normal carrying angle is considered to be between 5 and 15 degrees valgus.

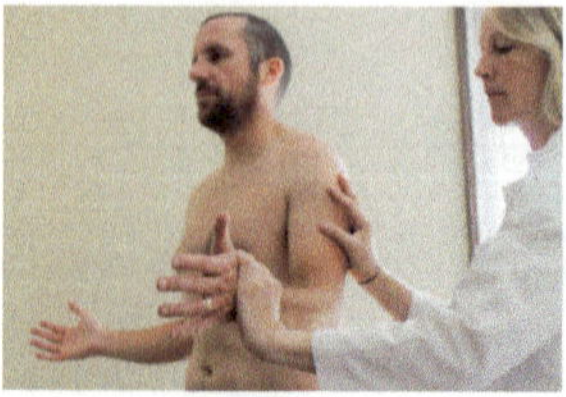

FIGURE 11.13 External rotation resistance test.

An increase in the angle is known as *cubitus valgus*. Cubitus varus is a decrease in that angle, also known as *gunstock deformity*; in children, this can be a sign of a fracture affecting the rotation of the distal end of the humerus. Also, look for edema at the tip of the elbow, over the olecranon fossa, as olecranon bursitis is a common complication of falling onto the tip of the elbow.

- Palpate the following bony landmarks: Medial and lateral epicondyles, origins for the wrist flexors and extensor bundles, medial and lateral supracondylar lines of the humerus, olecranon, olecranon fossa, ulnar border, and radial head (which is palpated an inch distal to the lateral epicondyle during pronation and supination).
- Palpate the medial side of the elbow, feeling for the origin of the flexor bundle (pronator teres, flexor carpi radialis, palmaris longus, and flexor carpi ulnaris) and the ulnar nerve. Palpate for any tenderness over the ulnar collateral ligament. On the lateral side, palpate the extensor bundle (brachioradialis, extensor carpi radialis longus, and the extensor carpi radialis brevis) and feel for any tenderness over the radial collateral and the annular ligaments. The hand should be moved anteriorly to find the insertion of the biceps tendon and the brachial artery, which lies just medial to the biceps insertion point. The median nerve is found medial to the brachial artery.
- Passive ROM normal values are noted in **Figure 11.14**.

Special Tests of the Elbow

- **Cozen test**: Identify lateral epicondylitis (tennis elbow). With elbow stabilized and hand pronated and in a fist, have the patient extend their wrist against resistance. Pain over the lateral epicondyle is considered a positive test.
- **Golfer elbow test**: Identifies medial epicondylitis (golfer's elbow). With elbow stabilized, have patient supinate their hand and close their fist. Next, have the patient flex their wrist against resistance. Pain over the medial epicondyle is considered a positive test.
- **Varus stress test**: Identifies injury to the radial (lateral) collateral ligament of the elbow. With wrist stabilized, apply a varus force to the medial side of the elbow while it is flexed to 20 or 30 degrees. Pain or excess motion compared to the contralateral side is considered a positive test.

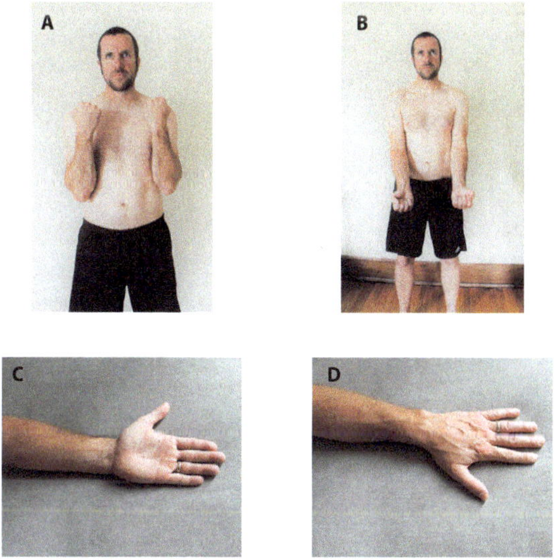

FIGURE 11.14 Elbow range of motion. (**A**) Flexion: 135 degrees. (**B**) Extension: 0–5 degrees hyperextension. (**C**) Supination: 90 degrees. (**D**) Pronation: 90 degrees.

- **Valgus stress test**: Identifies injury to the ulnar (medial) collateral ligament of the elbow. With the elbow flexed to 20 or 30 degrees and wrist stabilized, apply valgus force to the lateral elbow. Pain or excess motion compared to the contralateral side is considered a positive test.
- **Tinel's sign**: Identifies compression of the ulnar nerve. With elbow relaxed and wrist supported, tap the ulnar nerve as it courses through the ulnar notch (**Figure 11.15**). Tingling or pain along the ulnar distribution is considered a positive test.

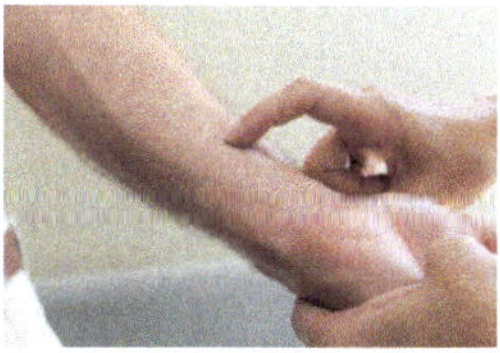

FIGURE 11.15 Tinel's sign.

Wrist/Hand

- Inspect the wrist and hand (**Figure 11.16**). Ensure all five fingers are present; missing digits or parts of digits are not always noticeable at first glance. Observe the creases on the hands.

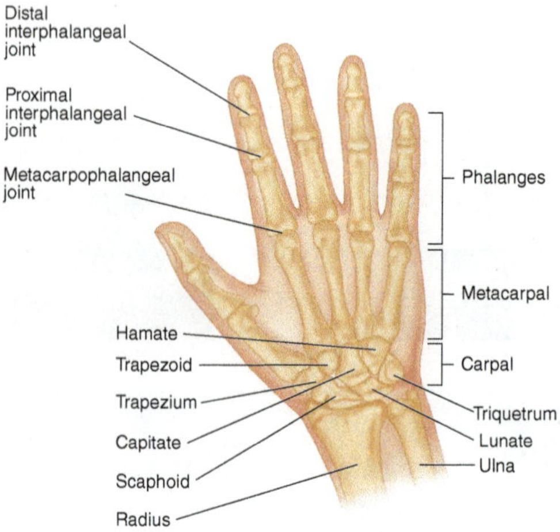

FIGURE 11.16 Bones of the hand and wrist.

Note the thenar eminence, thick muscle belly at the base of the thumb, and hypothenar eminence, at the base of the little finger.

- Inspection of the fingers and nails is essential for a thorough exam. With the fingers extended, look for rotation or crossing over of the fingers. This could be a sign of a phalange or metacarpal fracture. With a closed fist, fingers should lay next to each other and not cross one another.
- Palpate the styloid processes of both the radius and the ulna. Move to the anatomical snuffbox, the depression on the radial side of the wrist bordered by the abductor pollicis longus and the extensor pollicis brevis tendons (**Figure 11.17**). Tenderness is a sign of a possible scaphoid fracture. Feel for fullness and good muscle tone in the thenar and hypothenar eminences.
- Palpate the entire length of each metacarpal, feeling for any tenderness or deformity. Finish the bony palpation at the fingers with each phalange and interphalangeal joint.
- Passive ROM normal values: Wrist extension, 70 degrees; wrist flexion, 80 degrees; radial deviation, 20 degrees; ulnar deviation, 30 degrees; MCP flexion, 80 to 90 degrees; MCL extension, 30 to 45 degrees; PIP flexion, 100 degrees; PIP extension, 0 degrees; DIP flexion, 90 degrees; DIP extension, 20 degrees; finger abduction, 20 degrees; finger adduction, 0 degrees; thumb MCP flexion, 50 degrees; thumb MCP extension, 20 degrees; thumb abduction, 70 degrees; thumb adduction, 0 degrees.

Special Tests for the Wrist and Hand

- **Finkelstein test**: Identifies tenosynovitis of the abductor pollicis longus and extensor pollicis brevis tendons, also known as *De Quervian's syndrome*. With the forearm stabilized, have the patient grasp their thumb in their fist then perform ulnar deviation of the hand (**Figure 11.18**). Pain over the tendons is considered a positive test. Be sure to slowly deviate the hand, as this test, when positive, can be exquisitely painful.
- **Phalen test**: Identifies median nerve pathology, particularly carpal tunnel syndrome. Have the patient sit with the dorsum of their hands touching, in maximal wrist flexion, applying force through the wrists for 1 minute (**Figure 11.19**). Numbness or tingling in the median nerve distribution is considered a positive test.
- **Varus/valgus test**: As with the elbow, the collateral ligaments in the fingers can be tested with a varus or valgus force applied while the joint is relaxed and supported. Pain or excess motion compared to the contralateral side is considered a positive test. This test is particularly useful at the MCP joint of the thumb to identify skier's thumb, or a tear of the ulnar collateral ligament at the base of the thumb with increased motion or pain with a valgus force.

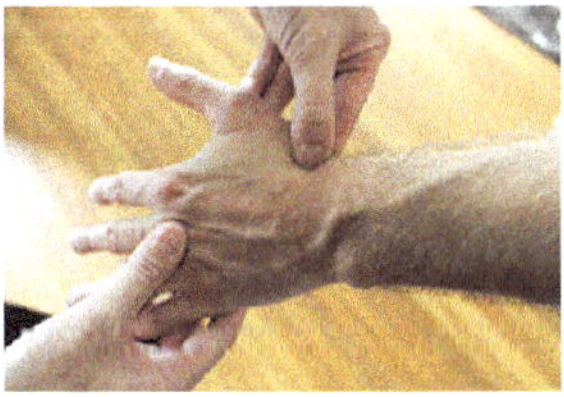

FIGURE 11.17 Area of snuffbox tenderness.

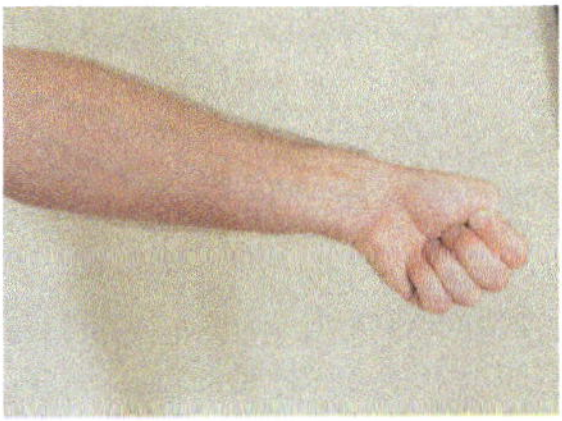

FIGURE 11.18 Finkelstein test.

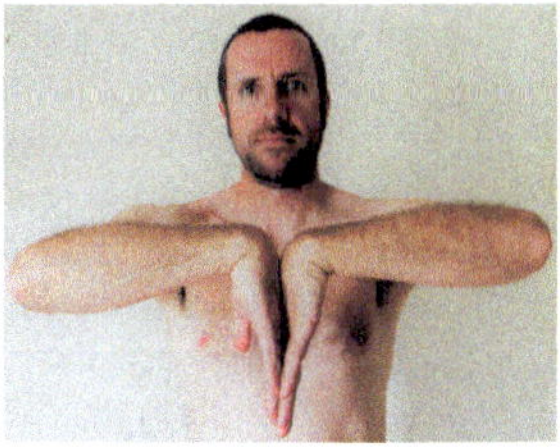

FIGURE 11.19 Phalen's test.

Lower Extremities

Hip

- Inspect the hips. Assess gait patterns. Look for altered gait patterns as these can be a clue to a variety of lower extremity conditions. A Trendelenburg gait could be a sign of weak abductors.

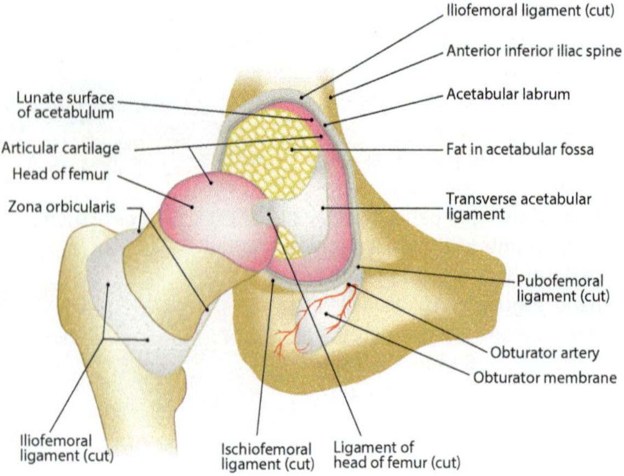

FIGURE 11.20 Hip anatomy.

Shuffling of the feet or a wide base gait can be signs of Parkinson's or cerebellar disease.

- Inspect the bony landmarks, including the levels of the iliac crests, PSIS, ASIS, gluteal folds, and medial malleoli to determine the symmetry of the lower limbs, leg length, or possible pelvic obliquity (**Figure 11.20**). Note the bony landmarks while the patient is standing and laying supine.
- A measurement from the ASIS to the medial malleolus is considered a true leg-length measurement and should be done bilaterally for comparison. A measurement from the umbilicus to the medial malleolus is considered an apparent leg length measurement and can be compared to the true leg length measurement to help identify possible soft tissue adaptations that can result in apparent leg length differences even when true ones do not exist.
- Palpate the hip. True hip joint pathology typically presents as pain and tenderness in the groin. Pain on the lateral hip, over the greater trochanter, is more commonly a trochanteric bursitis or abductor tendinitis, possibly related to a tight IT band or gluteal musculature.
- Palpate the ischial tuberosities deep in the gluteal folds as this is the origin of the hamstrings and a common area of injury.
- Passive ROM normal values are noted in **Figure 11.21**.

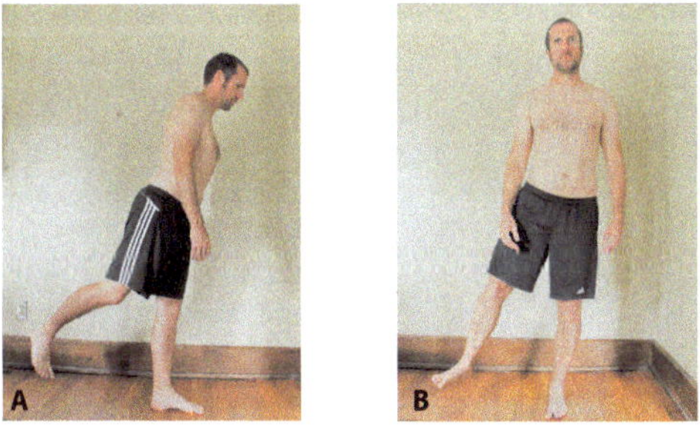

FIGURE 11.21 Hip range of motion. (**A**) Extension: 20–30 degrees. (**B**) Abduction: 40 degrees.

Special Tests for the Hip

- **Thomas test**: Identifies hip flexor contracture and tightness. With the patient supine, have them bring one knee to their chest. When completing this maneuver, it is imperative for the clinician to control for lumbopelvic movement (i.e., pelvic tilt). Passive flexion in the contralateral leg is considered a positive test on the contralateral side.
- **FABER test**: Identifies hip flexor, sacroiliac, or hip intra-articular pathology. FABER stands for **F**lexion, **AB**duction, and **E**xternal **R**otation. With the patient supine, have them flex, abduct, and externally rotate the hip until the ankle rests upon the contralateral knee. Apply downward pressure, moving the knee closer to the table (**Figure 11.22**). Pain or decreased ROM is considered a positive test.
- **Log roll**: Identifies intra-articular pathology, particularly symptomatic arthritis. With the patient supine, hold the ankle or knee and passively internally and externally rotate the leg. Pain in the groin is considered a positive test.
- **Stinchfield test**: Identifies intra-articular hip pathology. With the patient supine, have them flex the hip to 30 or 45 degrees. Apply a downward pressure on the ankle with the patient resisting. Pain in the groin is considered a positive test.
- **Trendelenburg test**: Identifies weakness of the abductor musculature. Have the patient stand on one leg for 10 seconds, then switch legs (**Figure 11.23**). Weakness of the gluteus medius on the

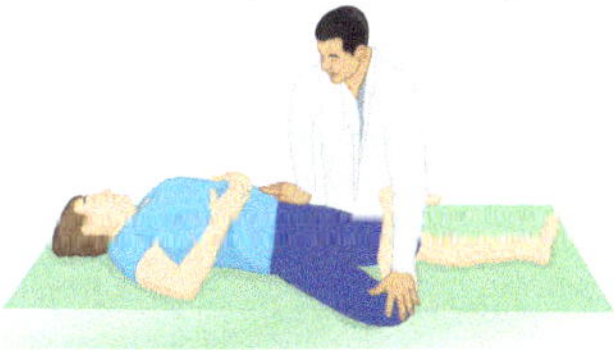

FIGURE 11.22 Flexion, abduction, and external rotation test.

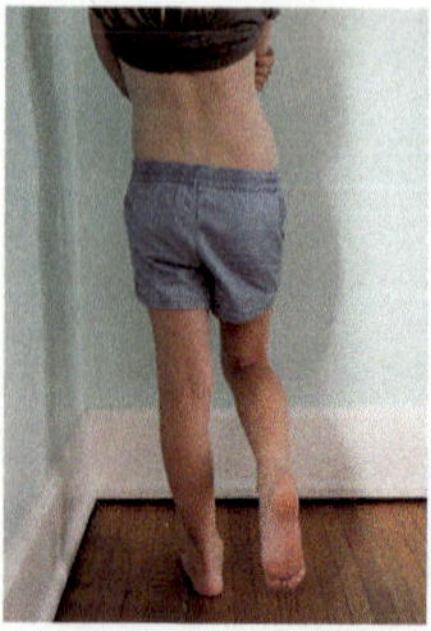

FIGURE 11.23 Negative Trendelenburg test. No dip of the pelvis noted on the unsupported side.

standing side will lead to a dip of the pelvis on the unsupported side—a positive test.

Knee

- Inspect the knee. Look for any deformity, asymmetry, and/or edema. Look for genu valgus (knock knee) and genu varus (bow legged). A prominent tibial tuberosity can be a sign of Osgood–Schlatter's disease, which is common in adolescence.
- Palpate the knee (**Figure 11.24**). On the lateral side of the knee, palpate the fibular head, lateral joint line, lateral femoral condyle, IT band and insertion on Gerdy's tubercle, biceps femoris insertion, and lateral collateral ligament. On the medial side, palpate the medial joint line, MCL origin and insertion, pes anserine, and muscle bellies of the semitendinosus and semimembranosis. Feel

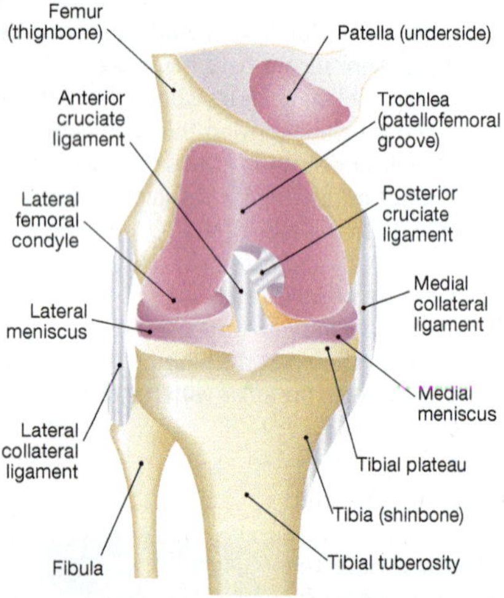

FIGURE 11.24 Knee anatomy. Frontal view of right knee (with patella reflected).

anteriorly for the patella and its borders, the tibial tuberosity, and patellar and quadriceps tendons. On the posterior side, feel in the popliteal fossa for a possible fluid collection (a Baker's cyst), a sign of a meniscus tear, which may refer pain to the popliteal fossa.

- Passive ROM normal values: Flexion, 130 to 140 degrees; extension: 0 to 5 degrees hyperextension.

Special Tests for the Knee

- **Valgus stress test** (**Figure 11.25**): Identifies injury to medial collateral ligament. With patient supine and relaxed, hold the ankle and apply valgus stress to the lateral knee. Test in full extension and 20 to 30 degrees of knee flexion. Pain/excessive laxity is considered a positive test.
- **Varus stress test** (**Figure 11.26**): Identifies injury to the lateral collateral ligament. With patient supine and relaxed, hold the ankle and apply varus stress to the medial knee. Test in full extension and 20 to 30 degrees of knee flexion. Pain/excessive laxity is considered a positive test.
- **Anterior drawer test** (**Figure 11.27A**): Identifies injury to the ACL. With patient supine, have them flex their hip to 45 degrees and flex knee to 90 degrees, resting their foot on the table. The clinician should sit on the patient's foot to stabilize the leg and place their hands behind the proximal tibia, resting their thumbs on the tibial tuberosity. Use the index fingers to ensure relaxation of the hamstring muscles. Apply an anterior force. Increased anterior translation is indicative of an ACL tear.
- **Posterior drawer test** (**Figure 11.27B**): Identifies injury to PCL. With patient supine, have them flex their hip to 45 degrees and flex the knee to 90 degrees, resting their foot on the table. Sit on the patient's foot to stabilize the leg. Hands should be placed behind the proximal tibia, resting the thumbs on the tibial tuberosity. Use the index fingers to ensure relaxation of the hamstring muscles. Apply a posterior force.

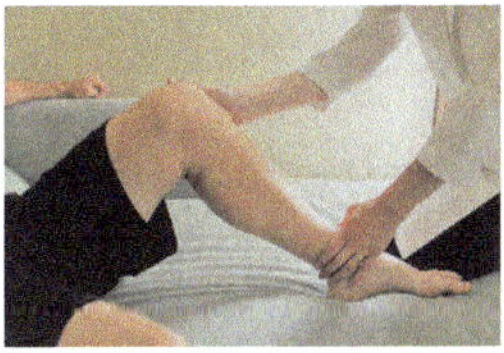

FIGURE 11.25 Valgus stress test.

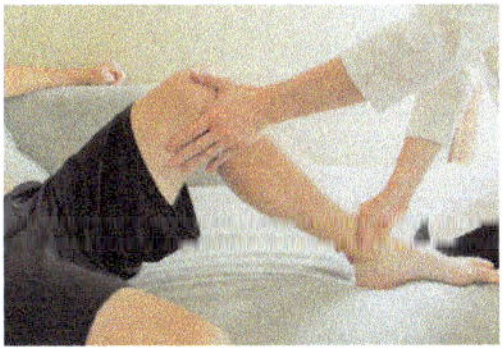

FIGURE 11.26 Varus stress test.

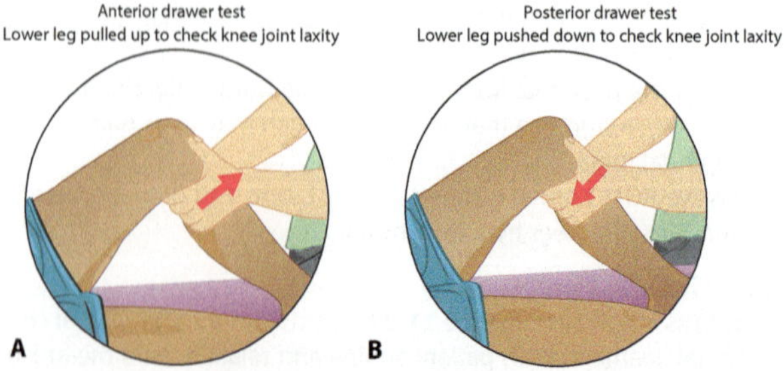

FIGURE 11.27 Drawer tests. (**A**) Anterior. (**B**) Posterior.

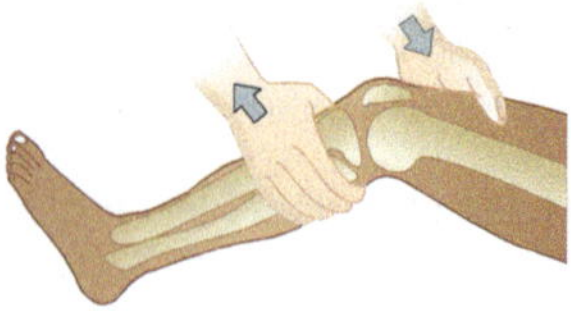

FIGURE 11.28 Lachman test.

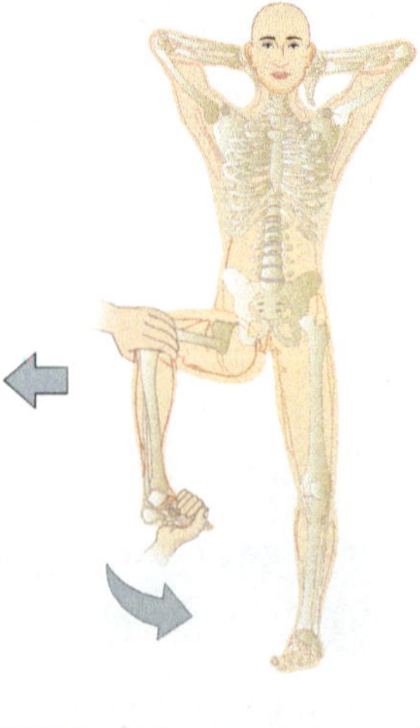

FIGURE 11.29 McMurray's test.

Increased posterior translation in indicative of a PCL tear.

- **Lachman test** (**Figure 11.28**): Identifies a tear to the ACL. With patient supine and relaxed, place outside or proximal hand over the distal thigh and inside hand (distal hand) over the proximal tibia. Allowing the hip to externally rotate can help ensure the patient is relaxed. Apply anterior translation force on the tibia with the distal hand while stabilizing the thigh with the proximal hand. Excessive anterior tibial translation is indicative of an ACL tear. This test can be challenging if the patient is guarding.
- **McMurray's test** (**Figure 11.29**): Identifies meniscus pathology. With patient supine, use one hand to grasp patient's ankle, the other hand to stabilize patient's knee. With the knee flexed, externally rotate the tibia and apply a valgus force while extending the knee.

Move the knee from flexion while internally rotating the tibia and applying varus force. Pain or clicking over the medial or lateral joint lines is considered a positive test.

- **Apprehension test** (**Figure 11.30**): Identifies patellar laxity or subluxations/dislocations. With patient supine and relaxed, place the knee in full extension. Apply a lateral force to the medial border of the patella. Pain or guarding is considered a positive test.
- **Ballottement test**: Identifies joint effusion in the knee, which is most commonly caused by trauma to the knee. Patient should lie in the supine position with legs extended. Clinician should place one hand superior to the patella and use the other hand to apply downward pressure in an anterior to posterior "milking" motion. If there is fluid, the clinician will feel it against their lower hand. Gently push down on the patella. If it can be depressed, it means that it was "floating" in fluid and signifies a positive test.

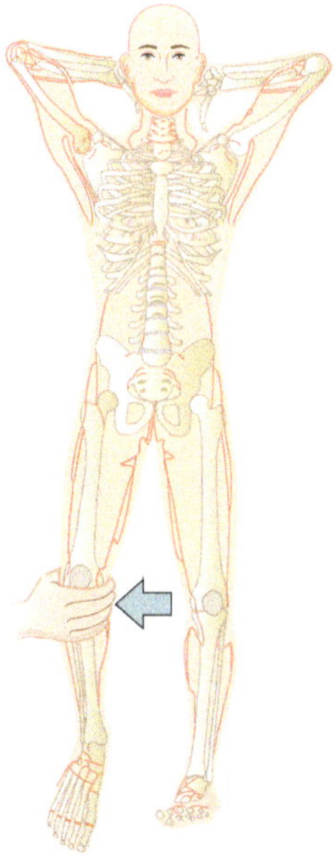

FIGURE 11.30 Apprehension test.

- **Bulge sign**: Commonly used to test for knee effusion. Gently press slightly medial to the patella, then move the hand in an ascending motion and apply pressure firmly on the lateral aspect of the knee. A positive test is a "bulge" seen on the medial aspect of the knee after lateral pressure was applied, which indicates that a moderate amount of fluid is present. A medial aspect that does not bulge but tensely reflects lateral pressure is consistent with a large amount of fluid.

Ankle/Foot

- Inspect the patient's footwear. Shoes can provide information on wear patterns and show where a person is putting pressure on their feet throughout their gait cycle, which provides information about possible foot deformities or gait patterns.

- Observe the foot and ankle of the patient both in standing and sitting positions. Look for deformities and asymmetries as with any other joint, as well as any areas of calluses or corn formations. Calluses can indicate abnormal weightbearing or improperly fitting shoes. The skin should be the thickest around the heel, at the lateral border, and over the metatarsal heads.
- Look at the arches in the patient's feet. The arches should be more pronounced when the patient is not bearing weight. Observe the metatarsals (**Figure 11.31**). Note toe deformities, including claw toes, hammertoes, and mallet toes, on inspection.
- Palpate the medial side of the ankle and foot. Palpate over the medial malleolus, then down the foot to the navicular bone (most prominent bone on the medial side). Palpate the medial head of the talus, which is just proximal to the navicular bone. Move down the foot to the first metatarsal, then distally to the first phalange and the IP joint. On the lateral side, start palpation at the lateral malleolus, then move inferiorly to palpate the peroneus longus and brevis. Just distal to the lateral malleolus is the area of the anterior talofibular ligament. Palpate down the foot and feel for the styloid process of the fifth metatarsal. This is a common area of avulsion or stress fractures. Lastly, palpate the shaft of the metatarsals and phalanges, feeling for the MTP and IP joints.
- On the posterior foot, palpate the Achilles tendon and its insertion site, feeling for any crepitus or nodularity. Then move to the plantar surface and the calcaneus. Continue moving distally and palpate the metatarsal shafts and heads, feeling for any tenderness.

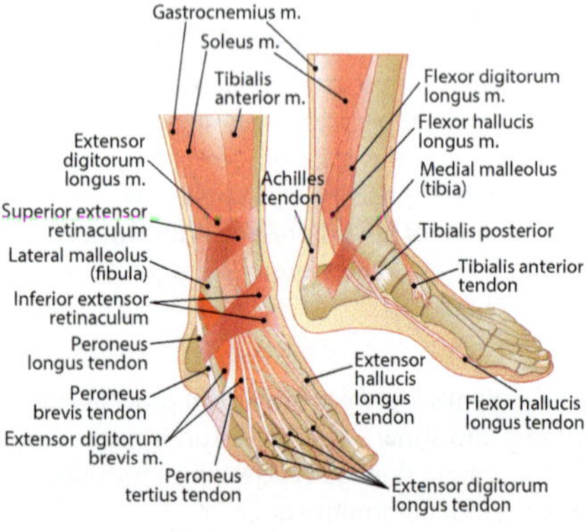

FIGURE 11.31 Foot and ankle anatomy.

- Palpating for pedal pulses. The posterior tibial artery can be palpated just posterior to the medial malleolus and the dorsalis pedis artery can be palpated between the extensor hallucis longus and the extensor digitorum longus tendons. Absent or diminished pedal pulses can indicate PVD, compartment syndrome, or other pathology.
- Passive ROM normal values: Dorsiflexion, 20 degrees; plantarflexion, 50 degrees; inversion, 30 degrees; eversion, 20 degrees; abduction, 10 degrees; adduction: 20 degrees; first MTP flexion, 45 degrees; first MTP extension: 70 degrees

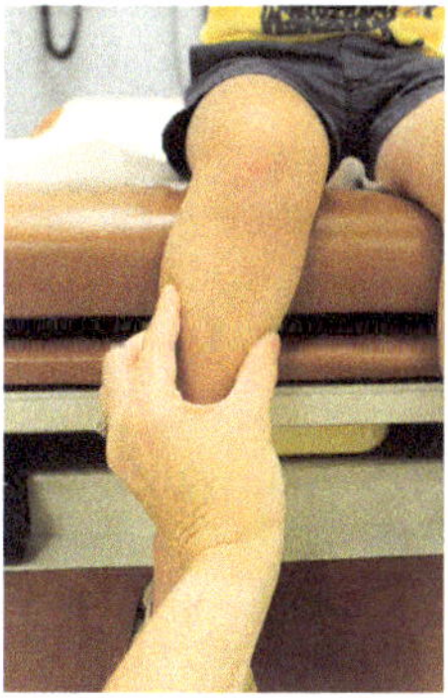

FIGURE 11.32 Squeeze test

Special Tests for the Ankle/Foot

- **Squeeze test** (**Figure 11.32**): Identifies syndesmotic (or high) ankle injuries or fractures. With patient relaxed, squeeze the proximal tibia and fibula together. Pinpoint or pain distally is considered a positive test.
- **Talar tilt**: Identifies ankle ligamentous injury. With patient relaxed and foot in a neutral position, passively move the foot into an adducted position; pain or increased motion is considered positive and a sign of damage to the lateral ankle ligaments. Passively move the foot into an abducted position. Pain or increased motion is considered a positive test.
- **Thompson test**: Evaluates the integrity of the Achilles tendon complex. With patient prone or seated with the foot unsupported, squeeze the belly of the gastrocnemius. With an intact complex, the foot should passively plantar flex when the calf is squeezed. No plantar flexion of the foot is considered a positive test.

RED FLAGS IN HISTORY AND PHYSICAL EXAM

- History of cancer
- Associated neurological deficits
- Saddle anesthesia
- Loss of bowel or bladder control
- Paralysis
- Weakness (especially unilateral with an acute onset or progressive)

- Gross deformity
- Associated unintended weight loss
- Point tenderness
- Extreme pain or pain that reoccurs over time
- Absence of pulses

PEDIATRIC CONSIDERATIONS

Barlow–Ortolani Maneuvers

- Designed to test for hip dislocations and subluxations in 0 to 1 year olds. With infant supine, flex the hips and knees to 90 degrees. Clinician's thumbs should rest on the medial side of the knees, fingers resting on the greater trochanters. Adduct the thighs and put gentle pressure through the femurs, trying to shift them out of the acetabulums. A clunk is considered positive. Slowly abduct the thighs and use the fingers to put pressure on the trochanters to guide the femoral head back into position. Again, a clunk is considered a positive test and could be a sign of hip subluxation or dislocation. If dysplasia is suspected within the first 6 months of life, an ultrasound evaluation is preferred to x-ray. If any tests are abnormal, refer to a pediatric orthopedic clinician for intervention(s) and/or treatment options.

Scoliosis

- Have the patient stand and observe them from the front. Note the symmetry of the patient's shoulders; the shoulders should be even. Uneven shoulder height can be a clue to scoliosis. Ask the patient to turn around and bend at the waist. Clinician should observe the patient from the rear. The spine should be straight without curvature and centered over the sacrum. Angles fewer than 10 degrees can often be followed with periodic radiographs. Angles of up to 30 degrees typically show no lasting effects into adulthood. Angles over 50 degrees will lead to complications later in life. In more severe cases, a unilateral rib hump may be present. Routine screening for scoliosis is not recommended. See **Figure 11.33**.

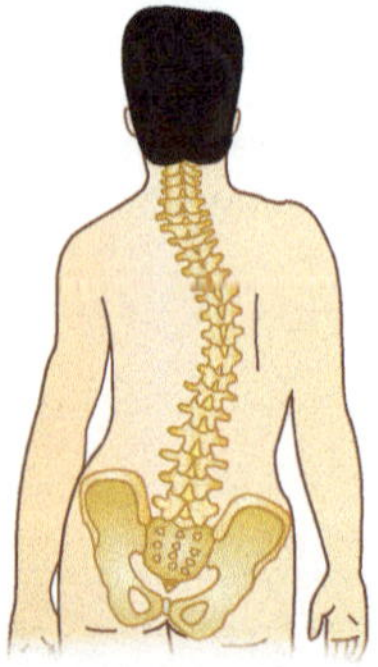

FIGURE 11.33 Scoliosis.

EVIDENCE-BASED RESOURCES

- **American Academy of Pediatrics' Orthopaedics Guidelines and Research:** https://pediatrics.aappublications.org/section-on-orthopaedics
- **American College of Rheumatology Clinical Practice Guidelines:** www.rheumatology.org/Practice-Quality/Clinical-Support/Clinical-Practice-Guidelines
- **American Medical Society for Sports Medicine position statements and guidelines:** www.amssm.org/Publications.html
- **North American Spine Association Guidelines:** www.spine.org/Research-Clinical-Care/Quality-Improvement/Clinical-Guidelines
- **The Choosing Wisely Initiative:** www.choosingwisely.org

ABNORMAL FINDINGS

The abnormal findings and differential diagnoses listed in this section are in alphabetical order, not in order of prevalence. The list is not exhaustive.

CARPAL TUNNEL SYNDROME

An inflammation and compression of the median nerve as it moves through the carpal tunnel of the wrist (**Figure 11.34**).

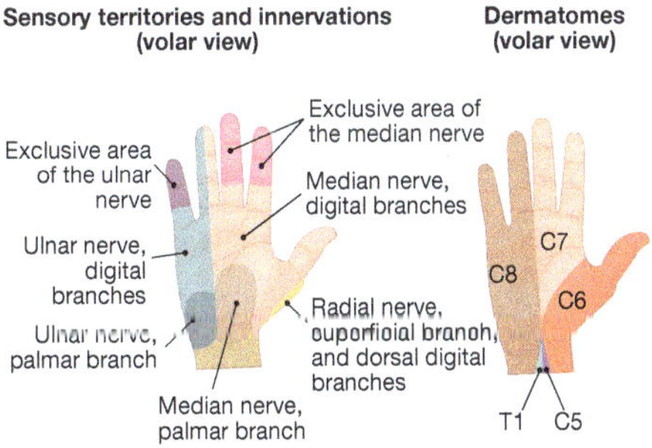

FIGURE 11.34 Median and ulnar nerve distribution (volar view).

History

- Numbness and tingling over the median nerve distribution into the hand (thumb and index, middle or ring fingers); numbness and pain is worse at night
- History of repetitive activity such as writing or typing
- Reports pain with gripping objects
- Pregnancy can induce symptoms

Physical Examination

- Decreased grip strength
- Atrophy of thenar eminence (later stages)
- Positive Phalen and Tinel tests
- Weakness of thumb strength and opposition

DE QUERVAIN'S SYNDROME

A tenosynovitis of the abductor pollicis longus and extensor pollicis brevis tendons.

History

- History of repetitive thumb movements
- Reports a "sticking" sensation in the thumb when moving it

Physical Examination

- Pain and edema over radial styloid; exacerbated with active wrist ulnar deviation
- Difficulty moving the thumb and wrist when performing activities that involve grasping or pinching
- Positive Finkelstein test

DUPUYTREN CONTRACTURE

A progressive nodularity and flexion contracture of the palmar fascia and digital flexors in the hand.

History

- Occurs slowly over years; is usually seen in people over the age of 50
- Use of tobacco and alcohol
- History of diabetes

Physical Examination

- Commonly seen in fourth and fifth digits
- Inability to completely straighten affected finger(s)
- Nodules on flexor tendons on palmar side of hand
- Without intervention, it can progress to skin puckering and flexion contracture of the MCP and PIP joints

GOUT

A form of arthritis that causes inflammation of joints due to excess uric acid.

History

- Commonly seen in middle aged men
- History of alcohol use and diets high in purines
- Acute onset with no known injury

Physical Examination

- Red, inflamed, exquisitely tender joint; most often the thumb, great toe, or knee
- Joint discomfort that lasts several weeks; limited ROM in the affected joint
- Joint aspiration analysis is positive for monosodium urate crystals
- Serum ESR and CRP may be elevated during acute attack

LATERAL EPICONDYLITIS (TENNIS ELBOW)

An inflammation and eventual chronic degeneration of the common extensor bundle on the lateral elbow.

History

- History of repetitive wrist extension
- Reports pain that may radiate from the lateral side of the elbow into the forearm and wrist

Physical Examination

- Pain over lateral epicondyle of humerus with activation of wrist extensors. Pain is worse when shaking hands, squeezing objects, holding the wrist stiff, or moving the wrist with force
- Decreased grip strength
- Positive Cozen test

LEGG–CALVE–PERTHES DISEASES

Occurs when the blood supply to the femoral head is temporarily severed, then eventually restored. Over time, this causes bone weakening and break-down, causing the round, ball-like femoral head to lose its shape.

History

- Typically affects boys aged 4 to 10
- Pain in the groin, hip, thigh, or anterior knee
- Reports stiffness in the hip joint

- Family history of Legg–Calve–Perthes

Physical Examination

- Limited ROM in the hip joint
- Patient limping

Considerations

- The cause of Legg–Calve–Perthes is unknown. On imaging, the femoral head will appear mottled and sclerosed.
- Treatment can vary depending on the patient's age and the progression of the disease. Treatments can range from bracing and observation to femoral osteotomy.

MUSCULAR DYSTROPHY

A rare group of diseases that cause muscle weakening.

History

- Family history of MD
- Males
- Usually starts in early childhood (before age 5)
- Learning to walk late (older than 18 months)
- Muscle weakness and degeneration are progressive

Physical Examination

- Decreased muscle strength
- Difficulty walking; waddling gait, or walking on the toes or balls of the feet
- Difficulty running or jumping because of weakness in leg muscles
- Frequent falls, stumbling, and difficulty climbing stairs
- Difficulty standing from a lying or sitting position
- Reduced endurance
- Enlarged calf muscles
- Gower's sign (**Figure 11.35**)
- May gradually lose the ability to walk and do other everyday activities

Considerations

- Conditions are sex-linked (X-linked) disorders that typically pass from a mother (who has no symptoms) to her son. Girls are rarely affected.
- The average life expectancy in the early 30s.

OSGOOD–SCHLATTER DISEASE

An apophysitis injury that occurs when the growth plates are still open and excess force is generated through the tibial tuberosity.

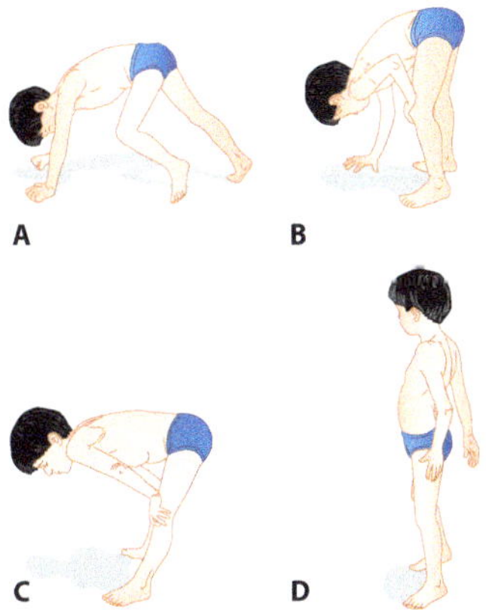

FIGURE 11.35 Gower's sign. In a positive test, the child will move from hands and knees (**A**) to hands and feet (**B**), then move hands to knees (**C**) to help push themselves to a standing position (**D**).

History

- Common in children and adolescents during puberty
- Report anterior knee pain, centered over tibial tubercle or distal patellar tendon
- History of sports participation that involves running, jumping, and swift changes of direction
- Can last from weeks to months
- Pain is often worsened during activity and resolves with rest
- Typically unilateral

Physical Examination

- Painful, bony bump on the tibia just below the knee
- Pain and edema just below the patella on palpation

Consideration

- Similar injuries can be seen at the inferior pole of the patella (Sinding–Larsen–Johansson disease) and at the calcaneus (Sever's disease).

OSTEOARTHRITIS

Wear of the articular cartilage at the end of the long bones or between spinal processes, leads to joint space narrowing, osteophyte formation, and sclerosis of the bones.

History

- Often found in older adults
- History of previous trauma or injury
- Pain isolated to single joint
- Pain worse in the morning and improves throughout the day; will often improve with mild-to-moderate activity
- Worsens with prolonged activity

Physical Examination

- Pain typically with active and passive ROM
- Decreased ROM in affected joint(s)
- Tenderness to palpation over joint line (if applicable)
- Positive x-ray showing joint cartilage degeneration

OSTEOPOROSIS/OSTEOPENIA

A condition that causes bones to weaken and become porous and brittle, increasing fracture risk. Early stages of bone loss are considered osteopenia. As disease progresses, osteoporosis can develop.

History

- Typically asymptomatic in the beginning
- Diet low in calcium and/or vitamin D
- Females are affected more than males
- Menopausal women
- Lack of weight-bearing exercise
- Smoking history
- History of fractures
- Taking certain medications such as glucocorticoids, proton pump inhibitors, antiepileptic drugs, medroxyprogesterone acetate, aromatase inhibitors, and androgen-deprivation therapies

Physical Examination

- Loss of height over time
- Bone fracture, often with no associated trauma
- t-score <-2.5 (indicates osteoporosis); between -1.0 and -2.5 (indicates osteopenia) on DEXA scan

RADIAL HEAD SUBLUXATION (NURSEMAID'S ELBOW)

Partial dislocation of the head of the radius at the level of the radio-humeral joint.

History

- Seen in young children, aged 1 to 4

- History of arm jerking motion or history of a fall while holding onto an object, such as monkey bars

Physical Examination

- Pain palpated at the elbow or wrist
- Child will not want to move the arm
- Child is holding arm in a flexed and pronated position

Consideration

- Hyperpronation or a supination-flexion technique may be used to reduce a radial head subluxation. It is easier to reduce the subluxation soon after the injury occurs and can be more difficult to reduce after more time has passed.

Rheumatoid Arthritis

A chronic autoimmune inflammatory disease affecting the joints. It can lead to debilitating pain and deformity, most commonly of the MCP and PIP joints in the hands.

History

- More common in women
- Onset typically in middle age
- History of smoking
- Positive family history of rheumatoid arthritis
- Morning stiffness typically lasting more than 1 to 2 hours
- Symptoms ongoing (present for at least 6 weeks)
- Anorexia, fatigue
- Reports pain in three or more joints (smaller joints are typically affected first)

Physical Examination

- Tender, warm, edematous joints
- Commonly affects PIP and MCP joints first
- Firm lumps (rheumatoid nodules) under the skin that form close to joints
- Ulnar deviation of the fingers (later sign)
- Positive RF, ANA, and anti-CCP serum levels
- Possible short-term elevation of CRP, possible long-term elevation of ESR

ROTATOR CUFF TEAR

Tear in the rotator cuff muscles, the supraspinatus, infraspinatus, subscapularis, and teres minor.

History

- Risk increases with age
- History of traumatic injury or repetitive movements
- Reports pain and weakness with overhead activities
- Described pain as a dull ache
- Often causes significant deficits in completing ADLs

Physical Examination

- Typically seen in the dominant arm
- Decreased ROM, including forward flexion and internal and/or external rotation, in the affected arm
- Decreased shoulder strength in affected arm
- Positive empty can test, external rotation resistance test, and/or lag test

Consideration

- Degenerative tears can be exacerbated insidiously.

SLIPPED CAPITAL FEMORAL EPIPHYSIS

The femoral head of the femur slips backward at the growth plate, causing a shift in the normal alignment of the femoral head of the femur and the neck section of the femur.

History

- Affects males more often than females and African Americans more often than Caucasians
- Overweight or obese
- Typically occurs in adolescents
- Reports pain in the hip, thigh, or knee
- Usually develops gradually
- Pain worsens with activity

Physical Examination

- Typically unilateral pain in the groin, knee, or hip during ROM
- Limited ROM in the hip—especially limited internal rotation
- Involuntary muscle guarding and muscle spasms
- Foot/leg is turned outward
- Walking with a limp
- One leg may appear shorter than the other

Consideration

- X-rays will have the appearance of ice cream falling off a cone. Treatment is surgical unless disease is significantly progressed and growth plates closed. Referral to orthopedics is necessary.

PHYSICAL EXAMINATION DOCUMENTATION

Documentation should include results of inspection, palpation, ROM, strength, reflexes (and/or applicable neuro exam components), and the results of any special tests completed.

EXAMPLE OF NORMAL FINDINGS (BACK EXAM)

No visible deformity of spine, or upper or lower extremities. Scapulae, iliac crests, and gluteal crease are symmetric. No visible dermal cysts or hairy patches. No limp or alteration of gait or leg length abnormality. Muscle circumference is equal throughout the lower extremities bilaterally. No paraspinal musculature or spinal processes tenderness; no tenderness to percussion of spinous processes. Muscle strength: 5/5 with hip flexion, knee flexion, knee extension, plantar flexion, dorsiflexion. Toe and heel walking intact. Sensation: intact and equal bilaterally in lower extremities throughout to light touch, as well as sharp and dull stimuli. No saddle anesthesia. Spine: Flexion: 60 degrees, extension: 30 degrees, lateral bending: 20 degrees bilateral, lateral rotation: 10 degrees bilateral, straight leg test negative bilateral, patellar & Achilles reflexes 2+ symmetric bilaterally.

REFERENCES

References for this chapter draw from Chapter 15, "Evidence-Based Assessment of the Musculoskeletal System," of the textbook *Evidence-Based Physical Examination: Best Practices for Health and Well-Being Assessment*. The references may be accessed in the digital version of the handbook at https://connect.springerpub.com/content/book/97808-0-8261-6466-7/chapter/ch11

12

Evidence-Based Assessment of the Abdomen and Gastrointestinal and Urological Systems

CLINICAL CONSIDERATIONS

- Assessment of the abdomen requires an understanding of the bony and muscular architecture of the abdomen and the organs, muscles, and structures contained within it.
- Abdominal pain is one of the most common subjective CCs. Most individuals with abdominal pain have a benign or self-limiting condition. The initial goal of assessment is to identify individuals with a serious etiology.
- Abdominal pain can be challenging to diagnosis due to the non-specific neuroreceptors found in the visceral cavity.
- Abdominal pain can be referred pain from outside the GI/GU system, so other systems should always be considered and ruled out.
- Any painful areas of the abdomen should be examined last to prevent muscle guarding and decrease patient anxiety due to fear of pain.

SUBJECTIVE HISTORY

COMMON REASONS FOR SEEKING CARE

- Abdominal pain
- Nausea and vomiting
- Diarrhea or constipation
- Urinary problems (dysuria, incontinence)

HISTORY OF PRESENT ILLNESS

- **Onset:** When did the symptoms start? What was the individual doing when they became symptomatic? Did this occur suddenly, or has it been developing gradually?
- **Location:** Does the symptom have associated pain or discomfort? If so, where is the discomfort located? Does the pain radiate anywhere?
- **Duration:** How long do symptom(s) last? Over what period of time has the abdominal/GI/GU symptom developed? Have these symptoms occurred in the past?
- **Characteristics:** How would you describe the pain? Is it aching, burning, sharp, cramping, squeezing, dull, shooting, stabbing? Does the vomitus have undigested food, partially digested food, bile, or blood? What is the frequency, volume, and consistency (hard/watery/soft/unformed) of the stool? Would you describe the stool as greasy, bulky, foul-smelling, or bloody?
- **Associated symptoms:** Is there any associated fever, nausea/vomiting, diarrhea/constipation, arthritis/arthralgias, rashes, headaches, anorexia, passage of flatus, jaundice, dysuria, urgency and/or frequency of urination, hematuria, straining, bloating, sense of incomplete evacuation, urinary infection, urinary incontinence, heartburn, early satiety, or weight loss/gain?
- **Aggravating factors:** What actions, activities, types of food, or body positions make the symptoms worse?
- **Relieving factors:** What actions, activities, or body positions decrease the symptoms? If relieved, how long does the relief last?
- **Treatment:** What medications has the individual taken to help with the symptoms, including acid-suppressives, laxatives, or OTC pain relief? Clarify dosage and frequency of any medications.
- **Severity:** How severe are the symptoms on a scale of 0 to 10? Do the symptoms interfere with sleep or daily function? Are the symptoms worsening? How often are the symptoms causing you to miss work/school?

HEALTH HISTORY

Past Medical History

- History of GI/GU illnesses throughout their life span:
  - History of abdominal or urological surgeries
  - History of *Helicobacter pylori*
  - Last colonoscopy (results, interventions)
  - History of UTI and/or pyelonephritis (any untreated UTIs)
  - Incontinence—current, acute, chronic

  - Recent, previous, or traumatic vaginal childbirth
  - Pelvic or rectal prolapse
  - Benign prostatic hypertrophy
  - Hematuria
- Comorbidities or risk factors related to gastrointestinal or urological diseases:
  - Chronic diseases (cancers, congenital disorders, autoimmune disorders)
  - CV disease (history of myocardial infarction)
  - Mental health conditions including substance abuse
  - Diabetes and/or HTN
  - Disability related to mobility
  - Neurological disease or disorders, including neurogenic bladder
  - Dementia and/or confusion
  - Overweight/obesity
  - Recent illness, trauma, or travel

Medications

- Prescribed and OTC medications or supplements, including dose and frequency
- Recent antibiotic use

Allergies

- Allergies to medications or seasonal, environmental, and/or food allergies. If yes to being allergic to any substance or environmental trigger, clarify reaction:
  - Nausea, intestinal upset? Vomiting?
  - Skin rashes, itching? Hives?
  - Swelling of tongue, lips, face?

Immunizations

- Risks for vaccine-preventable illnesses; vaccine status (rotavirus, hepatitis A, hepatitis B)

Pediatric Considerations

- **Neonate.** Birth history, meconium passage, intolerance of eating (e.g., vomiting, diarrhea, little interest in eating)
- **Infants:** Breast/bottle-fed, type of formula (frequency and amount per feeding), introduction of solid food (what kind, when given), other fluid intake

- **Toddlers/young children:** Diapers or toilet trained, difficulty with toilet training (e.g., methods used, challenges), overflow soiling, retentive posturing during stooling, known food sensitivities, current diet, liquid intake, change in eating patterns
- **All ages:** Where does the child fall for growth and development based on pediatric growth charts? Has the trend been stable or has there been a recent change in the trajectory?

FAMILY HISTORY

- Family history of GI disease (celiac disease, IBD, GERD, EoE, liver disease, IBS, PUD, Barrett's esophagus, or hepatobiliary disease)
- Cancer (esophageal, gallbladder, liver, pancreatic, gastric, small intestine, colon, rectal)
- Autoimmune disorders (thyroid disease, diabetes mellitus type 1, IBD)
- Polyposis syndromes (including Lynch syndrome)
- CF
- Migraines
- Mental health disorders (mild, moderate, or severe anxiety, depression, or mental illness)

SOCIAL HISTORY

- Current dietary patterns, including fiber intake
- Recent change in diet
- Access to healthy food, clean water
- Family dynamics/environment
- Life event stress
- Emotional/behavioral symptoms
- Recent travel out of the country
- Exposure to lakes/streams
- Contact with animals
- Caffeine intake (type, amount, frequency)
- Sexual activity and practices
- Water/fluid intake
- Smoking history/history of tobacco use
- Substance use, including alcohol

REVIEW OF SYSTEMS

- **General:** Fever, fatigue, malaise, anorexia, weight loss, weight gain
- **CV**: Chest pain, ankle edema, dyspnea

- **Respiratory**: Shortness of breath, pain with inhalation, cough, history of pneumonia
- **GI**: Abdominal pain, nausea, vomiting, constipation, diarrhea, heartburn, increased abdominal girth, irritable bowel symptoms, and/or dysphagia
- **GU:** Dysuria, urinary frequency and/or urgency, suprapubic pain, lower back pain (flank pain), hematuria, turbid or cloudy urine, foul-smelling urine, concentrated or dilute urine, nocturia
- **Reproductive**: Vaginal or urethral discharge, dyspareunia, recent or current pregnancy, menstrual history
- **Neurologic**: Memory loss, confusion, disorientation, mental/physical disability, decreased sensation of lower extremities or perineum, decreased reflexes in lower extremities
- **MSK**: Back pain, muscle aches, arthritic joints, arthritis pain, history of exercise or back strain
- **Mental health**: Mild, moderate, or severe anxiety, depression, or mental illness

PHYSICAL EXAMINATION

In the abdominal exam, the sequence is inspection, auscultation, percussion, and palpation. Palpation should occur last since there is the possibility that pain can be elicited during this aspect of the exam and can alter the clinical findings that occur following the occurrence of pain.

PREPARATION FOR THE EXAM

- Ensure adequate lighting. Ensure patient has been adequately draped with the abdomen exposed while maintaining privacy of the genitalia and breasts.
- Ask the patient to empty their bladder prior to the exam, which can help relax the abdominal musculature, maintain comfort, and assist in all elements of the abdominal exam, especially palpation.
- Place the patient in a supine position with arms at the side and knees bent. Positioning the patient with arms above the head can cause tension in the abdominal muscles, making the exam difficult.
- Use of a warm room and stethoscope can also help to relax tense abdominal muscles.

GENERAL SURVEY

- **Vital signs:** Temperature, pulse rate, respiratory rate, blood pressure
- Posture and position

- Presence of abdominal guarding and/or evidence of pain (facial expressions, body movements, vital signs)
- Toxic versus nontoxic appearance

INSPECTION

- Use tangential lighting while seated next to the patient to highlight skin characteristics/color, as well as the contour of the abdomen and any underlying organs or masses.
- Inspect the abdomen from the side as well as while looking down at the abdomen for symmetry and contour. Note any jaundice.
- Inspect the contour and the skin for bruises, discoloration, spider angiomas, scars, or lesions. Look for any visible pulsations, dilated abdominal veins, edema, or ascites (**Figure 12.1**).
- Ask the patient to take a deep breath and hold it; this helps to lower the diaphragm and move abdominal organs downward to better assess bulges or masses that may not have been previously noted. Ask the patient to raise their head off the exam table, which allows the abdominal muscles to contract and the clinician to assess for previously undetected masses, bulges, or nodules.

AUSCULTATION

- The majority of available evidence does not recommend auscultating bowel sounds.
- Auscultate the abdomen for bruits over the aorta, renal, and femoral arteries (**Figures 12.2 and 12.3**). Normally, no bruits are auscultated. Abdominal bruits (during systole) heard in the epigastric region of the abdomen are likely a normal finding in a healthy person; however, continuous bruits (across systole and diastole) or a bruit heard away from the midline are more concerning and deserve a more focused assessment.

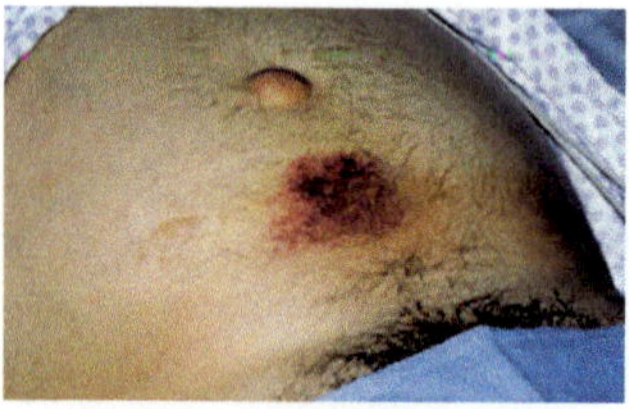

FIGURE 12.1 Cullen's sign.
Source: Image courtesy of Herbert L. Fred, MD and Hendrik A. van Dijk.

PERCUSSION

- Percussion helps to assess the size, density, and location of abdominal organs and structures. In addition, percussion can help to detect fluid or air in the abdomen. To percuss, place the distal joint and tip of the middle finger of the nondominant hand firmly on the abdomen, avoiding the ribs. Do not place any other portion of the hand on the abdomen as this will dampen percussion notes. Use the middle finger of the dominant hand to strike the distal IP joint of the stationary finger on the abdomen (**Figure 12.4**). Use short, quick motions while listening for the percussion tone produced from vibration of underlying organs and structures.

- Percuss lightly in all four quadrants of the abdomen. Generalized tympany is found over the majority of the abdomen due to gas. Dullness occurs over fluid, organs, masses, or distended bladder.

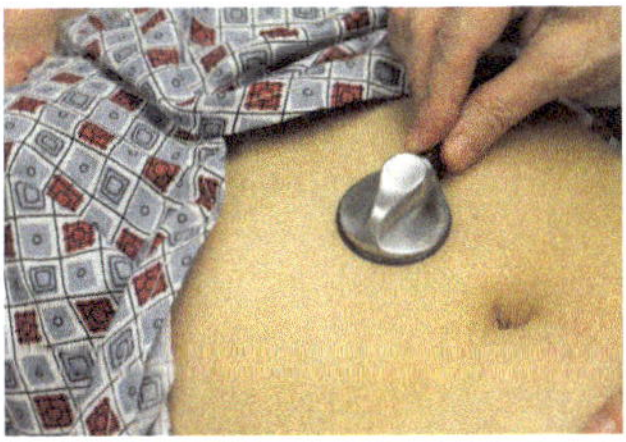

FIGURE 12.2 Auscultation of abdominal aorta.

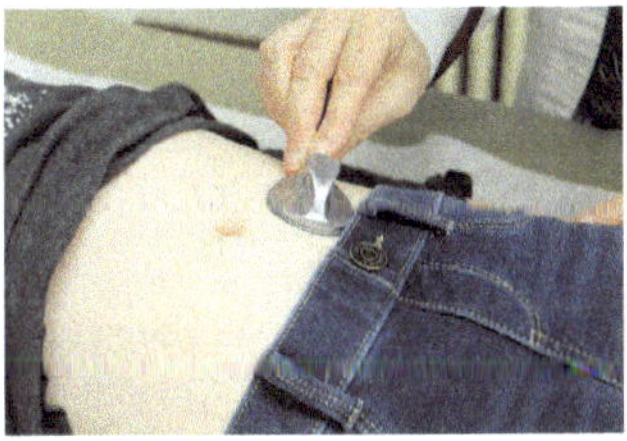

FIGURE 12.3 Auscultation of renal arteries.

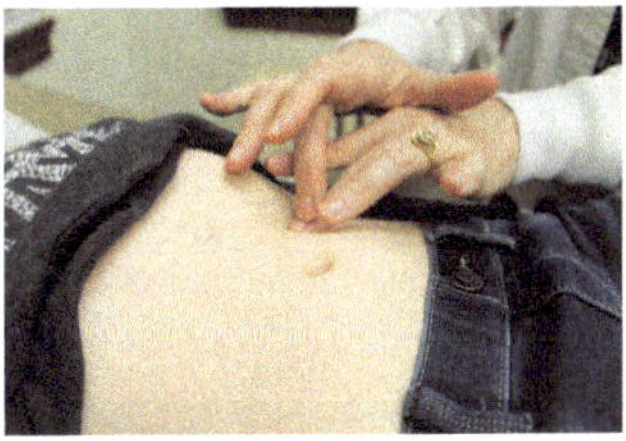

FIGURE 12.4 Abdominal percussion technique.

Percussion of the Liver

- Percussion can be used to estimate liver size; however, this technique is a general estimation of the size of the liver, or the liver span. It is often inaccurate due to difficulty of technique, especially in females due to the presence of breast tissue. Enlargement of the liver associated with hepatitis or ascites may be easier to detect than normal liver size. While percussion of the liver may be useful in determining the location of the lower border of the liver, percussion findings should be interpreted with caution.
- Dullness is typically heard over the liver when percussed. To estimate the size or span of the liver, percussion should be used

to determine both the lower and upper borders. Start percussion at the right midclavicular line over an area of lung resonance. Percuss at the interspaces between the ribs and move down the right midclavicular line, listening for a change in percussion tones from resonance to dullness. Mark this change in tone associated with the upper border of the liver, typically at the fifth ICS, with tape or an appropriate writing device. Start percussion at an area of tympany in the abdomen at the right midclavicular line. Percuss upward along the midclavicular line, noting the change from tympany to dullness and mark this spot associated with the lower border of the liver. Measure the distance between the two marks; the normal liver span at the right midclavicular line is 6 to 12 cm (2–5 inches) at the right midclavicular line.

Percussion of the Spleen

- The spleen is difficult to percuss due to the stomach and intestine, which lie in the abdominal cavity. Listen for the dullness of the spleen while percussing just posterior to the left midaxillary line. Splenic dullness may be heard from the sixth to tenth rib. Dullness at Traube's space (**Figure 12.5**) has been shown to have moderate sensitivity and specificity in association with splenomegaly; however, this finding is less accurate when patients are overweight or obese. There is limited evidence for the use of spleen percussion techniques to rule out splenomegaly (specificity 32.6%–87%, sensitivity 22%–85.7%).
- The spleen can also be assessed by percussing the lowest intercostal space in the left anterior axillary line before and after the patient takes a deep breath. Using this method, the area should

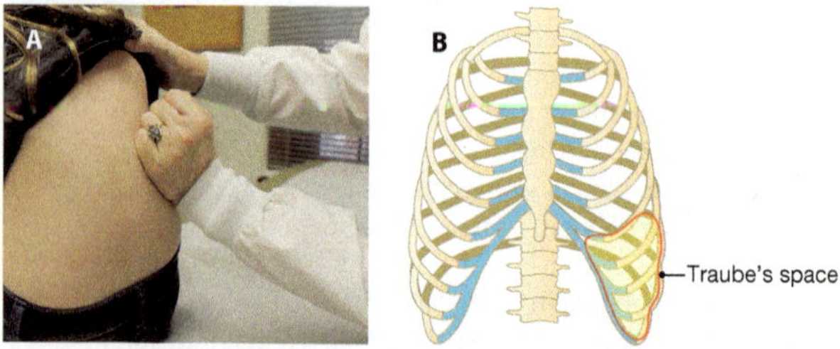

FIGURE 12.5 (**A**) Percussion of the costovertebral angle to assess for tenderness. (**B**) Traube's space. Surface markings: left sixth rib, left midaxillary line, left costal margin.

remain tympanic with the patient's breathing. If the spleen is enlarged, tympany changes to dullness as the spleen moves forward and down with inspiration.

Percussion of the Kidneys

- Percuss the right and left costovertebral angle to assess for tenderness or pain, indicating kidney inflammation or musculoskeletal problems. Direct fist percussion, when the clinician directly strikes the costovertebral angle using the ulnar surface of the fist, can be used (see Figure 12.5). Conversely, indirect fist percussion may be used by placing the palm of the right hand on the back and striking this hand with the ulnar surface of the fist of the left hand.

PALPATION

- Similar to percussion, palpation can be used to assess for masses, tenderness, and fluid in the abdomen. In addition, abdominal organs can be evaluated for size, shape, mobility, and consistency using palpation techniques (**Figure 12.6**).
- Remember to review techniques that allow the patient to relax, especially during the palpation portion of the exam. Pressing too firmly, having cold hands, and/or having used a cold stethoscope may cause the abdominal muscles to tense or cause voluntary guarding to occur, which may interfere with deep palpation. Palpate the painful areas last as examining these areas will cause pain and muscle tension that skew palpation findings.

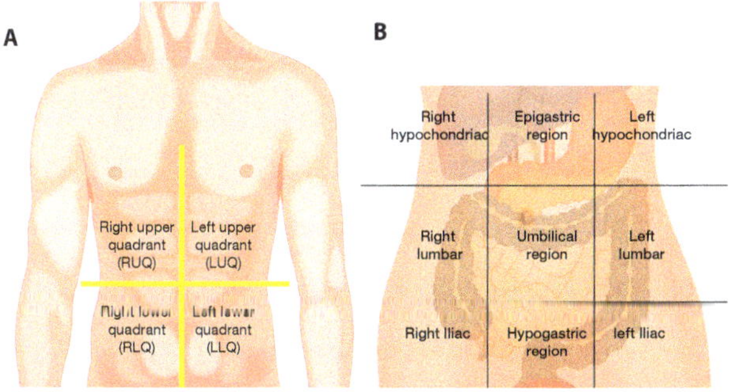

FIGURE 12.6 Quadrants of the abdomen to describe the location and symptoms of pain. (**A**) Four quadrants. (**B**) Nine quadrants.

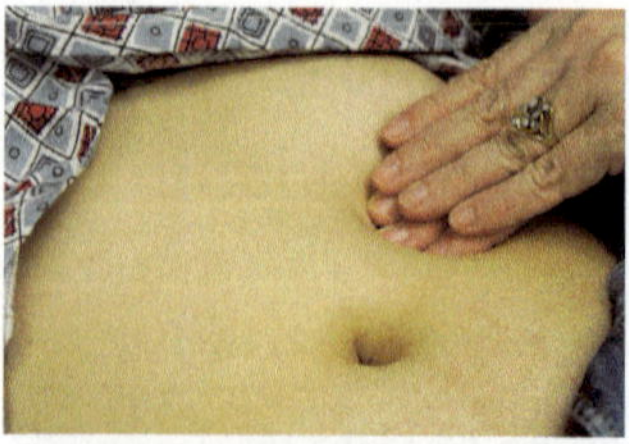

FIGURE 12.7 Abdominal palpation.

Light Palpation

- Start with light palpation of the abdomen, moving in a systematic way through all four quadrants (see Figure 12.6). The clinician should place the palmar surface of their hand lightly on the abdomen with fingers outstretched and close together (**Figure 12.7**). Press down on the abdominal wall no more than one centimeter with light palpation. Keep hands low and parallel to the abdomen; keeping the hands high and pointing downward increases the likelihood of the patient tensing the abdomen. Use a light and circular motion, avoiding disjointed, jabbing, or hurried motions. Pick up the hand when moving to the next area of the abdomen; do not drag the fingers. The abdomen should normally feel soft and smooth.

Deep Palpation

- Deep palpation requires the clinician to depress the abdomen 5 to 8 cm. Similar to light palpation, move in a systematic way through all four quadrants of the abdomen. Deep palpation can help determine abdominal organs and masses that may not be large enough to detect with light palpation. It also may reveal tenderness not evident with light palpation. When performing deep palpation, note any masses, tenderness, and pulsations.
- Exam findings of guarding, rigidity, rebound tenderness, percussion tenderness, and pain with coughing nearly double the likelihood of peritonitis. Review the "Special Tests of the Abdomen" section for information on how to elicit rebound tenderness. Rigidity alone makes the diagnosis of peritonitis almost 4 times as likely.

Liver Palpation

- Because the rib cage covers most of the liver, it is difficult to palpate. Place your left hand under the patient at the 11th and 12th ribs while pressing up in order to elevate the liver toward the abdominal wall. The right hand should be placed on the abdomen, fingers parallel to the midline. Using the right hand, push deeply under the right costal margin. Ask the patient to take a deep breath while trying to feel the edge of the liver as the diaphragm brings it down to the fingertips of the clinician's right hand. Normally, the liver is not palpable, although it may be palpated in thin patients without any underlying disease and in children. If the liver edge is palpated, it should feel smooth, nontender, and without nodules. A palpable liver edge below the costal margin significantly increases the likelihood of detecting hepatomegaly (+LR = 233.7).

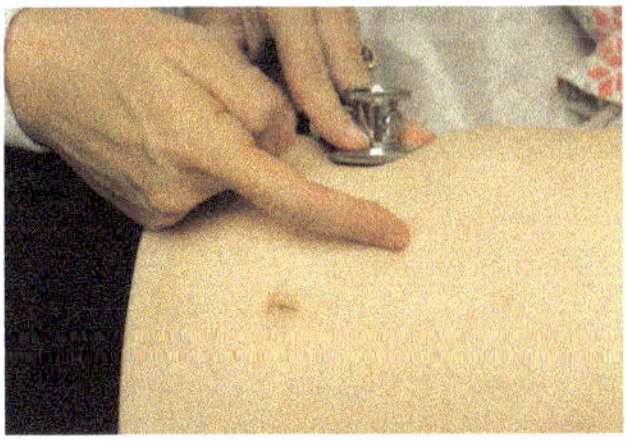

FIGURE 12.8 Scratch test.

- **Scratch test**: To perform this technique, place a stethoscope on the xiphoid process while using a finger to scratch the abdominal surface (**Figure 12.8**). Note differences in sound transmission over solid and hollow organs. When the liver is reached, the sound of the finger scratching the abdominal surface becomes louder. This test has shown high reproducibility and moderate agreement between scratch test findings and ultrasound; obesity can jeopardize results.

Palpation of the Spleen

- There is moderate evidence for the use of palpation tests to confirm an enlarged spleen (specificity 82%–93%, sensitivity 31%–85.6%). The clinician places their left hand across and behind the patient's left side at the costovertebral angle, lifting up the spleen (**Figure 12.9**). The right hand is placed on the patient's abdomen below the left costal margin, pressing the fingers toward the spleen. Ask the patient to take a deep breath while attempting to feel the spleen as it comes toward the clinician's fingers. Normally, the spleen is not palpable, although approximately 3% of the population have a palpable spleen tip. If the spleen is palpable, it is considered an abnormal exam if it is greater than 2 cm below the costal margin. A palpable spleen increases the likelihood of

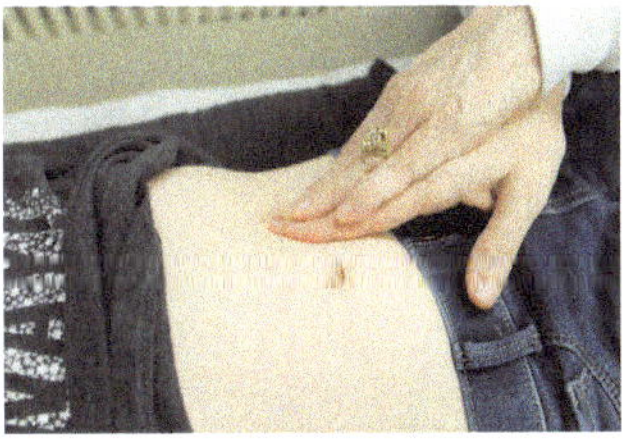

FIGURE 12.9 Palpation of the spleen.

TABLE 12.1 Hackett's Grading System for Palpable Splenomegaly

Grade 0	Normal impalpable spleen
Grade 1	Spleen palpable only on deep inspiration
Grade 2	Spleen palpable on midclavicular line, halfway between umbilicus and costal margin
Grade 3	The spleen expands toward the umbilicus
Grade 4	The spleen goes past the umbilicus
Grade 5	The spleen expands toward the pubis symphysis

Note: Modest correlation ($r \leq 0.62$, $p < .001$).

detecting splenomegaly (+LR = 8.5). The spleen must be enlarged three times before it is palpable. See **Table 12.1** for Hackett's grading system for a palpable spleen.

Palpation of the Kidneys

- To palpate the right kidney, stand at the right side of the patient and place one hand on the patient's right flank and the other hand at the right costal margin. Press the two hands together and ask the patient to take a deep breath (**Figure 12.10A**). The kidney edge may be felt between the fingers or not palpated at all; both findings are normal. To palpate the left kidney, reach across the patient and behind the left flank with the left hand. Press the right hand into the abdomen while asking the patient to inhale (**Figure 12.10B**). Press firmly between the two hands; there should be no change with inhalation.

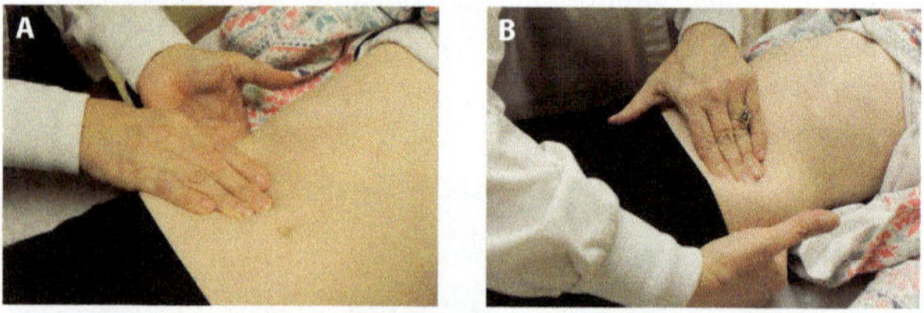

FIGURE 12.10 Palpation of the (**A**) right kidney and (**B**) left kidney.

Palpation of the Aorta

- Palpate the aorta with the opposing thumb and fingers slightly left of the midline in the upper abdomen. As an alternative, assess the width of the aorta by pressing on either side of the aorta in the upper abdomen with one hand on each side of the aorta. The ability to palpate the aorta is related to the size of the aneurysm, but the inability to palpate the aorta is not efficient at ruling out an aneurysm in obese patients or in those who cannot relax their abdomen to facilitate the examination. The normal aorta is 2.5 to 4.0 cm wide in the adult.

Palpation of the Gallbladder

- If a gallbladder is palpable during an abdominal exam, this is an abnormal finding. A palpable and tender gallbladder suggests acute cholecystitis and has a positive likelihood of detecting obstruction of the bile ducts (+LR = 26.0). If enlarged, the gallbladder can be felt behind the smooth liver border in the RUQ of the abdomen. Compared with the smooth liver, an enlarged gallbladder feels like a firm mass. If palpable, an inflamed gallbladder is exquisitely tender, making palpation difficult due to abdominal muscle guarding.

SPECIAL TESTS FOR THE ABDOMEN

The following tests are typically considered positive when pain is associated with the maneuver. Therefore, these specialized tests need to be completed last since the pain response may cause peritoneal irritation and could jeopardize any future exam findings. Similar to other clinical exam tests, combinations of findings from the clinical examination are **more powerful** than any single finding.

McBurney's Point

- Pain with palpation of the RLQ of the abdomen indicates a positive McBurney's point (sometimes called *McBurney's sign*).
- A positive test can be associated with the diagnosis of appendicitis.

Rebound Tenderness or Blumberg's Sign

- Palpate the abdomen by applying slow and steady pressure to the suspected area, followed by abrupt removal of the pressure.
- Test is considered positive if pain is worsened upon release of the hands (versus application of the pressure) when the underlying structure(s) shift back into place. A positive sign indicates

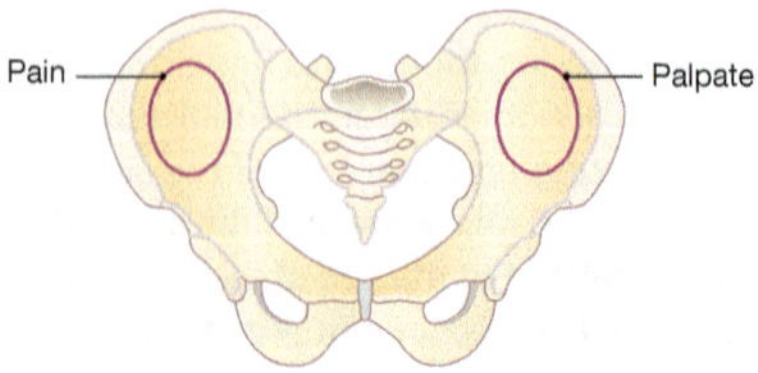

FIGURE 12.11 Rovsing sign. Location of the iliac fossa and eliciting the Rovsing sign.

peritoneal irritation. The odds of appendicitis triple in children who exhibit rebound tenderness (LR, 3.0; 95% CI, 2.3–3.9) and reduce the likelihood of its occurrence if rebound tenderness is absent (summary LR, 0.28; 95% CI, 0.14–0.55). The results do not appear as favorable for adults (LR+, 1.59; 95% CI 1.22–2.06; LR- 0.65; 95% CI 0.54–0.61).

Rovsing Sign

- Deeply palpate the left iliac fossa. If pain is felt, this is considered a positive sign (**Figure 12.11**). Historically, a positive Rovsing sign has been associated with acute appendicitis; it has a sensitivity of 30.1% and specificity of 84.4%.

Psoas Test

- With the patient in the supine position, place one hand just above the patient's right knee. Ask the patient to raise their leg while applying downward pressure on the leg (**Figure 12.12**).
- Pain indicates irritation of the psoas muscle due to inflammation of the appendix. Some sources advise that a positive test can indicate a retrocecal (behind the cecum) appendicitis presentation due to retroperitoneal inflammation (LR+ 2.38, 95% CI 1.21–4.57; LR- 0.90, 95% CI 0.83–0.86).

Heel Drop Test (Also Called the Markle Test *or* Heel Jar Test*)*

- Have the patient stand on their toes and then abruptly release back onto their heels, creating a jarring sensation to the body. Pain in the RLQ is a positive test and contributes information toward possible diagnosis of appendicitis (LR+ 1.95,95% CI 1.51–2.52, LR- 0.48, 95% CI 0.38–0.61).

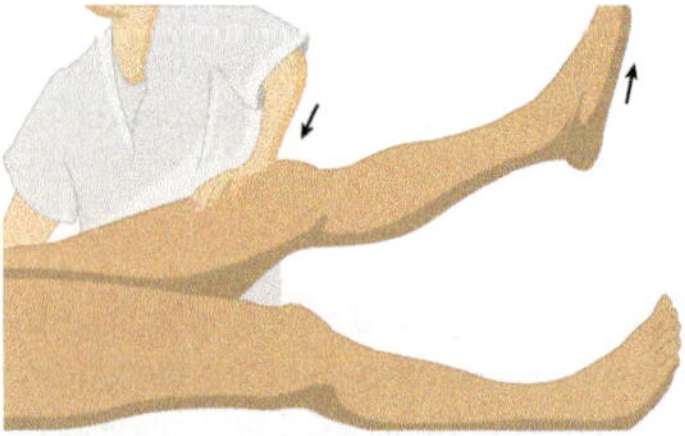

FIGURE 12.12 Psoas test.

Digital Rectal Examination

- DREs are warranted when a patient has a gastrointestinal or urinary concern. See Chapter 13, "Evidence-Based Assessment of Male Genitalia, Prostate, Rectum, and Anus."

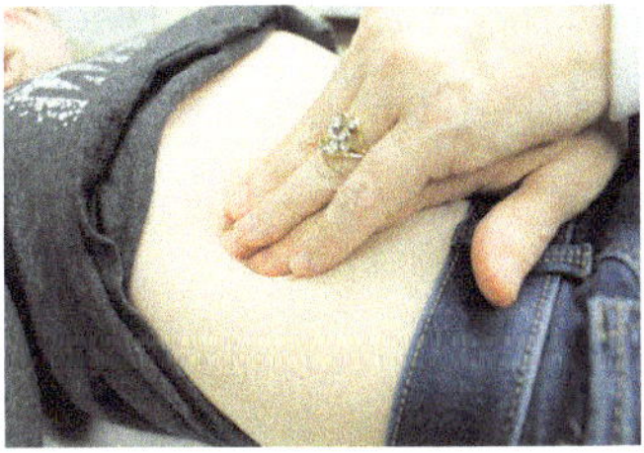

FIGURE 12.13 Murphy's sign.

Murphy's Sign

- Place one hand at the costal margin in the RUQ and ask the patient to breathe in deeply (**Figure 12.13**). If the gallbladder is inflamed, the patient will experience RUQ pain upon palpation and will have abrupt cessation of breath (i.e., catch their breath) due to pain as gallbladder descends and contacts the palpating hand.
- Murphy's sign (positive LR, 2.8; 95% CI, 0.8–8.6) is considered positive when the patient experiences RUQ pain with palpation. Sensitivity is 80% for diagnosis of cholecystitis.

PEDIATRIC CONSIDERATIONS

- In the infant, the contour of the abdomen is protuberant because of undeveloped abdominal musculature and may reveal respiratory movement and peristalsis. The liver predominates in the RUQ, and the liver edge may be palpated at the right costal margin or slightly below. The spleen, kidneys, and bladder may be palpated in the infant.
- In children 4 years and older, the liver is still palpable as is the spleen. The liver span is 3.5 cm at age 2 years, 5 cm at age 5 years, and 6 to 7 cm during adolescence. The right and left kidney may also be palpated. Modifications in how the abdominal exam is performed may be necessary in young children.

CONSIDERATIONS FOR THE OLDER ADULT

- Palpation of the abdominal organs may be easier due to thinning of the abdominal wall and weakness of the abdominal musculature.
- The liver is easier to palpate and may be found 1 to 2 centimeters below the costal margin with inhalation.
- Decreased motility occurs with aging, which in turn means symptoms of gas and distention, as well as tympany upon percussion.

RED FLAGS IN HISTORY AND PHYSICAL EXAM

- Arthritis
- Bilious emesis
- Deceleration of linear growth
- Delayed onset of puberty
- Dysphagia
- Family history of IBD, Lynch syndrome, celiac disease, PUD, Barrett's esophagus, or hepatobiliary disease
- Hematuria
- Hematemesis
- Hepatosplenomegaly
- Nighttime pain or diarrhea
- Oral ulcers
- Perianal skin tags/fissures
- Persistent RUQ or RLQ pain
- Persistent vomiting or diarrhea
- Recurrent unexplained fever
- Rectal bleeding or melena
- Severe flank pain or groin pain
- Unexplained anemia
- Unintentional weight loss

EVIDENCE-BASED RESOURCES

- **American Gastroenterological Association Guidelines:** https://gastro.org/guidelines
- **American Society of Nephrology:** www.asn-online.org/publications
- **American Urogynecologic Society:** www.augs.org/clinical-practice/guidelines
- **American Urological Association:** www.auanet.org/guidelines
- **Choosing Wisely Initiative:** www.choosingwisely.org
- **Society of American Gastrointestinal and Endoscopic Surgeons:** www.sages.org/publications/guidelines
- **U.S. Preventive Services Task Force:** https://uspreventiveservicestaskforce.org/uspstf/recommendation-topics

ABNORMAL FINDINGS

CONSTIPATION

Abnormal transport mechanisms of the GI tract that cause slow motility in the intestinal lumen, which leads to infrequent, hard, and difficult-to-pass stools.

History

- Diets with high refined carbohydrates and low fiber intake
- History of prolonged laxative use
- Drug usage (e.g., opiates)
- Decreased physical activity
- At least a 3-month duration of symptoms
- Straining with bowel movements
- Hard stool
- Incomplete evacuation
- Fewer than three bowel movements a week

Physical Examination

- Dried, hard, small stools palpated in rectal cavity
- Mass palpated in left lower quadrant

Considerations

- Most often, the decreased motility is noted in the large intestines.

DIARRHEA

Abnormal and rapid transport of chyme in the gastrointestinal tract, causing increased intestinal motility and changes in the osmotic mechanism that results in abnormal absorption. This leads to loose, watery stools.

History

- Reports loose, watery stools
- Frequent bowel movements
- Cramping due to inflammation
- Increased intestinal motility of the GI tract
- Gas formation
- Can cause dehydration
- Underlying etiology will determine if other symptoms are present but can include vomiting, fever, lethargy/malaise, diffuse abdominal pain

Physical Examination

- Abdominal tenderness on palpation of the affected area

Considerations

- The rapid transport can be triggered by numerous causes that include bacterial, viral, organic, or functional. Viral gastroenteritis is the most common cause of diarrhea.
- Most often, the episodes are self-limited and resolve within a few days without intervention.
- When the diarrhea is accompanied by high fever and intractable vomiting, dehydration can occur. This complication occurs particularly frequently in children and older adults and can require hospitalization.

ABNORMAL FINDINGS BASED ON LOCATION OF ABDOMINAL PAIN

The location of abdominal pain and tenderness often provides the clinician with valuable insight into possible gastrointestinal and urological differential diagnoses (**Figure 12.14**).

RIGHT UPPER QUADRANT PAIN: DUODENUM/ LIVER/GALLBLADDER/PANCREAS

The RUQ of the abdomen has several underlying organs whose dysfunction can cause pain and pathology. RUQ pain encompasses a

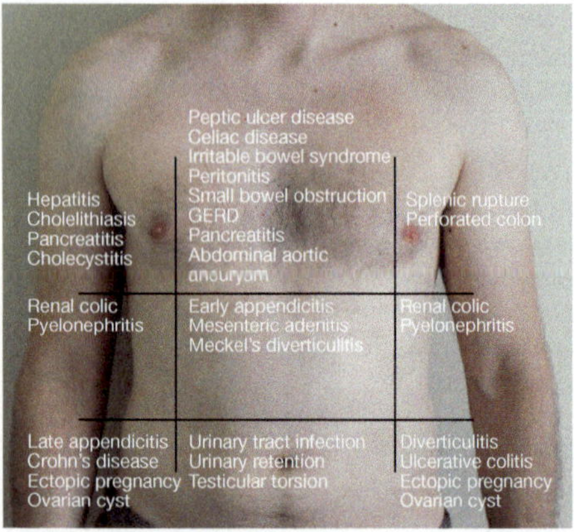

FIGURE 12.14 Differential diagnoses according to localization of abdominal pain.
GERD, gastroesophageal reflux disease.

variety of diagnostic possibilities. The most common etiologies are diseases of the liver, gallbladder, or pancreas. A careful history and physical exam can help the clinician differentiate the etiology of the pain, but all underlying structures need to be considered.

Acute Pancreatitis

Inflammation of the pancreas. It can be acute or chronic with symptoms ranging from mild to severe.

History

- RUQ or epigastric abdominal pain that is described as piercing/penetrating
- Pain radiating to the back
- Reported nausea and vomiting

Physical Examination

- Fever
- Tachycardia
- Shallow respirations
- Postural hypertension
- Diaphoresis

Consideration

- It can be the result of a variety of disorders including gallstones, biliary disease, alcohol abuse, cystic fibrosis, autoimmune diseases, certain heredity diseases, or as a side effect of medication administration.

Cholecystitis/Cholelithiasis

An occlusion of the bile duct due to either infection or stones. The term *cystitis* implies infection as a result of bacteria, whereas *lithiasis* refers to any obstruction as a result of stones.

History

- Affects females more than males; often occurs in the 40s
- Overweight/obese
- Acute, colicky RUQ pain with radiation to back or right shoulder or epigastric pain
- Anorexia
- Nausea and vomiting
- Sudden and rapidly intensifying pain

Physical Examination

- RUQ abdominal pain and/or epigastric pain on palpation
- Positive Murphy's sign
- Low-grade fever
- Jaundice can occur if obstruction is present

Hepatitis

An inflammatory condition of the liver that often occurs from a viral infection or, in some cases, occurs as a secondary result of medications, drugs, toxins, and alcohol. There are five types of viral hepatitis (A, B, C, D, and E). A different virus is responsible for each type of virally transmitted hepatitis. The history and physical exam findings are different based on the type of hepatitis that is contracted. The signs and symptoms in the list that follows are general for most types of hepatitis but can vary.

History

- Fatigue, flu-like symptoms
- Nausea/vomiting
- Anorexia
- Clay-colored bowel movements
- RUQ abdominal pain
- Dark urine

Physical Examination

- Jaundice
- Low-grade fever
- RUQ pain with palpation
- Palpable liver border on abdominal exam
- Abnormal liver function tests (ALT, AST, alkaline phosphatase elevations)
- Thrombocytopenia
- Jaundice
- Hepatomegaly on ultrasound

RIGHT LOWER QUADRANT PAIN: APPENDIX/ASCENDING COLON

Important to consider in the evaluation of RLQ pain is the potential for radiated or referred pain from a different site or to another part of the body. Pain referred to the back is commonly associated with RLQ pain. Always consider a female GU etiology when a female patient presents with LLQ pain. See Chapter 14, "Evidence-Based Assessment of Breasts, Female Genitalia, and Reproductive System."

Appendicitis

An inflammation of the appendix that can result from a variety of elements that can obstruct the appendix lumen and cause subsequent bacterial growth.

History

- Most common between the ages of 10 to 30 years
- Pain is initially vague and around umbilicus but migrates within hours to RLQ (LR+ = 4.81, 95% confidence interval [CI] = 3.59–6.44)
- Feeling of constipation
- Nausea/vomiting

Physical Examination

- Low-grade fever* (LR+ 3.4; 95% CI, 2.4–4.8)
- Positive McBurney's point tenderness (RLQ pain)
- Cough/hop pain (LR+ = 7.64, 95% CI = 5.94–9.83)
- Rovsing sign tenderness (LR+ = 3.52, 95% CI = 2.65–4.68)
- Rectal tenderness
- Elevated white blood cell count
- Positive Psoas sign

*Applicable for children only

Consideration

- Appendicitis is a surgical emergency and can cause significant morbidity and mortality if not identified early. Perforation, gangrene, and peritonitis can result within the first 36 hours.

Regional Ileitis/Crohn's Disease

An autoimmune, inflammatory bowel disease of the terminal ileum, characterized by a subacute or chronic necrotizing inflammation and intermittent exacerbations of mucosal inflammation and ulceration.

History

- Intermittent, cramping abdominal pain
- Severe diarrhea usually with blood, pus, and mucus
- Fatigue and malaise, arthralgias

Physical Examination

- Fever, weight loss
- Decreased hemoglobin and hematocrit
- ESR is usually high during exacerbations
- Skip lesions on colonoscopy
- Other body systems can be affected

LEFT UPPER QUADRANT PAIN: SPLEEN/ STOMACH/CARDIAC

LUQ pain can be associated with splenic, gastric, or cardiac diseases. Always rule out a cardiac etiology when a patient presents with LUQ pain. See Chapter 3, "Evidence-Based Assessment of the Heart and Circulatory System."

Perforated Colon

An opening that occurs anywhere in the intestinal tract that results in stool contents leaking into the viscera or peritoneal cavity.

History

- History of trauma, an abdominal surgery, or swallowing a foreign object (should always be a consideration in young children)
- Possible complication from various disease states such as diverticulitis, IBD, PUD, strangulated hernia, or toxic megacolon
- Reports gradual onset, but worsening, abdominal pain
- Nausea/vomiting
- Chills

Physical Examination

- Abdominal pain on palpation (location can vary based on affected area)
- Board-like abdomen distention
- Fever

Consideration

- A perforated colon is a surgical emergency.

Splenomegaly/Ruptured Spleen

Enlargement of the spleen due to infections, inflammatory diseases, or neoplasms. Motor vehicle accidents, sports injuries, and fighting are common causes of splenic rupture. Splenic rupture is a medical emergency that causes life-threatening internal bleeding.

History and Physical Findings

Splenomegaly

- Asymptomatic in some
- Pain and/or fullness in LUQ that can radiate to the left shoulder
- Fatigue
- Frequent infections
- Anemia

Splenic Rupture

- Often occurs due to blunt trauma or injury
- Reports lightheadedness and dizziness
- Sudden onset abdominal pain
- Splenomegaly and/or tenderness in LUQ on abdominal exam
- Hemodynamic instability
- Confusion

LEFT LOWER QUADRANT PAIN: DESCENDING COLON

LLQ pain is usually associated with diseases originating in the descending colon or sigmoid colon region.

Sigmoid Diverticulosis/Diverticulitis

Diverticulosis is the herniation or out-pouching of the walls of the colon. This herniation creates small pouches. When these pouches fill with food particles, or feces, it causes inflammation and/or the bacteria count to increase, causing infection.

History

- LLQ pain, occasionally abdominal pain can be in RLQ
- History of chronic constipation or, less commonly, diarrhea
- Nausea/vomiting

Physical Examination

- Fever
- Tenderness to the LLQ abdominal quadrant with palpation
- Leukocytosis

Ulcerative Colitis

An autoimmune disorder that can affect any area of the large colon that is characterized by intermittent inflammation and ulceration of the colon mucosal lining.

History

- Periods of exacerbations and remissions
- Urgency when having bowel movement
- Abdominal pain, often in the LLQ
- Diarrhea with blood or pus
- Other systems can be affected (symptoms include arthralgias, eye irritation, rashes)

Physical Examination

- Weight loss
- LLQ abdominal pain with palpation
- Rectal pain and bleeding
- Anemia
- Stool cultures have white blood cells
- Colonoscopy shows cobblestoning
- In severe cases, signs of systemic toxicity including fever, tachycardia, anemia, elevated ESR, and rapid weight loss

PERIUMBILICAL/EPIGASTRIC PAIN: STOMACH/TRANSVERSE COLON/AORTA

Epigastric or periumbilical pain is a very common concern of discomfort stemming from digestive structures but cardiac differentials should always be considered.

Abdominal Aortic Aneurysm

AAA should be considered and ruled out when abdominal pain is in the epigastric area as it can be a life-threatening condition. See Chapter 3, "Evidence-Based Assessment of the Heart and Circulatory System."

Celiac Disease

An autoimmune disorder with strong genetic predisposition where the ingestion of gluten leads to damage of the small intestinal wall, eventually leading to malabsorption of all nutrients.

History

- Constipation, diarrhea, bloating, flatulence
- Depression
- Fatigue
- More than half the adults with celiac disease have signs and symptoms unrelated to the digestive system, including arthralgias; loss of bone density (osteoporosis) or softening of bone (osteomalacia); itchy, blistery skin rash (dermatitis herpetiformis); mouth ulcers; headaches and fatigue; nervous system injury, including numbness and tingling in the feet and hands, possible problems with balance, and cognitive impairment.

Physical Examination

- Weight loss
- Iron-deficiency anemia
- Pain with palpation of the abdomen (diffuse or in the epigastric region)

Consideration

- Children with celiac disease are more likely than adults to have digestive problems.

GERD/Dyspepsia

A condition in which stomach acid flows back into the esophagus due to the inadequate closure of the lower esophageal sphincter. It is often called *heartburn, ingestion, reflux,* or *sour stomach*.

History

- A burning sensation in the chest (heartburn), usually after eating; symptoms are worse at night with laying supine; worse after meals and with certain foods and medications
- Chest pain
- Difficulty swallowing, globus sensation
- Abdominal bloating, regurgitation of food or sour liquid
- Certain medications: Theophylline, dopamine, diazepam, calcium channel blockers, anticholinergics, and opioids
- Triggers may include caffeine, alcohol, chocolate, or fatty foods
- Relieved with antacids
- Tobacco use
- Pregnancy
- Hiatal hernia

Physical Examination

- Pain with palpation of epigastric area
- Negative *H. Pylori* test
- Cough, hoarseness

Irritable Bowel Syndrome

A functional bowel (motility) disorder characterized by intermittent, mild to severe abdominal pain with a change in bowel habits.

History

- Recurrent abdominal pain, at least 1 day/week in the last 3 months, with an altered bowel pattern
- Diarrhea, constipation, alternating diarrhea and constipation
- Bowel movements generally occur during waking hours, most often in the morning or after meals
- Abdominal bloating, increased gas production (belching and/or flatulence)
- Exacerbated with emotional stress and/or eating
- Abdominal pain relieved with defecation
- Periods of exacerbations and remissions
- Mucus in the stool
- History of food intolerances or sensitivities

Physical Examination

- Diffuse abdominal pain with palpation

Considerations

- The cause is unknown but can be associated with other conditions; celiac disease, parasitic infection, or inflammatory bowel diseases.
- The Rome IV criteria are the most widely used diagnostic criteria.

Peptic Ulcer Disease

An inflammation and ultimate ulceration of the stomach or duodenal lining.

History

- History of chronic use of NSAIDs
- Asymptomatic in some
- Abdominal pain, often in epigastric region, but can be in the LUQ or RUQ of the abdomen
- Pain described as gnawing or burning; can radiate to back; worsens with immediate food intake (gastric) or 2 to 5 hours after food intake (duodenal)
- Heartburn, belching, bloating, nausea

Physical Examination

- Pain with palpation of epigastric area of abdomen
- Positive guaiac test and *H. pylori* testing
- Gastroduodenal lesions found on endoscopy

Considerations

- Some patients may initially present only with complications like GI bleeding, gastric outlet obstruction, fistulas, and perforation.
- In rare cases, PUD can be due to Zollinger–Ellison syndrome.

Peritonitis

An inflammation to the peritoneal lining of the abdomen as a result of bacterial infection from a perforation in the bowel or as a result of surgical contamination.

History

- History of advanced cirrhosis
- Diffuse abdominal pain

Physical Examination

- Fever
- Guarding; rebound tenderness

- Rigidity and distention of abdomen
- Altered mental state
- Leukocytosis

Consideration

- Spontaneous bacterial peritonitis primarily occurs in patients with advanced cirrhosis. It usually manifests with severe abdominal pain and is considered a medical emergency, requiring immediate intervention. If it is not found early in the course of infection, shock ensues, rapidly followed by multisystem organ failure.

Small Bowel Obstruction

A condition that occurs when the normal flow of intraluminal contents is interrupted, causing partial or complete blockage of GI contents.

History

- History of previous abdominal surgery, postoperative adhesions, and hernias
- Stools that have decreased in diameter and frequency
- Abrupt onset of periumbilical abdominal pain; paroxysmal, cramping abdominal pain
- Nausea/vomiting
- Abdominal distention
- Obstipation

Physical Examination

- Dehydration, causing tachycardia, orthostatic hypotension, and reduced urine output
- Abdominal/inguinal hernias on exam

ABNORMAL FINDINGS OF THE URINARY SYSTEM

LOWER URINARY TRACT INFECTION

Infection of the lower urinary tract including the bladder and urethras.

History

- Women are more often affected, older adults can be more susceptible
- Sexually active
- Having a urinary catheter
- Incomplete bladder emptying due to an enlarged prostate, prolapsed bladder or uterus, kidney stones, or pregnancy

- Dysuria (pain is often worse at the end of urination); nocturia
- Urinary frequency or urgency
- Suprapubic or lower back pain

Physical Examination

- Gross hematuria
- Appearance of turbid urine
- Low-grade fever
- Urethral discharge (primarily in men)
- Mild abdominal tenderness over bladder with palpation
- No CVA tenderness
- Positive nitrites, pyuria, and hematuria on urinalysis (sensitivity of 74.02%)
- Positive urine culture result

Consideration

- Gram-negative organisms are most commonly the causative agent in UTIs with strains of *E. coli* accounting for the majority of cases.

PYELONEPHRITIS

An inflammation and infection of the upper urinary tract involving the renal pelvis and kidney.

History

- History of untreated lower UTI
- Sudden onset of systemic symptoms (fever, chills, malaise)
- Urinary frequency or urgency; dysuria
- Unilateral flank pain; abdominal pain
- Nausea/vomiting

Physical Examination

- Gross hematuria
- Unilateral CVA tenderness
- Enlarged kidney (palpable on exam)
- Urinalysis showing pyuria, bacteriuria, and nitrites
- White blood cell casts on microscopy
- Urine culture (>10,000 colony-forming units of a uropathogen/mL)

Considerations

- An infection of the upper urinary tract is more severe and can have more serious implications than an infection of the lower urinary tract.
- Acute pyelonephritis will classically present as a triad of fever, unilateral flank pain, and nausea or vomiting, but not all symptoms have to be present.

RENAL COLIC (UROLITHIASIS, URETEROLITHIASIS)

An obstructing calculus (renal/kidney stone) within the urinary system that causes severe pain.

History

- Sudden-onset, unilateral, severe pain in the flank
- Intermittent, colicky pain (comes in waves and fluctuates in intensity)
- Pain can radiate to the lower abdomen, groin, or genitals
- Nausea/vomiting
- Urinary frequency or urgency; dysuria
- Low voided volumes (distal ureteric stones)

Physical Examination

- Positive CVA tenderness
- Pink, red, or brown urine
- Tachycardia
- Patient often paces and is constantly moving due to pain
- Microscopic hematuria

Considerations

- The pain from renal colic is caused by dilation, stretching, and spasm of the ureters.
- Most kidney stones are formed from calcium oxalate. Kidney stones are treated in different ways depending on the location and size of the stones.

URINARY INCONTINENCE

The involuntary leakage of urine. The four main types of incontinence are: stress incontinence, urge incontinence, overflow incontinence, and functional incontinence. There can be overlap of two or more of these conditions called mixed incontinence. See **Table 12.2** for the Historical Symptom Assessment tool.

History

- **Stress incontinence**: History of vaginal childbirth; being overweight or obese; history of pelvic prolapse; pregnancy; loss of urine when sneezing, laughing, coughing, jumping, exercising, or increasing abdominal pressure
- **Urge incontinence**: History of neurological disease or injury, history of diabetes, urinary frequency, intense urinary urgency immediately followed by the involuntary loss of urine
- **Overflow incontinence**: History of benign prostatic hypertrophy, neurogenic bladder, diabetes, or any other condition that can damage the nerves or bladder; constant or frequent dribbling of urine

TABLE 12.2 Urinary Incontinence: Historical Symptom Assessment

	Types of Incontinence			
Symptom	**Stress**	**Urge**	**Mixed**	**Overflow**
Leak with cough, sneeze, exercise	+	–	+	–
Leak with urgency	–	+	+	–
Frequent urination	–	+	+	–
Continuous leakage	–	–	–	+

- **Functional incontinence**: Dementia, disabilities related to mobility, history of arthritis, diuretic medications, any physical or mental impairment that causes difficulty in effectively getting to the bathroom

Physical Examination

- Exam findings can be highly variable based on the individual, their medical/surgical history, and the type of incontinence they are experiencing.

PHYSICAL EXAMINATION DOCUMENTATION

Documentation should include results of inspection, auscultation, percussion, palpation, and special tests (if applicable).

EXAMPLE OF NORMAL FINDINGS

Abdomen is flat. No visible pulsations, masses, or distention. Skin is without rashes, lesions, ecchymoses, or scars. No bruits over aorta, renal, or femoral arteries. Tympany noted on percussion and abdomen is non-tender to light and deep palpation of all four quadrants. No splenomegaly or hepatomegaly. No inguinal lymphadenopathy. Right and left kidneys are nonpalpable. No CVA tenderness bilateral.

EXAMPLE OF ABNORMAL FINDINGS

Abdomen appears slightly distended. No visible pulsations or masses. Skin is without rashes, lesions, ecchymoses, or scars. No bruits over aorta, renal, or femoral arteries. Tympany noted on percussion over gastric bubble. Patient exhibits abdominal guarding upon the start of palpation. Abdomen is tender to light palpation, which triggers tenderness at the right lower quadrant between the iliac crest and umbilicus (McBurney's point). Unable to tolerate deep palpation. Muscle rigidity noted, positive rebound tenderness, and Rovsing sign. Positive psoas test, positive heel drop test. No splenomegaly or hepatomegaly. No inguinal lymphadenopathy. Kidneys nonpalpable, nontender with direct percussion.

REFERENCES

References for this chapter draw from Chapter 16, "Evidence-Based Assessment of the Abdominal, Gastrointestinal, and Urological Systems," of the textbook *Evidence-Based Physical Examination: Best Practices for Health and Well-Being Assessment*. The references may be accessed in the digital version of the handbook at https://connect.springerpub.com/content/book/97808-0-8261-6466-7/chapter/ch12

13

Evidence-Based Assessment of Male Genitalia, Prostate, Rectum, and Anus

CLINICAL CONSIDERATIONS

- Owing to the personal nature of discussions about sexual and reproductive health, there are populations who are vulnerable to disparities in care related to implicit or unconscious bias and/or related to reluctance to share information for fear of bias. Care should be taken to provide sensitive assessment and counseling for individuals with respect for gender identity and sexual orientation.
- Gender identity can be determined only by the individual; therefore, it is imperative that individuals be given the opportunity to provide their preferred name and gender pronouns. Correct gender pronouns and the name that the patient chooses to use must be used during all encounters with each patient.
- Sexual orientation must be assessed to determine what preventive care should be recommended and/or what specific health risks an individual may have.
- Maintain neutrality in history taking with all patients to ensure that individuals are not misidentified (gender identify or sexual orientation), which limits the quality of the history, and creates barriers to care. Gender and ethnic disparities are significant related to men's health and wellness.
- As part of a well visit, assess for normal functioning of GU and reproductive systems, health maintenance, and health-promotion needs.

- Clinical examination of the adult male genitalia is not typically done as part of routine wellness examinations. However, a thorough examination is done for any individual presenting with GU concerns. In addition, genital exams should be performed during all infant and child wellness examinations, with a caregiver present.
- Male GU and anogenital conditions may be inflammatory, infectious, neoplastic, or traumatic in nature, or can be associated with developmental changes. For example, sexual function and testosterone levels wane during older adulthood; the prostate enlarges throughout a man's lifetime.

SUBJECTIVE HISTORY

COMMON REASONS FOR SEEKING CARE

- Reproductive health and/or sexual health concerns, including exposure to sexually transmitted infections, penile discharge, or lesions; pubic area rash/itching
- Scrotal pain, swelling, or lesions
- Inguinal or groin swelling

HISTORY OF PRESENT ILLNESS

- **Onset:** When did symptoms start? Are symptoms recent? How did symptoms begin?
- **Location:** Specific location of symptoms?
- **Duration:** Are symptoms persistent or transitory? Increasing or unchanged?
- **Characteristics:** How would you describe the symptoms? Is there itching, burning, discharge, pain, swelling, bruising, or redness?
- **Aggravating factors:** Worse with exercise, movement, activity, or straining? Are symptoms associated with sexual activity?
- **Relieving factors:** What actions or activities decrease the symptoms?
- **Treatment:** What medications has the individual taken to help with the symptoms? Clarify dosage and frequency of OTC and prescribed medications.
- **Severity:** How severe are the symptoms on a scale of 0 to 10?

HEALTH HISTORY

Clinicians who establish trust, remain open-minded, and are careful about using unassuming language find that patients willingly share the information needed to provide evidence-based, sensitive, high-quality care that supports their health and well-being.

Script for Health History Assessment

Key health and well-being assessments pertinent to sexual orientation and gender identity, including past medical history, family, and social history, are included in the script that follows. This script can be adapted for age and gender identity and is provided for assessment practice. Note that the information being assessed includes all components of a health history.

Hello, my name is _____. How do you like to be addressed?
All individuals should have the opportunity to state their name and preferred pronouns.

Tell me about your health history. Have you ever been diagnosed with a chronic condition? Have you had surgery? Any hospitalizations? Do you take any prescribed medications? Over-the-counter medications?
Assessing past medical and surgical history should be conducted in a similar way for all patients, regardless of sexual orientation and/or gender identity.

Where do you live? Does anyone live in the home with you? Is your housing safe and stable?
Assessing social determinants of health is imperative, especially for individuals who identify with vulnerable minority groups.

To understand whether you have any inherited health risks, could you tell me about your biological parents' health? Any cancers, heart disease, diabetes . . . ?
It may be important to ask specifically about genetic relationships, as many LGBTQ+ people have chosen families that are not genetically related.

How is your relationship with your family of origin? Are they supportive of you? Who are your best supports?
Assessing family and social support systems is a key component of health assessment.

Do you now or have you ever smoked tobacco? Do you drink alcohol? Any past or present drug use?
Screening all patients for tobacco, alcohol, and drug use is an evidence-based priority.

Tell me about your gender identity.
It is important to allow the person the space to explain their identity to you, but you may need to ask specifically whether the person identifies as female, male, nonbinary, or some other description.
These follow up questions are especially important for nonbinary, transgender, and gender fluid individuals:

Tell me about your gender journey. When did you first realize your identity differed from your sex assigned at birth? What steps have you taken to affirm your gender identity?
Allow the individual to share their history. Options include, but are not limited to, using a different name and/or gender pronoun, as well as changes in physical appearance, medical treatment, and/or surgical treatment; include dates of initiation of medical treatments such as puberty suppressors and hormones.

What organs were present at birth?
An organ inventory should be done to determine what organs the person has or had, including breast tissue, cervix, uterus, ovaries, penis, testes, prostate, and so forth. It should be performed for all patients, as cisgender people may also have had surgeries that alter their reproductive organs.

What organs are present currently?
Assess for surgical removal of the cervix, uterus, ovaries, breast tissue, penis, and testes.

Are organs enhanced with hormones?
Clitoral tissue, breast tissue

Are organs enhanced with surgery?
Breast augmentation, vaginoplasty, facial feminization, metoidioplasty, phalloplasty, testicular implants

Have you shared your identity with friends? Family? Partners? School? Work?
Responses to these questions provide information related to social, family, community, and professional support and/or concerns.

Do you have safe access to bathroom facilities?
Urinary stasis from holding the bladder for extended periods of time is a risk factor for UTIs. Also assess safety in environment.

Do you tuck?
Tucking is the process of moving the penis and testes between the legs to conceal the organs; this may be accomplished by wearing tight clothing or using some type of binder or strap. Sometimes, the testes are pressed up into the inguinal canal, risking incarceration/strangulation. *Escherichia coli* UTIs are more common in individuals who tuck.

Do you bind?
Binding is the process of flattening breast tissue so that the chest appears more masculine. This is typically achieved with medical-grade binders and can cause fungal infections and skin breakdown.

Do you need help changing legal documents to align with your identity?

Know where to refer patients, such as www.lambdalegal.org

Are you sexually active? Do you have a regular partner?

Sexual health screening is a key assessment for all individuals.

How do you identify sexually?

If the person does not understand, provide options, such as, "Do you identify as straight, gay, lesbian, bisexual, or something else?"

In order to know which screenings would benefit you, can you tell me with whom you have sex? What parts of your body do you use when having sex? How do your partners identify their gender and sexual orientation?

If the person does not understand, provide options, such as, "Do you have sex with women, men, both? Are your partners cisgendered? Do you participate in oral sex (receptive/insertive), oral–vaginal contact, oral–anal contact, anal sex (receptive/insertive), vaginal sex (receptive/insertive)? Do you use shared sex toys or have any type of genital-to-genital contact?" Note: For individuals who identify as transgender, it may be important to first ask about "triggering" labels for body parts; for example, an individual who identifies as transgender male may prefer to use the term *frontal canal* instead of *vagina*, and may find that the term *vagina* triggers feelings of gender dysphoria. Reflecting preferred labels or terms within sexual health history questions is most appropriate.

Are you in a relationship?

Not all people who are sexually active, even with regular partners, are in a relationship, and a relationship is not always exclusively between two people.

Is your relationship open or closed?

Some relationships have consensual agreements that partners have other sexual partners outside of the relationship. Some relationships are between multiple people, rather than two.

Are you satisfied with your sexual function?

Key assessment for all individuals.

How do you protect yourself from STIs?

If using barrier protection such as condoms, ask, "Do you wear protection 100% of the time? Are barriers used for oral–genital contact?"

When was the last time you had STI screening?

Key assessment related to sexual health for all individuals.

Do you use drugs or alcohol when having sex? Do you exchange sex for money, drugs, or a place to stay?
These questions are intended to identify behaviors and situations that increase risks to health and well-being.

Do you desire to have biological children? Do you desire pregnancy?
For transgender patients, also ask whether they desire to have preserved fertility, such as cryopreservation of sperm and eggs, prior to starting hormonal or surgical transition. This issue is especially complicated in individuals on puberty blockers as they are never exposed to natal hormones necessary for gamete development.

Have you felt isolated, trapped, or like you are walking on eggshells in an intimate relationship? Has someone pressured or forced you to do something sexual that you didn't want to do? Has someone hit, kicked, punched, or otherwise hurt you?
Screen for intimate partner violence, as well as past and/or current history of physical, sexual, emotional, economic, or verbal abuse.

REVIEW OF SYSTEMS

- **General/dermatologic:** Recent illness, weight loss, lesions or rashes, fever, chills
- **HEENT:** Oral lesions, eye drainage or redness, pharyngitis
- **Lymphatic:** Lymphadenopathy, tender lymph nodes in groin area
- **CV/respiratory:** Chest pain, edema, dyspnea, cough
- **GI:** Localized pain, change in bowel habits, blood in the stool, pain with defecation, dyschezia
- **GU:** Urinary frequency, dysuria, weak urinary stream, "dribbling," urinary frequency, nocturia, hematuria, rectal bleeding, rectal pain, anal itching
- **MSK**: Back pain, myalgias
- **Neurologic/mental health**: Worry; sadness, helplessness, hopelessness; fatigue or insomnia; change in mood, stress, coping; healthy lifestyle behaviors

RED FLAGS IN SUBJECTIVE HISTORY

- Testicular torsion occurs when a testicle rotates, twisting the spermatic cord and causing ischemia. Emergency surgery is required to preserve the viability of the testicle. **Box 13.1** includes a summary list of symptoms.

BOX 13.1 Red Flags in Subjective History That Indicate Possible Testicular Torsion

- Sudden onset of testicular pain and swelling
- Transverse testicular lie
- Nausea, vomiting
- Acute abdominal pain (which may be the presenting symptom in children and adolescents)

PHYSICAL EXAMINATION

- Maintain patient modesty by exposing the patient's groin and anogenital region only as required.
- Genital examination can be performed with patient supine or sitting; ideal approach is patient standing with clinician in a sitting position to best assess for hernia or testicular abnormalities.
- Anorectal examination can be performed with the male in a side-lying position with hips and knees flexed.

INSPECTION

- Inspect the skin of the groin, pubis, penis, scrotum, and perineum for rashes, lesions, discoloration, or swelling. Note whether penis is circumcised or uncircumcised. When adults present with GU concerns, retract the prepuce (foreskin) of the uncircumcised penis to inspect the glans and urethral meatus. Phimosis, inability to retract the foreskin, is normal during infancy and childhood and should not be forcefully retracted.
- Gently compress the glans penis between the thumb and first finger to inspect for patency, inflammation, or urethral discharge.
- Following the genital examination, inspect the anus for skin tags, fissures, hemorrhoids, or other skin lesions.

PALPATION

- Palpate the shaft of the penis for nodules, plaques, or other soft-tissue masses. The index or middle finger of the clinician's hand should be placed posteriorly while the thumb of the same hand is placed anteriorly.

- Testis should be gently palpated for nodules, hard masses, and abnormal shape. A normal testis should feel smooth, ovoid, and nontender. Palpate the epididymis along the posterior aspect of the testis and up along the spermatic cord. Note any swelling or soft tissue masses within the scrotal sac, epididymis, or spermatic cord.
- Palpate inguinal nodes for enlargement and/or tenderness, especially when evaluating for concern of infection or malignancy of the genitalia.

ADDITIONAL ASSESSMENTS FOR SPECIFIC CONDITIONS

Cremasteric Reflex

- Attempt to elicit the cremasteric reflex when evaluating for certain testicular concerns that cause scrotal pain. The reflex is triggered by stroking the inner thigh with the index and middle finger. An intact reflex will cause the ipsilateral cremaster muscle to contract, thereby raising the testis. In some conditions, like testicular torsion, the cremasteric reflex will be negative because the cremaster muscles surrounding the spermatic cord are twisted and unable to contract.
- The absence of the cremasteric reflex for patients presenting with scrotal pain is a useful sign, indicating the need for emergent evaluation.

Transillumination

- Transillumination evaluates the scrotal sac for concerns such as scrotal swelling. Perform the procedure by dimming the lights of the exam room and shining a bright light (e.g., penlight, otoscope) through the wall of the scrotum. Fluid will illuminate; soft tissue masses will not.

Assessment for Hernia

- A hernia is a protrusion of a body organ through the wall of the cavity that contains it.
- An inguinal hernia occurs when there is a fascial defect in the inguinal canal that allows bowel to protrude through the deep inguinal ring (indirect inguinal hernia; **Figure 13.1A**) and sometimes through the superficial inguinal ring (direct inguinal hernia; **Figure 13.1B**).
- When bowel protrudes through the deep inguinal ring and becomes entrapped, it is considered an *incarcerated inguinal hernia*. If the bowel cannot be reduced (pushed back into the abdominal

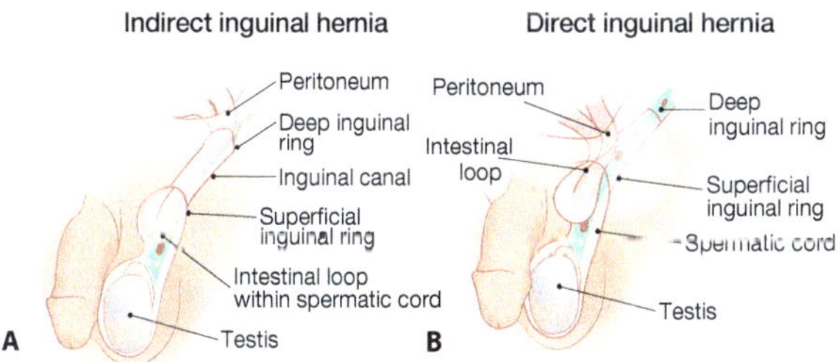

FIGURE 13.1 Inguinal hernias. (**A**) Indirect. (**B**) Direct.

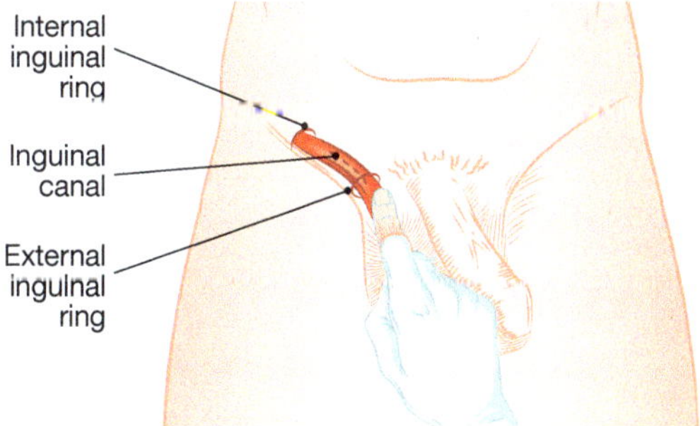

FIGURE 13.2 Technique for assessing inguinal hernias.

cavity), emergent surgery is required to preserve viability of the bowel. A femoral hernia, or direct inguinal hernia, enters the inguinal canal via a defect inferior to the deep inguinal ring.

- The examination for inguinal hernia should be performed with patient in standing position and clinician in a seated position facing the patient. With a gloved index or middle finger, gather loose skin from the scrotum and invaginate the scrotal sac with the finger upward along the inguinal canal until the external ring is reached (**Figure 13.2**).
- Ask the patient to cough or bear down as when making a bowel movement. If a hernia is present, a bulging sensation can be

palpated/felt at the tip of the finger. While the patient bears down, also observe the inguinal area for bulging over the femoral canal that can indicate a femoral hernia.

Digital Rectal Examination

- DRE can be performed to evaluate the lower rectum and prostate. DRE is typically performed for concerns of unexplained blood in the stool, abnormal mass in the anus or rectum, significant change in bowel or bladder habits, change in urinary stream, and/or urethral discharge or bleeding. Otherwise, DRE is not performed as a routine element of male wellness examinations.
- Patient should be unclothed from the waist down and in a gown and/or covered with a drape. Ideal positioning for the examination is either with the male standing with a forward bend at the waist or side-lying with knees to chest. Separate the buttocks and inspect for fissures, hemorrhoids, bleeding, skin tags, and rashes.
- Lubricate index or middle finger of a gloved hand. Inform the patient that a finger will be inserted into the rectum. Ask the patient to take a deep breath and relax and breathe out while gently inserting the examining finger into the anal canal.
- Palpate prostate anteriorly, noting size, symmetry, and texture. A normal prostate is walnut-sized, symmetrical, and smooth with a cartilaginous texture (similar to the tip of the nose). The prostate has a midline groove (sulcus) that should be palpable. The proximity of the prostate to the rectum during a DRE is depicted in **Figure 13.3**.
- Rotate finger 360 degrees to palpate the span of the rectal wall for masses or irregularities. Stool may be palpated in the rectal vault; note consistency (hard or soft). Assess anal tone by asking patient to tighten their anal sphincter on the finger. Once patient relaxes, withdraw the finger and inspect for blood, stool, or mucus. Re-drape the patient, provide tissues or cleansing cloths, and allow privacy so the patient can clean up and get dressed.

PEDIATRIC CONSIDERATIONS

- The anogenital examination of the infant or child should be performed with a caregiver present. If the caregiver is unable to be present, another healthcare clinician (chaperone) should be present. Some states have mandatory chaperone laws; it is important for clinicians to know their respective state laws. For adolescents, a chaperone can be a caregiver or another healthcare clinician, but this should be the adolescent's choice.

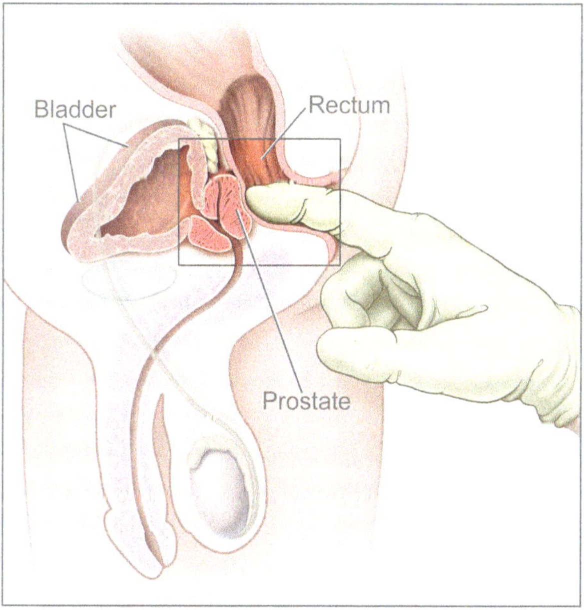

FIGURE 13.3 Digital rectal examination, including examination of the prostate.

- Routine GU exams should be performed during all infant and child wellness exams. The foreskin of uncircumcised newborns and young infants may be tightly adhered to the glans penis and should never be forcefully retracted. The newborn exam, in particular, should include inspection for congenital malformations, ambiguous genitalia, and placement and patency of the anus.
- The clinician should palpate the scrotal sac for soft tissue masses to ensure that both testes have descended and can be brought down into the lower third of the scrotal sac. If the testis cannot be palpated in the scrotum, the clinician should palpate the inguinal canal and upper scrotal sac for the testis. Some testes are "retractile," meaning they can move between the inguinal canal and scrotum. A retractile testis can be located and brought down into the lower third of the scrotum. Retractile testes should resolve by puberty.

- For adolescents, the genital examination can produce anxiety. Adolescents can be unsure whether their developing bodies are "normal," and they have a greater need for modesty and privacy. Assessment of adolescent genitalia is similar to that for adults, except the clinician should assess for sexual maturity (Tanner staging) while inspecting the genitalia. The sexual maturity rating for preadolescent and adolescent males uses a scale from 1 (prepubertal) to 5 (adult-like), based on changes in pubic hair distribution and growth of the penis and testes. The Tanner stages are:

  1. Testes more than 2.5 cm, no change in penis size, no pubic hair
  2. Enlargement of testes, pigmentation of scrotal sac; no change in penis size; pubic hair is long, downy, and variable in pattern
  3. Further enlargement of testes; significant enlargement of penis, especially in diameter; increase in amount and curling of pubic hair
  4. Further enlargement of testes and penis, pubic hair is adult in type but not distribution, development of axillary and facial hair begins
  5. Testes and penis are adult in size, pubic hair is adult in distribution, body hair continues to grow, overall growth (height/weight/muscle) velocity peaks

CONSIDERATIONS FOR OLDER ADULTS

- Although DRE may be a component of screening for prostate cancer, men >50 who are at average risk, >45 at high risk, and >40 at the highest risk (with more than one first-degree relative with prostate cancer at an early age) should discuss PSA testing with their primary care clinician.
- Recommendations must be individualized and evidence-based, as new recommendations about life expectancy and risks become available.

RED FLAGS IN OBJECTIVE EXAM

- Patients who present with urinary symptoms, including dysuria, frequency, straining, hesitancy, or urgency of urination, urinary incontinence, and/or erectile dysfunction should have an exam to evaluate for GU disorders, including bladder cancer, testicular cancer, prostatitis, and prostate cancer. Red flags indicating serious urologic disorders are listed in **Box 13.2**.

BOX 13.2 Red Flags in Objective Exam That Are Indications of Serious Urologic Disorders

- Hematuria
- Palpable bladder
- Fever and flank pain or tenderness
- Penile discharge and/or lesions
- Painless testicular lump
- Exquisite tenderness of a testicle
- Exquisite tenderness of the prostate
- Nodularity of the prostate
- Loss of anal reflex
- Loss of cremasteric reflex
- Loss of bowel or bladder control

EVIDENCE-BASED RESOURCES

- **American Cancer Society:** www.cancer.org
- **American Psychological Association:** www.apa.org/pi/lgbt/resources/guidelines
- **American Urological Association:** www.auanet.org/guidelines
- **Center of Excellence for Transgender Health:** http://transhealth.ucsf.edu/trans?page=guidelines-home
- **Centers for Disease Control and Prevention:** www.cdc.gov/std/tg2015/default.htm
- **Choosing Wisely Campaign:** www.choosingwisely.org
- **U.S. Preventive Services Task Force:** www.uspreventiveservicestaskforce.org

ABNORMAL FINDINGS

CONGENITAL OR DEVELOPMENTAL ABNORMALITIES

Anorectal Agenesis/Imperforate Anus

Congenital anorectal malformation in which there is an absence of or abnormal location of the anal opening. Not always readily evident on exam, the key finding is failure of the newborn to pass meconium within the first 24 to 48 hours following birth. Imperforate anus can be part of a cluster of findings of a more complex congenital syndrome. Surgical correction is required.

Epispadias and Hypospadias

Hypospadias is a congenital malformation of the male GU tract in which the urethral opening is abnormally located on the ventral aspect of the penis. Similarly, but less commonly, epispadias is an abnormal dorsal placement of the urethral meatus.

History

- Abnormal spraying during urination

Physical Examination

- Urethral meatus located on the glans, penile shaft, scrotum, or perineum

Consideration

- Severity varies

Hydrocele

A collection of peritoneal fluid in the scrotal sac resulting from a fascial defect in the inguinal canal. All males have this defect at some point during gestation, but when it persists, it allows peritoneal fluid to travel back and forth. This can be normal up to age 1 to 2 years.

History

- Painless scrotal swelling (unilateral or bilateral) that may fluctuate in size

Physical Examination

- Transillumination of the scrotum can be helpful for diagnosis. Peritoneal fluid will illuminate in the scrotal sac, while bowel tissue will not.

Considerations

- Hydroceles that persist beyond age 1 to 2 years require surgical correction.
- In older children and adults, a hydrocele can be idiopathic or develop secondary to infection, inflammation, trauma, or malignancy.

Phimosis/Paraphimosis

Phimosis is a condition in which the foreskin of an uncircumcised penis cannot be retracted over the glans. This condition can be physiologic or pathologic. Physiologic phimosis occurs in almost all newborn males due to naturally occurring adhesions between the foreskin and glans penis. The adhesions spontaneously resolve over time with intermittent erections and foreskin retraction. Physiologic phimosis is expected to resolve prior to puberty, but usually by age 3. Key findings of physiologic phimosis can vary from an inability to retract the foreskin far enough to view the urethral meatus to an inability to retract the foreskin fully past the corona of the glans penis. Pathological phimosis is acquired as a result of distal scarring of the prepuce due to infection or inflammation. The key finding is a contracted fibrous ring around the opening of the distal prepuce with an inability to retract the foreskin. Pathological phimosis requires medical treatment. Paraphimosis is a condition that results from forcefully retracting tight foreskin back over the glans penis. The foreskin becomes entrapped behind the corona of the glans. Key signs and symptoms include painful swelling of the distal glans penis with a constricted band of tissue proximal to the corona. Paraphimosis is a medical emergency because it will eventually result in tissue ischemia and necrosis.

Testicular Torsion

Occurs when a testicle rotates, twisting the spermatic cord and causing ischemia.

History

- Review "red flags" listed in Box 13.1
- Symptoms include sudden onset of testicular pain and swelling

Physical Examination

- Absent cremasteric reflex
- Transverse lie

Consideration

- Medical emergency, can result in testicular ischemia within 6 to 12 hours

Undescended Testes

History

- Testis fails to descend into the lower third of the scrotum by 4 months of age.

Physical Examination

- Testis may be located in the intra-abdominal space (cryptorchidism), the inguinal canal, or the upper third of the scrotum.

Consideration

- Surgical correction is required to preserve fertility and decrease risk of testicular cancer.

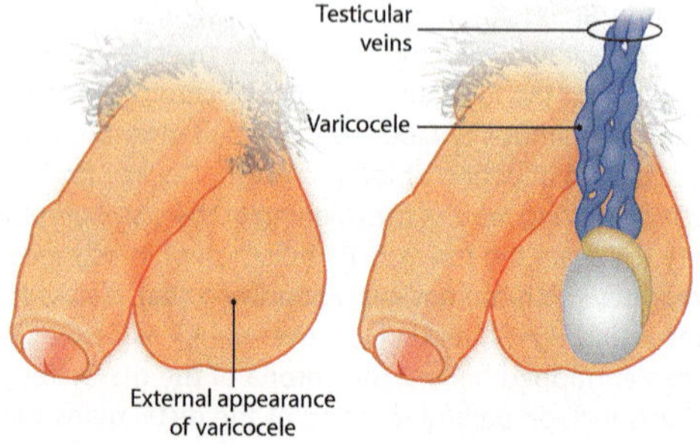

FIGURE 13.4 Varicocele.

Varicocele

A collection of dilated twisted veins surrounding the spermatic cord that typically occurs in the left hemiscrotum.

History

- Scrotal sac has "bag of worms" texture and appearance (**Figure 13.4**).
- Most are asymptomatic, but some will present with a dull ache.

Physical Examination

- Palpable testicular veins worsen with increased venous pressure (e.g., standing or performing Valsalva)

Consideration

- Does not require intervention unless there is atrophy of the testicle, which can lead to infertility

INFECTION OR INFLAMMATORY DISORDERS

Balanitis and Balanoposthitis

Balanitis describes an inflammation of the glans penis, while balanoposthitis describes an inflammation of the glans penis and foreskin in uncircumcised males. Key signs and symptoms can include genital itching, pain, dysuria, exudate, erythema, swelling of glans or the foreskin, foul odor, and phimosis. Causes include poor hygiene and infectious agents like STIs and other bacterial, fungal, and viral organisms.

Epididymitis, Orchitis, and Scrotal Cellulitis

Acute epididymitis is a clinical syndrome involving pain, swelling, and inflammation of the epididymis that can last up to 6 weeks. When the testis is also affected, it is referred to as *epididymo-orchitis* or *orchitis*. Scrotal cellulitis of the scrotum is an infection of the dermis of the scrotal tissue, which occurs from bacterial entry via a break in the integrity of the epidermal barrier. Scrotal cellulitis presents with scrotal pain, swelling, and inflammation (**Figure 13.5**). Urgent medical treatment is required to prevent an abscess or gangrene.

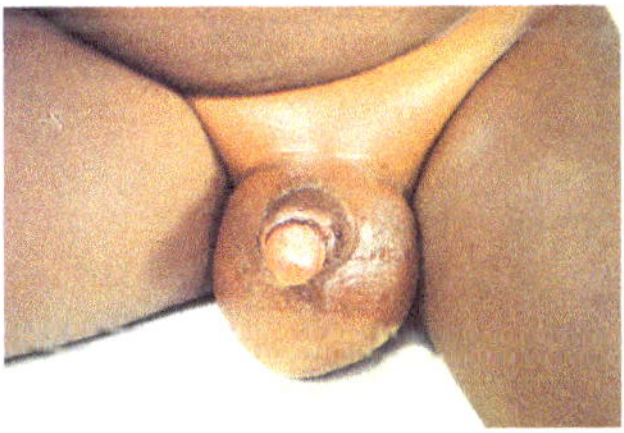

FIGURE 13.5 Scrotal cellulitis.
Source: Centers for Disease Control and Prevention/Robert S. Craig.

Male Genital Candidiasis

History

- Itchy genital rash caused by fungal or yeast infection

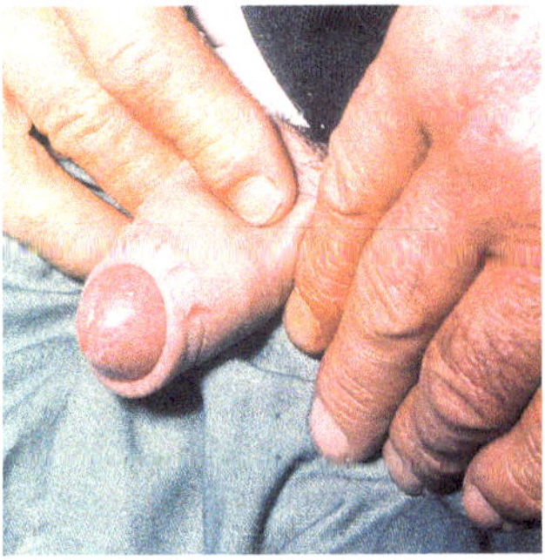

FIGURE 13.6 Male genital candidiasis.
Source: Centers for Disease Control and Prevention/Brian Hill.

Physical Examination

- Potentially fissured, erythematous rash (**Figure 13.6**)
- White, curd-like exudate is possible, especially in uncircumcised males
- Can affect the glans, foreskin, scrotum, thighs, gluteal folds, and buttocks

Consideration

- More common among men with diabetes, uncircumcised males, and males with female sex partners with recurrent vaginal yeast infections

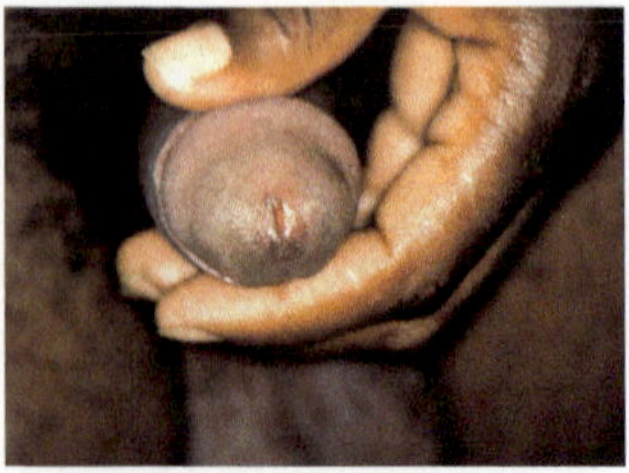

FIGURE 13.7 Nonspecific urethritis.

Nonspecific Urethritis

Urethritis describes an inflammation of the urethra. Urethritis can be caused by chemical irritants but is often a common indicator of STIs in males.

History

- Dysuria, itching, burning, and/or discharge
- Associated with unprotected sex; sexual activity with new partner

Physical Examination

- Erythema and/or discharge at the urethral meatus, which can be clear or purulent (**Figure 13.7**).

Considerations

- Purulent penile discharge is often associated with chlamydia and/or gonorrhea
- Although secondary causes may exist, infectious organisms are the most common cause

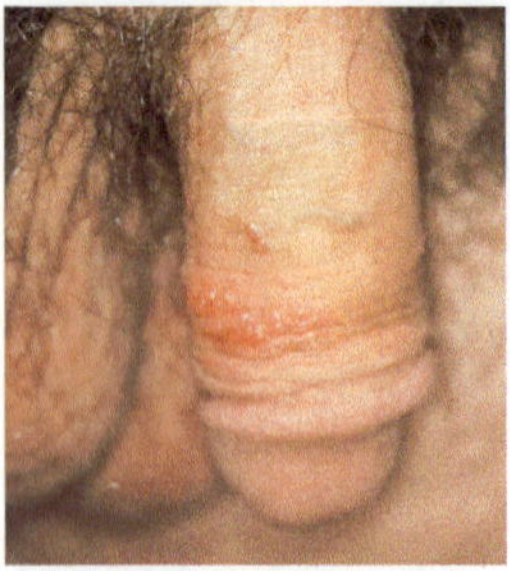

FIGURE 13.8 Condyloma. Note the presence of soft, wart-like growths about the penile shaft, known as *condylomata acuminate* or *anogenital warts*.
Source: Centers for Disease Control and Prevention/MF Rein, MD.

Sexually Transmitted Infections

History

- Discharge, burning with urination, itching
- May be asymptomatic
- Unprotected sex, less than 100% condom use increases risk

Physical Examination

- Urethritis, urethral discharge
- May have associated inguinal lymphadenopathy, tenderness
- May have skin changes, including inflamed, erosive papules (scabies), vesicles/ulcers (herpes), chancre (syphilis), or genital warts (HPV)

Considerations

- Gonorrhea and chlamydia are the most common bacterial causes of STIs.
- HPV is the most common STI. There are numerous types of HPV; many types are associated with cancers, some are associated with genital warts or condyloma (**Figure 13.8**).

OTHER ABNORMALITIES OF MALE GENITALIA

Manifestations of Systemic Conditions

Systemic conditions can cause dermatologic symptoms in the male genitalia. In particular, reactive arthritis can manifest in part as vesicles and crusted plaques on the penis. Chronic, generalized pruritus and dermatologic changes can signify an underlying systemic disease; disorders such as connective tissue disease, lichen planus, seborrheic dermatitis, lichen sclerosus, atopic dermatitis, and psoriasis cause cutaneous findings.

Peyronie Disease

A condition in which dorsal fibrous plaques alter penile anatomy and impair function; etiology is unknown but likely multifactorial and related to a post-inflammatory healing process.

History

- Penile curvature or deformity
- Erectile penile shortening
- Penile pain and sexual dysfunction
- Risk factors include genital injuries, urethral instrumentation, and prostatectomy

Physical Examination

- Penile curvature, nodules

Considerations

- Noncancerous, fibrous tissue causing curvature is likely scar tissue
- Pain during erections usually improves within 1 to 2 years

Skin Cancer

History

- First sign of penile cancer is often skin change of the foreskin, glans penis, or penile shaft
- Key symptoms may include thickening of skin, changes in skin color, ulcers

Physical Examination

- Well-defined, velvety red plaques
- Lesions or skin changes with or without lymphadenopathy

Consideration

- Initial assessment and evaluation should be guided on the likelihood of whether an infection or malignancy is more likely. While penile cancer is rare, 95% are squamous cell carcinomas.

Testicular Tumor/Malignancy

History

- Solid, firm lump within the testicle; often painless
- Males with history of cryptorchidism (undescended testicle) are at an increased risk

Physical Examination

- Solid, firm mass within the testes
- Scrotal ultrasound reveals testicular mass

Considerations

- Average age at time of diagnosis is 33 years old.
- Testicular cancer is not uncommon.

PROSTATE, RECTAL, OR ANAL ABNORMALITIES

Anal Fissures

An anal fissure is a small tear in the mucosal lining of the anus.

History

- Key symptoms can include bleeding or pain with bowel movements

Physical Examination

- Visible cracks in the skin around the anus

Considerations

- Risk increases with history of constipation or straining during bowel movements
- Risk increases with anal penetration during sexual intercourse

External and Internal Hemorrhoids

Enlarged, bulging veins of the distal rectum and anus.

History

- Painless, bright-red bleeding with bowel movements, anal itching, acute onset of perianal pain, and/or fecal soiling
- Risk factors include family history of hemorrhoids, obesity, pregnancy, chronic constipation, and straining with bowel movements

Physical Examination

- Rectal irritation, erythema; hemorrhoids may prolapse outside the anal sphincter.
- Internal hemorrhoids are located in the distal rectum.

- External hemorrhoids are located within the anus.

Consideration

- Acute onset of perianal pain may be indicative of a thrombosed hemorrhoid

Prostate Cancer

Cancer of the prostate gland is typically detected at an asymptomatic stage. Key signs of prostate cancer include abnormal finding of the prostate on DRE, that is, nodules or asymmetry, and/or elevated PSA levels. PSA is not specific for prostate cancer, however, and can be elevated in other conditions. Abnormal DRE or urinary/rectal symptoms warrant further investigation.

Prostatic Enlargement

An enlargement of the prostate gland, which becomes more common as men age (**Figure 13.9**).

History

- Urinary frequency, impaired flow, weak urine stream, nocturia, urinary dribbling post-urination

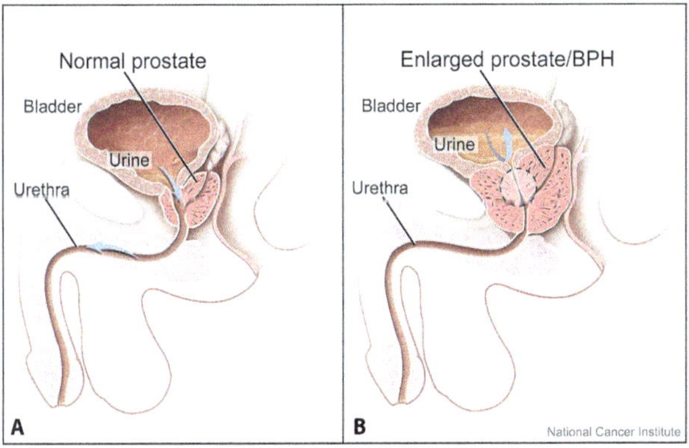

FIGURE 13.9 Benign prostatic hyperplasia. (**A**) Flow of urine with a normal prostate and (**B**) with an enlarged prostate/BPH.
BPH, benign prostatic hyperplasia.
Source: National Cancer Institute.

Physical Examination

- Normal anal sphincter tone
- Nontender prostate; no palpable distinct nodules

Considerations

- Medications may contribute to symptoms (e.g., antihistamines, decongestants, diuretics)
- Comorbidities also contribute to symptoms (diabetes, heart failure, prostate or bladder cancer)

Rectal Polyps and Rectal Cancer

Rectal polyps refer to a protrusion of the rectal mucosa into the lumen of the rectum. Hyperplastic polyps can be pre-cancerous. Nearly all colon and rectal cancers begin as polyps.

History

- Usually asymptomatic
- May have persistent bowel pattern changes (diarrhea, constipation, or narrow stools)

Physical Examination

- Palpable rectal mass
- Occult or frank blood in the stool

Consideration

- Polyps are usually asymptomatic but may ulcerate and bleed if they become enlarged and obstruct the colon. Polyps can be benign, inflammatory lesions or neoplastic lesions. Inflammatory polyps are an endoscopic physical finding of inflammatory bowel disease like Crohn's disease or ulcerative colitis. Neoplastic polyps are an endoscopic physical finding of rectal cancer.

PHYSICAL EXAMINATION DOCUMENTATION

Documentation should include results of inspection, palpation, and special tests.

EXAMPLE OF NORMAL FINDINGS

No palpable inguinal hernias or lymphadenopathy. Scrotal sacs pendulous without swelling, tenderness, palpable masses, discoloration, or lesions. Penis without erythema, lesions, tenderness, or urethral discharge. Anus: no hemorrhoids, fissures, or lesions. Rectal wall intact, no masses or tenderness. Prostate smooth, without palpable nodules or enlargement.

EXAMPLE OF ABNORMAL FINDINGS: ADOLESCENT MALE

Mild tenderness and lymphadenopathy of two inguinal nodes, right groin. No skin changes or lesions noted. Scrotum without tenderness or palpable masses. Mucopurulent penile discharge; lab specimen of urethral discharge obtained and sent for STI testing. No penile lesions or tenderness. Rectal exam deferred. Tanner stage 4.

REFERENCES

References for this chapter draw from Chapter 18, "Evidence-Based Assessment of Sexual Orientation, Gender Identity, and Health," and Chapter 19, "Evidence-Based Assessment of Male Genitalia, Prostate, Rectum, and Anus," of the textbook *Evidence-Based Physical Examination: Best Practices for Health and Well-Being Assessment*. The references may be accessed in the digital version of the handbook at https://connect.springerpub.com/content/book/97808-0-8261-6466-7/chapter/ch13

14

Evidence-Based Assessment of Breasts, Female Genitalia, and Reproductive System

CLINICAL CONSIDERATIONS

- The personal nature of discussions about sexual and reproductive health require recognition that populations are vulnerable to disparities in care related to implicit or unconscious bias. Care should be taken to provide sensitive assessment and counseling for individuals with respect for gender identity and sexual orientation.
- Consider conducting the health history while the patient's clothes are on. Sitting naked on an exam table under a flimsy gown increases the likelihood of the patient feeling vulnerable.
- Always carefully and fully listen when patients share concerns about breast lumps or masses, even when the clinical level of suspicion is low. Regardless of age, gender, or positive/negative family history of cancer, the presence of a breast mass should never be dismissed. All breast masses require imaging for full evaluation.
- Ideally, patients should have an opportunity to speak with a clinician privately, without anyone else in the room. Sometimes practices have a policy to meet with a patient alone.
- When a woman presents for a well-woman examination, advanced assessment includes a comprehensive, thorough, evidence-based history and physical examination. Testing to consider includes Pap and HPV testing; STI screening; wet prep; and breast, ovarian, endometrial, cervical, and colon cancer screening.
- For the woman who presents with reproductive or sexual health concerns, a sensitive, patient-centered, detailed history will inform what physical exam needs to be done; more specifically,

when breast and pelvic exams, or vaginal or cervical inspection, are warranted.

- Understanding anatomy and physiology of the female GU and reproductive systems, menstrual cycle, and reproductive life span is key to providing sexual and reproductive health guidance.

SUBJECTIVE HISTORY

COMMON REASONS FOR SEEKING CARE

- Well-woman exam
- Vaginal discharge, itching
- Menstrual cycle irregularities, including amenorrhea, heavy menstrual bleeding
- Pelvic pain, dysmenorrhea
- Breast lump, breast pain

HISTORY OF PRESENT ILLNESS

- **Onset:** When did symptoms start? Are symptoms recent? How did symptoms begin?
- **Location:** Specific location of symptoms—Vaginal, suprapubic, lower abdomen, adnexal, umbilical; highly localized (patient can point to one place) versus a more generalized discomfort or pain that moves around? Specific area of a breast or axilla, or bilateral breast symptoms?
- **Duration:** Are symptoms persistent or transitory? Increasing or unchanged?
- **Characteristics:** Describe the symptoms. Is there itching, burning, discharge, odor, changes in urination, changes in menstrual cycle, cramping, pain, and/or tenderness? If pain or tenderness, is the pain burning, stinging, sharp, dull, throbbing, or causing a feeling of heaviness or bloating? Any associated skin or lymph node changes?
- **Aggravating factors:** Are symptoms associated with sexual activity? Menstrual cycle? Traumatic event? Urination?
- **Relieving factors:** What actions or activities decrease the symptoms?
- **Treatment:** What medications has the individual taken to help with the symptoms? Clarify dosage and frequency of OTC and prescribed medications.
- **Severity:** How severe are the symptoms on a scale of 0 to 10? Do the symptoms limit participation in activities at work, school, or home?

HEALTH HISTORY

- Clinicians who establish trust, remain open-minded, and are careful about using unassuming language find that patients willingly share the information needed to provide evidence-based, sensitive, high-quality care that supports their health and well-being.
- Review the script provided in the previous chapter as an example of how to ask assessment questions related to reproductive and sexual health.
- For a complete woman's health history, include assessment of menstrual, gynecologic, obstetric, and sexual health, as well as past medical, family, and social history.

Menstrual History

- Date of last menstrual period: If cycles are irregular, date of last normal menstrual period
- Regularity of menstrual cycle: Describe any irregularities (e.g., spotting between cycles, missed periods); cycle length (from the first day of one to the first day of the next)
- Duration of flow: Irregularities related to bleeding (e.g., heavy bleeding, spotting)
- Symptoms that accompany menstruation: Breast tenderness or pain, dysmenorrhea or cramping, headaches, nausea
- Age of menarche (first episode of menstruation) and last menstrual cycle, if postmenopausal

Gynecologic History

- Breast history:
  - Current or previous malignant or nonmalignant conditions
  - Breastfeeding history
  - Presence of breast implants, including length of time, type, and complications
  - Self-breast exam concerns, practices
  - Last mammogram
- Gynecologic history:
  - Last pelvic examination
  - Last Pap test:

    - History of abnormal Pap testing
    - Treatment related to abnormal Pap testing (i.e., LEEP or cone biopsy)?
    - Last HPV testing and result
- History of STIs: Note when and how treated
- Gynecologic surgery, include year and rationale
- Fertility or infertility treatment
- Exposure to diethylstilbestrol

Obstetric History

- The obstetric history tells the story of every pregnancy that a woman has had. The clinician should document the year and duration of each pregnancy (in weeks), method of delivery, and any complications during or after the pregnancy for the mother and infant. It is important to obtain details about each child born (e.g., gender, weight, current condition of each child today). The GTPAL system is used to summarize these assessment findings.
    - G = Gravida: Number of pregnancies
    - T = Term: Number of full-term births (≥37 weeks' gestation)
    - P = Preterm: Number of preterm births (≥20 weeks', <37 weeks' gestation)
    - A = Abortions: Number of abortions (spontaneous, elective, ectopic) <20 weeks' gestation
    - L = Living: Number of living children

SEXUAL HISTORY

An opportunity for the clinician to acknowledge the importance of sexuality, relationships, and sexual behavior to one's overall health. This part of the exam should not be limited to a disease-oriented perspective, but should provide an opportunity to further the patient–clinician relationship and support behaviors that encourage sexual health across the life span. Assess the six P's as listed:

1. **Partners:** Currently sexually active, ever sexually active; number of recent partners, number of partners in the last year, lifetime partners; gender of partners
2. **Practices:** Genital (vaginal, penile), oral, anal
3. **Protection from STIs**: Use of condoms or other protection against STIs, typical use, comfort level in discussing protection with partner
4. **Past history of STIs**: Diagnosis, treatment, recurrent symptoms? Ever tested for STIs including HIV? Status of partner?

5. **Pregnancy prevention:** Assess reproductive life plan (i.e., desire for pregnancy, use of family planning methods, currently attempting to be pregnant or avoid pregnancy, partner support, and need for contraception or fertility counseling).
6. **Plus additional questions:** Allow time for questions about sexual health, which may include necessary screenings, intimacy, or sexual expression

Past Health History

- Hospitalizations, surgeries, emergency department visits
- Hypertension, cardiovascular disease, stroke, clotting disorders
- Cancer; treatment with chemotherapeutics, radiation
- Diabetes, insulin resistance, polycystic ovarian syndrome
- Endocrine or autoimmune disorders including thyroid disorders
- Anxiety, depression, trauma, or mental health disorders

Medications

- Prescribed and OTC medications or supplements, including dose and frequency

Allergies

- Allergies to medications or seasonal, environmental, and/or food allergies. If yes, clarify reaction.

Preventive Health Behaviors

- Physical activity and exercise
- Typical diet; nutritional concerns
- Sleep and rest; concerns or disorders
- Stress and coping
- Vaccine history

FAMILY HISTORY

- Breast, ovarian, cervical, colon cancers
- Genetic disorders or congenital malformations; recurrent pregnancy losses
- Diabetes, hypertension, heart disease
- Preeclampsia

SOCIAL HISTORY

- Home situation:
    - Married/single/divorced/widowed/partnered?
    - Who lives in the home? Is partner supportive?
    - Is housing/home/neighborhood safe? Risk or current victim of violence?
- Substance use:
    - Tobacco use? If yes, assess smoking history, readiness to quit
    - Alcohol use? If yes, screen for binge drinking, problematic use
    - Other substances (e.g., medications not prescribed, illicit drugs)?
- Occupation or school safety:
    - Exposure to hazards (e.g., fumes, radiation, chemicals, viruses)
    - Stress, anxiety, burnout related to workplace culture, school, or work expectations

REVIEW OF SYSTEMS

- **General/endocrine:** Recent illness, weight loss or gain, fever, chills, hair loss, acne, facial hair, night sweats, hot flashes
- **HEENT:** Headaches, changes in vision, congestion, pharyngitis, oral lesions
- **Lymphatic:** Lymphadenopathy, tender lymph nodes in axillae or groin area
- **CV/respiratory:** Chest pain, edema, dyspnea, cough
- **Breasts/dermatologic**: Nipple discharge, skin lesions or rashes, pruritus, palpable lumps, pain or tenderness, breast fullness
- **GI:** Nausea, vomiting, localized or generalized abdominal or pelvic pain, change in bowel habits, blood in the stool
- **GU:** Urinary frequency, dysuria, hematuria, dyspareunia, vaginal or anal itching, painful genital lesions
- **MSK**: Back pain, myalgias
- **Neurologic/mental health**: Worry; sadness, helplessness, hopelessness; fatigue or insomnia; change in mood, stress, coping; syncope

RED FLAGS IN SUBJECTIVE HISTORY

- Gynecologic cancers (ovarian, uterine, and cervical cancer) often present with vague and nonspecific symptoms, especially in early stages. Recognize red flag symptoms for prompt referral and treatment (**Box 14.1**).

BOX 14.1 Red Flags in Subjective History That Indicate Possible Gynecologic Cancer

- Abdominal distention or bloating
- Early satiety with loss of appetite
- Unexplained pelvic or abdominal pain
- Increased urinary urgency or frequency
- Postcoital bleeding
- Postmenopausal bleeding
- Unexplained weight loss or fatigue
- Unexplained change in bowel habits
- Over 50 years of age with new symptoms of irritable bowel syndrome

PHYSICAL EXAMINATION

- For a well-woman examination, a thorough head-to-toe examination is recommended. While this chapter reviews the breast and female genitalia exams only, components of the well-woman exam include assessing lymphatic, cardiac, respiratory, and integumentary systems, in addition to physical exam of the mouth, throat, thyroid, breasts, abdomen, pelvis, and genitalia.
- The presence of a chaperone during physical examination should be offered to all women, especially when performing breast and/or pelvic exams, which can be a source of anxiety for women. The clinician's approach should be respectful and caring.

CLINICAL BREAST EXAM

Despite the controversy regarding the population health benefit of CBE for the screening of breast cancer, it may identify a small proportion of breast malignancies not detected with mammography, may be requested by an individual as a component of their exam, and may be used to document the presence of palpable masses and cysts in young women who are not typical candidates for mammography. CBE includes visual inspection and palpation of the breasts and axillae.

Inspection of the Breasts

With the patient sitting and disrobed to the waist, note breast size, shape, and contour. Inspect the breasts and nipples for symmetry. Note any changes to the skin of the breasts, including dimpling, peau d'orange appearance, erythema, or edema. Have the patient raise her arms overhead, place her hands at the hips, and sit with her hands pressed together; observe for a shift in nipple position, as well as significant asymmetry or any unusual dimpling or bulging of breast tissue.

Palpation of Breasts and Axillae

- Palpate axillary lymph nodes while patient is still in a seated position; each arm should be supported while nodes are palpated. Palpation should be completed with the pads of the fingers, using a fluid, circular motion. Care should be taken to ensure the entire surface area of the lymphatic region is palpated, both lightly and deeply.
- Palpate each breast with the patient in the supine position with one hand above her head. The entire breast is examined from the second to sixth ribs and from the left sternal border to the midaxillary line. Imagine the breast divided into four quadrants with vertical and horizontal lines intersecting at the nipple (**Figure 14.1**). The upper outer quadrant encompasses

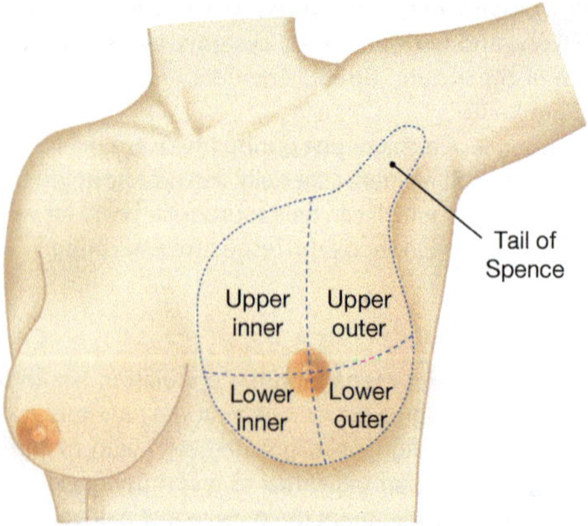

FIGURE 14.1 Breast quadrants. This figure shows the four quadrants of the breast. This anatomic system is commonly used to describe exam findings in breast conditions.

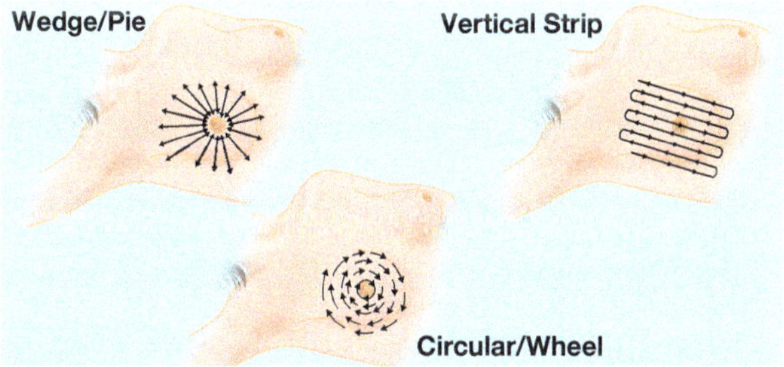

FIGURE 14.2 Breast palpation methods. Breast palpation should be completed in one of these three ways (*clockwise, left to right*): wedge/pie, vertical strip, or circular/wheel. These examination techniques provide a systematic way to ensure the clinician palpates the entire breast.

the axillary tail of breast tissue that extends into the axilla. Palpate in all four quadrants of both breasts by compressing breast tissue between the pads of the three middle fingers and the chest wall.

- Proper breast palpation technique entails the use of the finger pads in a continuous rolling, gliding circular motion in the vertical strip, circular, or wedge pattern (**Figure 14.2**). Pressure of the fingers should be varied from light to medium to deep palpation. Areolas and nipples are included inherently in the palpation of the breast; however, nipple expression to assess for nipple discharge is not recommended unless the patient describes spontaneous discharge that requires evaluation.

PHYSICAL EXAMINATION OF FEMALE GENITALIA

- Most commonly performed with the patient in the lithotomy position, a supine position with the legs separated, flexion at the hips and knees, and feet resting in foot rests. Use of optional positioning may be helpful in patients with mobility limitations.
- Regardless of the chosen positioning, attention should be paid to the appropriate draping of the patient during the examination. Care should be taken to preserve modesty and warmth. Ideally, clinician should drape the patient to ensure eye contact with the patient throughout the examination.

Inspection and Palpation of External Genitalia

- Begin with a thorough exam of the external genitalia. Starting with the mons pubis, evaluation should include the pattern and quality of hair distribution on both the mons and the labia majora. Inspect for signs of infection. Proceed to inspection of the skin of the mons and perineum. The skin inspection should evaluate for discoloration or hypopigmentation, erythema, and excoriation. Note any visible ulcerations, pustules, vesicles, growths, lesions, nevi, varicosities, or scars.
- Evaluate labia and clitoris for development or atrophy. Inspect the introitus, noting its shape—closed or gaping—in the lithotomy position. The Bartholin and Skene glands should be inspected for swelling and purulent exudates. The perineal body should then be assessed. This area begins with the posterior aspect of the labia and extends to the anus. The inspection of the perineal body should include the items previously described.
- The perianal area should be examined. Inspect for injury, lesions, warts, hemorrhoids, or other abnormalities. Evidence of trauma should prompt further investigation.

Internal Inspection: Speculum Examination

- Performing a speculum examination allows for direct visualization of the cervix and surrounding vaginal walls. A speculum examination for the sole purpose of screening for STIs is not necessary, as other methods for sample collection are available. The appropriately sized speculum should be chosen prior to starting the examination.
- By convention, the speculum examination is performed first, followed by the bimanual examination. The speculum should be warmed with warm water or a warming device. Current recommendations suggest that a small amount (dime-sized) be applied to the introitus and bills of the speculum for ease of insertion.
- Begin by separating the labia with the thumb and first finger of the nondominant hand for visualization of the introitus. The traditional approach to insertion of the speculum recommends holding the speculum with the bills completely closed facing the lateral aspects of the vagina. With the speculum angled slightly downward, apply gentle pressure toward the coccyx and direct the speculum inward. Avoid a severe angle downward as this will cause the base of the speculum to compress the sensitive structures of the upper genitalia. Upon full insertion of the speculum, rotate the handle of the speculum downward so the bills are in the inferior/superior position and open the speculum for

visualization of the cervix. Open the speculum only as wide as needed for visualization. It is not necessary to open it completely.

- An alternative method involves inserting the speculum directly into the vagina with the bills in the inferior/superior position. Application of a gentle downward pressure on the vaginal wall aids in the insertion of the speculum.
- If the clinician has difficulty finding the cervix or determining the appropriately sized speculum to use, consideration should be given to performing a bimanual examination first for assessment of anatomy and position of the cervix.
- Vaginal tissue should be inspected during both insertion and removal of the speculum. If using a plastic speculum, the bills are clear, which can aid in visualization. Use of a metal speculum will require tilting the position of the bills, so visualization of the entirety of the vaginal vault can be performed. The vagina should be inspected for color, tissue appearance, moisture, discharge, moles, or lesions, and any unusual odors should be noted.
- The speculum should be positioned to allow for visualization of the entire surface of the cervix (**Figure 14.3**). Inspection should include the size/shape of the os, color, bleeding or discharge, evaluation of the squamocolumnar junction, and assessment for any lesions or growths.
- Carefully complete the collection of endocervical and cervical cells (**Figure 14.4**) by meticulously following the technique recommended. This is required if an adequate specimen is to be evaluated for cellular changes. These techniques vary depending on the collection tools used.
- Upon completion of the inspection of the cervix and collection of necessary specimens, the speculum lock should be released and the speculum should be opened slightly while simultaneously drawing upward with the handle of the speculum, following the same plane used with insertion. This allows the bills of the speculum to release the cervix. A final inspection of the vaginal walls should be performed if needed. The bills of the speculum should be allowed to fall closed naturally, which avoids pinching the vaginal tissue and labia in the bills. Gently remove the speculum from the vagina.

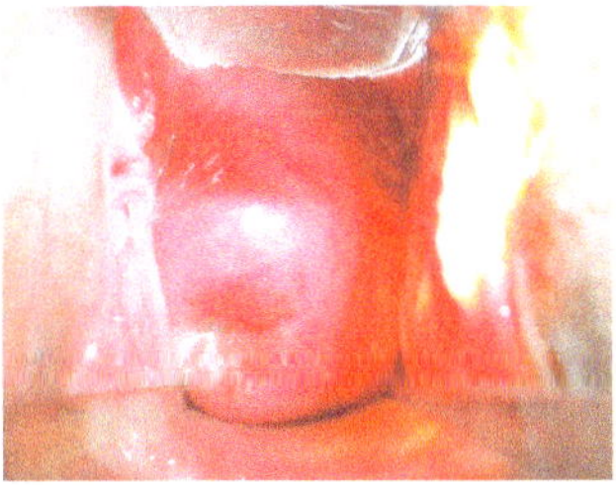

FIGURE 14.3 Cervix as viewed using a speculum.

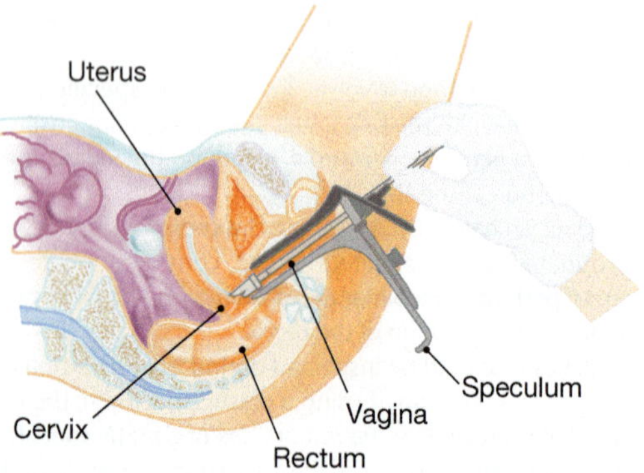

FIGURE 14.4 Collection of cervical specimen for Pap testing.

Palpation: Bimanual Exam

- The bimanual examination is performed to assess the uterus and adnexa. The index and middle finger of the dominant hand are lubricated with a water-soluble lubricant and inserted into the vagina until the cervix is palpable, moving fingers to the posterior fornix, located below the cervix. Take care to tuck the thumb out of the way to avoid compressing the sensitive structures of the pubic symphysis, mons pubis, and clitoris.
- The clinician should place the same leg as the dominant hand on the step of the examination table, leaning forward slightly so weight is shifted forward a bit. The nondominant hand is placed on the lower abdomen, above the pubic symphysis. Using the flat surface of the fingers, a sweeping downward motion toward the internal fingers is used to isolate the uterus. The internal fingers direct the uterus up to the fingers, gently compressing the uterus. This procedure allows for palpation of the uterine size and position in the pelvis
- Size, shape, and symmetry of the uterus should be documented, as well as the position and consistency of the uterus. In normal circumstances, palpation of the uterus is not painful; any discomfort should be noted and may warrant further evaluation.
- See **Figure 14.5** for a cross-sectional view of a bimanual examination and **Figure 14.6** to review normal variations in uterine position.
- Palpation of the adnexa serves to assess the ovaries and fallopian tubes. To assess the right adnexa, shift the internal fingers to the

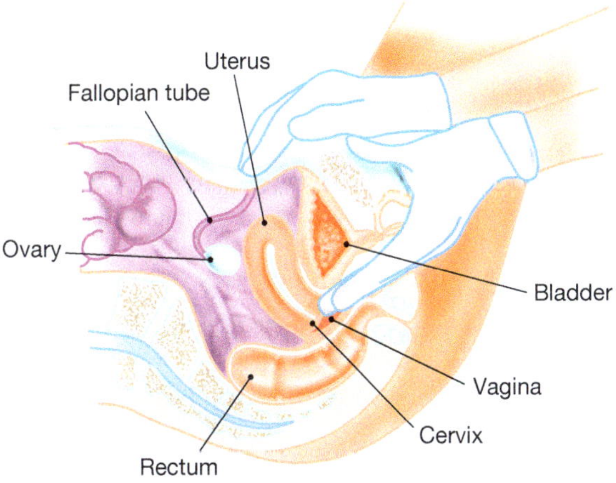

FIGURE 14.5 Bimanual examination.

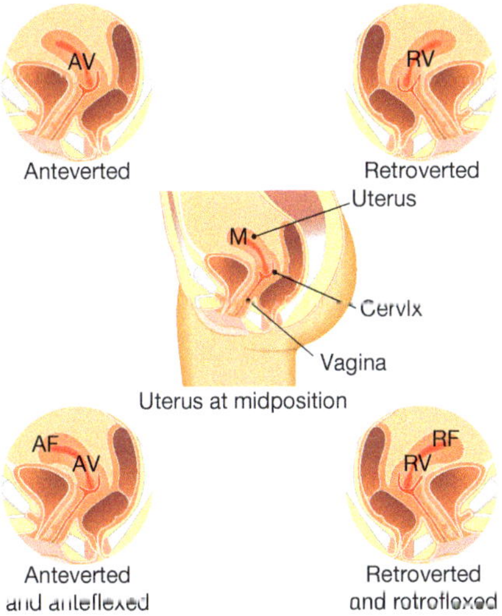

FIGURE 14.6 Normal variations in the position of the uterus. AF, anteflexed; AV, anteverted; M, midposition; RF, retroflexed; RV, retroverted.

patient's right side, moving the fingers to the right vaginal fornix. The flat surface of the fingers of the nondominant hand are placed just medial to the right anterior superior iliac spine and directed downward to meet the internal fingers. The goal is to capture the adnexa between the internal and external fingers for palpation. The ovary is approximately 3 × 2 cm and is often compared with the size of a walnut. This maneuver is repeated on the left side for assessment of the left adnexa. Documentation should include a description of the size and mobility of the adnexa, as well as consistency.

- Palpation of the ovaries in postmenopausal women is not considered a normal finding; if this should be identified on examination, it requires further evaluation.
- CMT is found in several pathologic conditions (e.g., PID, appendicitis, and ectopic pregnancy). It is performed by placing the index and middle fingers on either side of the cervix and gently pulling the cervix to one side, then the other. Pain with traction on the adnexa is a positive CMT. Inter-rater reliability for CMT is low, but there is still evidence that suggests its clinical significance in assisting with diagnosis of PID.

Rectovaginal Examination

- RVE can be used for additional evaluation, if needed, and is typically performed after bimanual examination is completed. It is used to further assess the uterus, uterosacral ligaments, and rectovaginal septum.
- Clean gloves should be donned prior to completing the RVE. The first finger of the dominant hand is placed into the vagina and middle finger of the same hand is placed into the rectum. Gentle upward pressure of the middle finger allows for the assessment of the rectovaginal septum. The uterosacral ligaments can be palpated by locating them along the posterior wall of the cervix, lateral to the sacrum. A retroverted uterus can be examined using this method. Examination should evaluate for any abnormalities, including tenderness, nodules, or apparent thickening or thinning.

LIFE-SPAN AND SPECIAL POPULATION CONSIDERATIONS

Pediatric and Adolescent Exams

- Routine GU exams should be performed during all infant and child wellness examinations. The newborn examination, in particular, should include inspection for congenital malformations, atypical or ambiguous genitalia, and placement and patency of the anus. The pediatric anogenital examination should be performed with a caregiver present.

- For adolescents, a chaperone can be a caregiver or another healthcare clinician, but this should be the adolescent's choice. Assess the Tanner state of sexual maturity for female adolescents:
  - **Stage 1**: Small nipples with no breast tissue; no pubic hair.
  - **Stage 2**: Breast and nipples have just started to grow. The areola has become larger. Breast tissue bud feels firm behind the nipple. Initial growth of long pubic hairs. These are straight, without curls, and of light colors.
  - **Stage 3**: Breast and nipples have grown additionally. The areola has become darker. The breast tissue bud is larger. The pubic hair is more widespread. The hair is darker and curls may have appeared.
  - **Stage 4**: Nipples and areolas are elevated and form an edge toward the breast. The breast has also grown a little larger. More dense hair growth with curls and dark hair. Still not entirely as an adult woman.
  - **Stage 5**: Fully developed breast. Nipples are protruding and the edge between areola and breast has disappeared. Adult hair growth. Dense, curly hair extending toward the inner thighs.

Trauma-Informed Care

- Approximately 45% of women in the United States have experienced sexual violence (i.e., rape, sexual coercion, and/or unwanted sexual contact). Before midadolescence, one out of every five girls has been sexually abused. Nearly one in three adult women experience at least one physical assault by a partner during adulthood. Given the significance of this problem, clinicians caring for women of all ages should be aware of the potential for a history of violence or other trauma.
- Trauma-informed care provides a framework for engaging with individuals who have had a history of trauma. There are four basic principles that direct trauma-informed care: an awareness of the prevalence of traumatic events, an ability to recognize the signs and symptoms of trauma, development of policies and practices that integrate knowledge regarding trauma, and avoiding re-traumatizing the individual during the history and patient examination.
- The pelvic exam can be an anxiety-inducing experience and is often more problematic for women who have experienced sexual

violence. It is important to have an open dialogue with the patient during all portions of the exam. Obtain permission to perform each part of the exam, explaining what the examination entails and the purpose for doing it. Give her permission to stop the exam at any time. Identification and a sensitive approach to individual concerns and needs will strengthen the clinician–patient relationship and allow for appropriate referrals for further assessment, support, and treatment.

Postmenopausal Considerations

The decrease in estrogen levels during the menopause transition results in thinning of the vaginal tissue. This thinning causes decreased elasticity of the tissue, a paler appearance, and more fragile tissue, which can result in vaginal dryness and petechiae. These changes can range from asymptomatic to moderate-to-severe dyspareunia, vaginal discomfort, and irritation. As a result of these changes, speculum examination may be uncomfortable for the postmenopausal patient. Consider use of water-based lubrication and a smaller size speculum.

RED FLAGS IN OBJECTIVE EXAM

- Red flags indicating possible breast malignancy are listed in **Box 14.2**. All breast masses require imaging for full evaluation. Regardless of age, gender, or family history of cancer, the presence of a breast mass should never be dismissed.
- The primary screening imaging modality for breast cancer is mammography. Other imaging should be considered on the basis of current evidence available, patient presentation, and breast specialist recommendation.

BOX 14.2 Red Flags in Objective Exam Indicating Possible Breast Malignancy

- Mastitis in nonpregnant, nonbreastfeeding female
- Axillary or supraclavicular lymphadenopathy
- Breast lump or mass palpated with indistinct, irregular borders
- Breast lump with hard, asymmetric texture
- Painless, immobile breast lump (fixed to adjacent structure)
- Skin dimpling associated with breast lump

(*continued*)

BOX 14.2 Red Flags in Objective Exam Indicating Possible Breast Malignancy (*continued*)

- Palpable mass with localized thickening of surrounding tissue
- New onset of nipple retraction
- Unilateral nipple discharge in nonpregnant individual
- Unilateral, spontaneous, bloody nipple discharge, originating from one breast duct with or without a breast mass

EVIDENCE-BASED RESOURCES

- **Agency for Healthcare Research and Quality:** www.ahrq.gov/professionals/prevention-chronic-care/healthier-pregnancy/preventive/trauma.html
- **American Cancer Society:** www.cancer.org
- **American College of Obstetricians and Gynecologists:** www.acog.org
- **American Psychological Association:** www.apa.org/pi/lgbt/resources/guidelines
- **American Urological Association:** www.auanet.org/guidelines
- **Center of Excellence for Transgender Health:** http://transhealth.ucsf.edu/trans?page=guidelines-home
- **Centers for Disease Control and Prevention:** www.cdc.gov/std/tg2015/default.htm; www.cdc.gov/cancer/breast/basic_info/risk_factors.htm
- **Choosing Wisely Campaign:** www.choosingwisely.org
- **National Cancer Institute:** www.cancer.gov/types/breast/hp
- **U.S. Preventive Services Task Force:** www.uspreventiveservicestaskforce.org

ABNORMAL FINDINGS OF THE BREAST AND AXILLAE

ACCESSORY BREAST TISSUE

Accessory or additional mammary tissue remote from the primary breast tissue can occur along "milk lines" anywhere from the axilla to the groin.

History

- May present as a soft subcutaneous lump near or in the axillae
- May present as a supernumerary or "third" nipple; may be mistaken for a freckle or mole

Physical Examination

- Accessory tissue present with/without an observable accessory nipple
- Area of the accessory breast tissue can be tender and enlarged in response to the hormonal fluctuations of the normal menstrual cycle, and can become full and active with pregnancy and lactation.

Consideration

- Accessory breast tissue is benign; this finding is common.

BENIGN BREAST MASS OR LUMP

- The self-detection of a breast mass or lump is the most common reason for women presenting for clinical breast evaluation in reproductive healthcare practices. The goal in evaluating any breast abnormality or patient concern is to exclude the presence of a malignancy and to find the most efficient path to an accurate diagnosis and management. Most breast lumps are benign. However, the presence of a breast mass should never be dismissed based solely on physical exam.
- Breast tissue can be rope-like or lumpy in texture as a result of glandular or fibrocystic breast tissue. More than half of women experience fibrocystic breast changes at some point in their lives. Benign breast disorders encompass a large group of nonmalignant conditions; most of these conditions are not pathologic and stem from exaggerated physiology of normal breast development and involution. The two most common benign conditions that are associated with distinct, palpable masses or lumps are fibroadenomas and breast cysts.

Breast Cyst

Fluid-filled, round-to-ovoid structures, and are nonproliferative lesions with a minimal breast cancer risk.

History

- Tender breast lump that is round and mobile
- Can be unilateral or bilateral

Physical Examination

- Palpable cysts vary greatly in size, present as single or multiple entities

Considerations

- Breast cyst formation can be related to hormonal changes induced by hormone fluctuations of the menstrual cycle, hormone replacement therapy, or medications
- More common in women over the age of 40 years old

Fibroadenoma

Fibroadenomas are composed mainly of parenchymal/stromal tissue, and are proliferative lesions that have the propensity to change over time.

History

- Palpable lump; may be tender to touch

Physical Examination

- Single well-defined mobile ovoid and discrete mass palpable on exam

Considerations

- Multiple fibroadenomas can be present
- More common in women younger than 25 years old

BREAST CANCER

Breast cancer is the most common female cancer and the second leading cause of cancer death in women in the United States. Invasive breast cancers constitute a heterogeneous group of lesions that differ with regard to their clinical, radiographic, and histologic features. The most common histologic type of invasive breast cancers are invasive (infiltrating) ductal carcinoma, and invasive lobular carcinoma.

Inflammatory Breast Cancer

A rare, highly aggressive malignant breast condition.

History

- Sensation of fullness/heaviness, burning, or tenderness
- Unilateral presentation of an erythematous or purplish, edematous, or inflamed appearing breast involving one third or more of the breast area
- Rapid change in breast size (<3 months)

Physical Examination

- Axillary or supraclavicular lymphadenopathy
- Breast mass may or may not be palpable

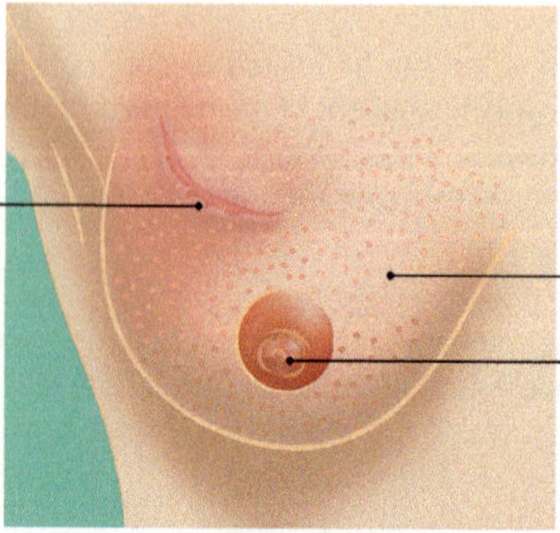

FIGURE 14.7 Inflammatory breast cancer.

- Breast changes may include inverted nipple, unilateral, localized area of erythema and edema, and peau d'orange skin changes of the affected breast (**Figure 14.7**).

Considerations

- Risk factors include race/ethnicity, younger age at menarche, and obesity.
- Metastatic disease present in one third of patients at diagnosis

Invasive Ductal Carcinomas

History

- Often presents as a discrete firm mass on palpation

Physical Examination

- There are no clinical characteristics that are specific to invasive ductal carcinomas
- More likely to present as an abnormality such as speculated mass on a mammogram

Consideration

- Prognosis varies and depends on tumor size, histologic grade, hormonal receptor expression, lymph node status, and whether lymph-vascular invasion has occurred

Invasive Lobular Carcinomas

History

- May present as a palpable mass or a mammographic abnormality similar to those of invasive ductal carcinoma, but findings often more subtle and underestimated

Physical Examination

- On exam, there may be only an area of thickening or induration, without distinct margins
- Mammogram may show no more than a poorly defined area of asymmetric density with architectural distortion, even in the presence of a palpable mass

Consideration

- Prognosis is similar and reliant on the same factors as with ductal carcinoma

Paget's Disease of the Breast

A rare type of breast cancer affecting the skin, nipple, and areola; it can occur in men or women from adolescence through the eighth decade of life.

History

- Itching, tingling, or erythema of the nipple and/or areola

Physical Examination

- Thickening, flaking, or crusting of the skin on/around the nipple
- Flat nipple
- Yellowish or bloody nipple discharge
- Breast lump(s) in the same breast

Consideration

- Owing to the benign appearance of Paget's disease in early stages, this cancer is often initially mistaken for dermatitis or eczema.

BREAST PAIN: MASTALGIA OR MASTODYNIA

Extremely common; the majority of all women experience this symptom during their reproductive years. Mastalgia is not correlated with malignancy, and is correlated with hormonal fluctuations. Breast pain, tenderness, and fullness are often early signs of pregnancy.

History

- Bilateral breast pain, often cyclic, that is, associated with menstrual cycle
- Often generalized and described as heaviness and tenderness
- If unilateral, more likely associated musculoskeletal strain, injury, or overuse

Physical Examination

- Tenderness of breast and/or of chest wall

- Nodularity may be palpable is pain is associated with normal fibrocystic breast changes

Considerations

- If the breast pain is cyclical, it is more likely to be related to hormonal fluctuations
- Noncyclical pain is more likely to be musculoskeletal in origin; the pain may originate from the breast or the chest wall since the pectoral muscle lies beneath the breast.

MASTITIS

An infection in the breast that occurs in up to 10% of women who are lactating. Note that mastitis is not common in women who are not breastfeeding and not pregnant; breast tissue that appears infected or inflamed in non-lactating women should be evaluated for conditions other than mastitis, including malignancy.

History

- Fever (over 100 °F)
- Fatigue, chills, arthralgia, myalgias, malaise, and/or poor appetite
- Unilateral presentation most likely
- Abrupt onset of symptoms

Physical Examination

- Warm, tender, erythematous, firm area of the breast
- Possibly complicated with a palpable abscess

Considerations

- May result from trauma/chafing to the nipple associated with breastfeeding, piercings
- Breast engorgement that is prolonged is a risk factor

NIPPLE DISCHARGE, GALACTORRHEA

- Discharge from the nipple is a relatively common occurrence in women and may represent either benign or pathologic conditions. Physiologic (normal) nipple discharge is often characterized as occurring with breast manipulation (not spontaneous), from more than one duct, and associated with pregnancy or breastfeeding, thyroid disease, or medications including antidepressants and contraceptives.
- Nipple discharge is suspicious for an underlying malignancy if it is unilateral, occurs spontaneously, persists, appears to be coming

from one duct, or is clear/colorless, or bloody. Milky nipple discharge (galactorrhea) in a nonbreastfeeding woman is likely associated with certain pharmacologic agents or pituitary/hypothalamic disease, warranting further evaluation. Any nipple discharge in males is considered abnormal and requires prompt evaluation. Pituitary tumors are the most common pathologic cause of galactorrhea; for the woman with amenorrhea and nipple discharge who is not pregnant, assessment of their prolactin level is an imperative.

ABNORMAL FINDINGS OF THE FEMALE GENITALIA

SEXUALLY TRANSMITTED INFECTIONS

Gonorrhea

An STI caused by the bacterium *Neisseria gonorrhoeae*, which most commonly infects the cervix, uterus, fallopian tubes, and urethra. Gonorrhea is transmitted by sexual contact via the mouth, penis, vagina, or anus of an infected partner and is the second most commonly reported STI.

History

- Asymptomatic in majority of women
- Midcycle vaginal bleeding
- Vaginal discharge
- Dysuria

Physical Examination

- Vaginal discharge
- Cervicitis

Consideration

- In severe or untreated cases, may develop PID infertility, increased risk for ectopic pregnancy, and chronic pelvic pain

Chlamydia

The most commonly reported bacterial STI. Caused by the bacterium *Chlamydia trachomatis* and transmitted through sexual contact similar to gonorrheal infections, Chlamydia is a common cause of cervicitis in women

History

- Asymptomatic in majority of women
- Vaginal discharge
- Dysuria, pyuria, urinary frequency

Physical Examination

- Vaginal discharge
- Friable cervix (i.e., easily induced endocervical bleeding)

Consideration

- Severe or untreated infections can result in PID, infertility, increased risk for ectopic pregnancy, and chronic pelvic pain

Trichomonas

Caused by an infection with the protozoal parasite *Trichomonas vaginalis.*

History

- Asymptomatic in majority of women
- Vaginal discharge and itching
- Dysuria
- Irritation and itching of the vulva

Physical Examination

- Greenish-yellow, frothy, and malodorous vaginal discharge
- Erythematous vulvar tissue and vaginal mucosa
- "Strawberry cervix" is a rare but pathognomonic finding that results from punctate hemorrhages on the cervix and vaginal tissue (**Figure 14.8**).

Consideration

- Trichomonads may be noted on microscopy

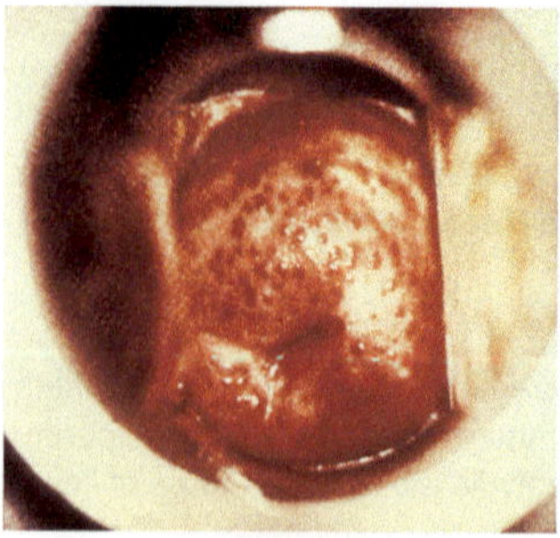

FIGURE 14.8 *Trichomonas vaginalis* infection and characteristic strawberry cervix.
Source: Centers for Disease Control and Prevention.

Syphilis

An STI caused by the bacterium *Treponema pallidum* that can present in a variety of ways depending on the stage of infection. Syphilis is spread by direct contact with a painless sore, known as a *chancre.*

Primary Stage

- Chancre (raised lesion, with an indurated margin, approximately 1–2 cm in size)
- Painless chancre may be found on the genitals, mouth/throat, anus, or vagina

- Typically occurs 21 days after exposure

Secondary Stage

- Palmar rash on the hands and bottoms of the feet; typically appears rough and red and does not usually cause itching (**Figure 14.9**)
- Fatigue, fevers, lymphadenopathy
- Hair loss, weight loss, myalgias
- Symptoms will eventually resolve even without treatment

Latent Stage

- Time when no symptoms are present that can last for years
- Continues to be contagious

Tertiary Stage

- Typically occurs 10 to 30 years after initial infection and can be fatal
- Symptoms of tertiary syphilis depend on the organ system affected; can cause infection in the nervous system, eyes, vascular and cardiac system, liver, bones, and joints

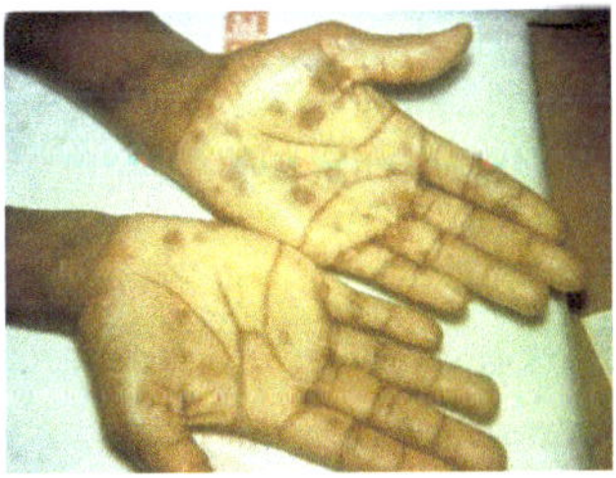

FIGURE 14.9 Palmar rash on palms of hands due to secondary syphilis. *Source:* Centers for Disease Control and Prevention.

Genital Warts (Condyloma Acuminata)

HPV types 6 and 11 are the most common cause of genital warts. As noted in this chapter, HPV is the most common STI. There are numerous types of HPV; many types are associated with cancers, whereas some are associated with genital warts or condyloma.

History

- Nonitchy, nontender lesions may appear as flesh tones, white, pink, or red
- Can appear as single lesions or grouped together, as depicted in **Figure 14.10**.

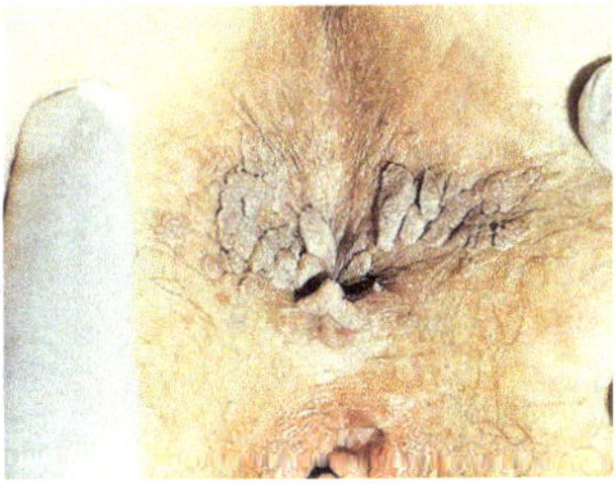

FIGURE 14.10 Genital warts found on perineum. *Source:* Image courtesy of SOA-AIDS Amsterdam.

Physical Examination

- Flat, papular, or pedunculated growths on the genital mucosa and surrounding skin of the perineal area, including the groin, suprapubic or perianal region, and vulva

Consideration

- HPV vaccines have significantly reduced the incidence of genital warts.

Genital Herpes

A viral STI caused by the herpes simplex virus type 1 or type 2. HSV infections can be transmitted via contact with infected herpes lesions, genital and oral secretions, or mucosa.

History

- Painful "blister" lesions located around the mouth or genital area
- May have flu-like symptoms, including body aches, fever/chills, headache, and lymphadenopathy during a primary infection
- If symptoms recur, the outbreaks usually have shorter duration and less severe symptoms.

Physical Examination

- Vesicular lesions; one or more may be ulcerated

Considerations

- A primary herpes infection occurs when a patient without antibodies to HSV develops an infection.
- The virus can be shed from normal appearing skin/tissues, and many people are not aware they are infected and have no symptoms.
- Although there is no cure for a viral herpes infection, there are treatment options available to help manage outbreaks.

Pubic Lice (Pediculosis Pubis)

Translucent parasites that are usually spread through sexual contact; transmission through fomites (e.g., towels, clothing, or linens) is possible, but much less likely.

History

- Itching in the pubic area

Physical Examination

- Visible live lice and/or nits in the pubic hair

Consideration

- Condoms do not provide protection against pubic lice infestation

Pelvic Inflammatory Disease

Involves infection and inflammation of the upper genital tract organs, including the uterus and/or fallopian tubes. Gonorrheal and chlamydial infections account for almost half of all cases of PID.

History

- Lower abdominal/pelvic pain
- Vaginal discharge
- Pain with intercourse
- Frequent urination

Physical Examination

- Fever, abdominal tenderness, rebound tenderness
- Tenderness on bimanual examination, including cervical motion tenderness
- Positive culture for gonorrhea, chlamydia, trichomonas, and/or bacterial vaginosis

Consideration

- The symptoms of PID range from mild to severe; infertility can result from damage to the upper genital tract organs.

VAGINITIS/VAGINOSIS

Bacterial Vaginosis

A vaginal infection caused by an imbalance in the vaginal flora; it is the most common vaginal infection in women aged 15 to 44 years.

History

- Often asymptomatic
- Vaginal itching or irritation
- Strong fishy odor that is particularly noticeable after intercourse

Physical Examination

- White or gray vaginal discharge with pH >4.5
- Positive whiff test
- Clue cells on microscopy

Consideration

- Known risk factors for bacterial vaginosis include having a new sexual partner or multiple sexual partners and douching.

Candidiasis

Vulvovaginal candidiasis is an inflammation of the vulvar and vaginal tissues owing to an infection with *Candida* yeast. Approximately half of all women will experience a yeast infection at least once during their lifetime. There are several different species of *Candida* that cause VVC; however, *Candida albicans* is by far the most common.

History

- Vulvar itching/irritation
- Thick, white discharge
- Dysuria
- Dyspareunia

Physical Examination

- Curd-like discharge adherent to the vaginal walls
- Erythematous vagina and vulvar tissue
- Blastospores and pseudohyphae on microscopy

Consideration

- Risk factors include sexual debut, pregnancy, immunosuppression, and uncontrolled or undiagnosed diabetes

Genitourinary Syndrome of Menopause

A constellation of symptoms that affect the vulvovaginal and urethra areas during menopause or postmenopause as a result of decreased levels of estrogen.

History

- Genital symptoms: Vaginal dryness, burning, and irritation
- Sexual symptoms: Dyspareunia, lack of lubrication, postcoital bleeding
- Urinary symptoms: Dysuria, urgency, frequent or recurrent urinary tract infections

Physical Examination

- Thinning of the epithelial tissue of the vagina, pallor, loss of rugae
- Labia minora resorption, introital retraction
- Decrease in elasticity and vascularity of vagina, tissue fragility

Consideration

- Care should be taken to use water-soluble lubrication when performing a speculum exam, as insertion of the speculum can be painful

VULVAR/VAGINAL/URETHRAL LESIONS

Lichen Planus

A chronic, inflammatory autoimmune condition of unknown etiology that affects the skin and mucous membranes, including the vulva and vagina.

History

- Dysuria
- Irritation of vulvar area, itching
- Dyspareunia, postcoital bleeding
- Itchy rash likely to affect other areas of the body

Physical Examination

- White papules, plaques, and erosions
- Vagina can be friable; speculum exam painful

Consideration

- Most common type, erosive lichen planus, causes painful ulcers and scarring

Lichen Sclerosus

One of the most common vulvar dermatoses. Similar to lichen planus, it is an autoimmune-mediated, chronic, and inflammatory disease; however, lichen sclerosus is progressive, most often occurs postmenopause, and vaginal involvement almost never occurs.

History

- Vulvar itching, typically worse at night
- Dysuria
- Urine/stool retention

Physical Examination

- Initial appearance of skin may be white, thickened, excoriated, and edematous.
- As disease progresses, skin loses pigmentation, becomes very thin with wrinkled appearance, and anatomic features of external genitalia become distorted.
- May have anal fissures, ulcerations, lichenification, scarring

Consideration

- Women with lichen sclerosis are at increased risk of squamous cell carcinoma of the vulva

Intertrigo

An inflammatory condition of the skin in warm moist areas; occurs in places where two skin surfaces rub together. Common skin rash that occurs throughout life span.

History

- Between skin folds or in genital areas, skin surfaces are irritated, red, macerated
- Typically occurs in larger skin fold areas such as the axilla, groin folds, inner thighs, and breast and abdominal folds

Physical Examination

- Cracked or crusty skin, erythema, edema

Considerations

- Intertrigo is susceptible to secondary infections.
- Factors increasing risk for development include hot and humid conditions, obesity, diabetes, incontinence, malnutrition, and poor hygiene.

Vulvar Cancers and Vulvar Intraepithelial Neoplasia

Vulvar cancers are relatively rare; most are squamous cell carcinomas. VIN is a premalignant condition of the vulva.

History

- Chronic vulvar itching
- Dyspareunia
- Burning, tingling, or soreness in the vulvar region

Physical Examination

- Change in appearance including lesions or areas of redness or white, discolored skin
- Slightly raised skin lesions; some may appear darkened like a mole or freckle

Considerations

- Squamous cell carcinomas of the vulva associated with HPV infections are found more commonly in younger women, whereas those associated with differentiated VIN are typically found in older women.
- Risk factors associated with vulvar cancer include HPV infection, cervical cancer history, smoking, and chronic vulvar skin conditions.

Urethral Caruncle

A benign lesion located at the posterior urethral meatus.

History

- May be asymptomatic or might note a bump at the urinary meatus
- May cause dyspareunia, dysuria, or bleeding if irritated

Physical Examination

- Bright-red, vascular lesion located on the posterior lip of the urinary meatus

Consideration

- Commonly found in postmenopausal women and premenarchal girls and suspected to be a result of decreased levels of estrogen.

Bartholin Gland Cyst

Bartholin gland cysts develop when the gland becomes blocked, which is a common gynecologic problem, especially in reproductive-aged women. An uninfected cyst is typically painless and presents as a palpable, nontender lump or swelling. Bartholin cysts can become infected and cause significant pain. Visible erythema and acute tenderness are suggestive of an inflamed cyst and possible abscess (**Figure 14.11**).

PELVIC SUPPORT ISSUES

Pelvic Organ Prolapse

A condition in which there is failure of the anatomic supportive structures to adequately support the organs of the pelvis. It is a common and most often asymptomatic problem that does not require intervention for most women. Symptoms vary depending on the severity of the defects in the supportive structures. Types of pelvic organ prolapse include:

- **Cystocele:** Loss of pelvic support in the anterior vaginal wall causes the bladder to prolapse into the vaginal canal.

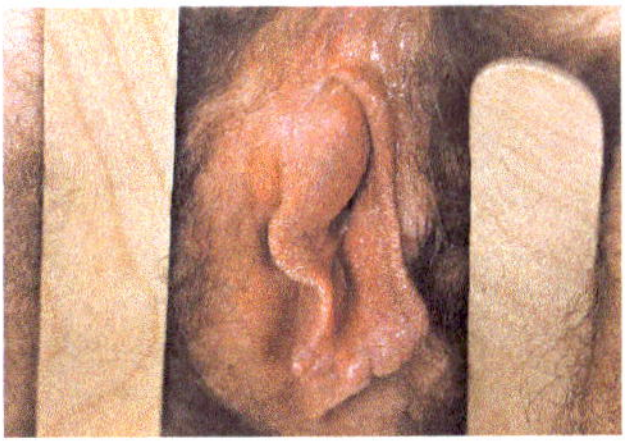

FIGURE 14.11 Infected Bartholin cyst. *Source:* Centers for Disease Control and Prevention/Susan Lindsley.

- **Rectocele:** Loss of pelvic support in the posterior vaginal wall allows the small bowel and/or rectum to prolapse.
- **Uterine prolapse:** Loss of pelvic support allows the uterus and cervix to prolapse through the vaginal canal; often associated with a concurrent cystocele and rectocele.

History

- May be asymptomatic, or may have pelvic pressure
- Urinary urgency, feeling of incomplete bladder emptying
- Difficulty with defecation

Physical Examination

- Bulging in the vulvar or vaginal areas
- May have visible tissue at the introitus

Consideration

- Risk factors for development include pregnancy, vaginal delivery and delivery-related injury, family history, obesity, and connective tissue diseases

GENITAL LESIONS/MASSES: MALIGNANT AND NONMALIGNANT

Cervical Intraepithelial Neoplasia and Cervical Malignancies

CIN is a premalignant condition of the squamous epithelial cell of the cervix. Infection with HPV is the most common cause of CIN lesions. There are two common types of CIN: low-grade squamous intraepithelial lesion and high-grade squamous intraepithelial lesion.

History

- History of abnormal Pap testing, HPV infection
- Unusual vaginal bleeding (i.e., after intercourse, between periods, or postmenopause)
- Pelvic pain, dyspareunia

Physical Examination

- May be unremarkable
- Cervix may have erosion, ulcer, or mass

Consideration

- Several risk factors have been identified in the development of HSIL and cervical cancer, including the subtype of HPV infection, the persistence of the HPV infection, cigarette smoking, and immunosuppressed state.

ADNEXAL MASSES

Adnexal masses have many etiologies, most of which are benign. Appropriate evaluation and monitoring of women with an adnexal mass is important to differentiate between benign, malignant, or emergent causes or conditions. **Figure 14.12** depicts adnexal masses, including ovarian cysts, ectopic pregnancy, ovarian cancer, and uterine fibroids.

Ovarian Cyst

Fluid-filled sacs that form in or on a woman's ovaries, most often during ovulation. They are a common ultrasound finding, and typically resolve without intervention.

History

- Often asymptomatic; however, can cause acute, unilateral pelvic pain
- Irregular menstrual periods, bloating

Physical Examination

- Ovarian cysts may be palpable during the bimanual physical exam.

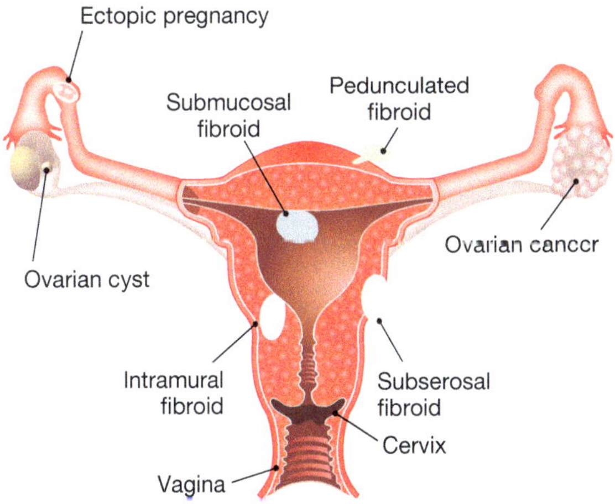

FIGURE 14.12 Adnexal masses, including ovarian cysts, ectopic pregnancy, ovarian cancer, and uterine fibroids.

Consideration

- More common in premenopausal women

Ectopic Pregnancy

A potential life-threatening emergency that results from the implantation of a fertilized egg outside of the uterus, most commonly in the fallopian tube.

History

- Vaginal bleeding
- Increasing unilateral pelvic pain
- Altered menstrual cycle

Physical Examination

- Positive pregnancy test
- Palpable adnexal mass on bimanual examination
- CMT

Consideration

- Failure to diagnose an ectopic pregnancy in a timely fashion can result in rupture of the fallopian tube, leading to hemorrhage and possible death.

Ovarian Cancer

The second most common gynecologic cancer, most often occurring in women aged 55 to 64 years. Refer to Box 14.2 for signs and symptoms.

History

- Abdominal distention or bloating
- Early satiety with loss of appetite
- Unexplained pelvic or abdominal pain
- Increased urinary urgency or frequency
- Postcoital bleeding; postmenopausal bleeding
- Unexplained weight loss, fatigue, or change in bowel habits
- Over 50 years of age with new symptoms of irritable bowel syndrome
- Family history of breast, ovarian, or colon cancer

Physical Examination

- No specific findings
- May palpate mass on pelvic exam, or adnexal fullness

Consideration

- Women with suspected ovarian cancer based on clinical presentation or a pelvic mass should undergo transvaginal ultrasonography

Uterine Fibroids

Benign growths arising from the smooth muscle (myometrium) of the uterus. They occur in more than half of all women, develop after menarche, and regress post menopause.

History

- Depending on size and location of fibroid, symptoms vary
- Can be asymptomatic or cause heavy menstrual bleeding
- Pelvic pain, dyspareunia, bladder dysfunction

Physical Examination

- Lump or mass on abdominal examination
- Enlarged uterus in a nonpregnant woman on bimanual examination
- Irregular contour of the uterus on bimanual examination

Consideration

- Management is individualized; considerations include desire to preserve fertility

OTHER DISORDERS CAUSING MENSTRUAL IRREGULARITIES

Polycystic Ovary Syndrome

A complex endocrine disorder of unknown etiology. Thought to be genetically linked, it is a common cause of menstrual irregularity and infertility and is associated with insulin resistance.

History

- Presentation is variable; can be asymptomatic
- Irregular menstrual cycles
- Infertility
- Weight gain

Physical Examination

- Signs of hyperandrogenism: Acne, hirsutism, acanthosis nigricans
- May have male pattern baldness, thinning hair
- Polycystic ovaries on ultrasound

Consideration

- Women with PCOS are at increased risk for metabolic syndrome, type 2 diabetes, dyslipidemia, and cardiovascular disease

Endometriosis

The implantation and abnormal growth of endometrial cells outside of the uterus. The endometrial cells induce inflammatory reactions, secrete prostaglandins, and infiltrate tissues and nerves, causing secondary dysmenorrhea, scars, traction, and fibrosis.

History

- Dysmenorrhea, lower abdominal pain, dyspareunia
- May have infertility
- Pain is most often cyclic, or intensified during menstrual cycle

Physical Examination

- No specific findings

Consideration

- Visual inspection by laparoscopy is the gold standard for diagnosing endometriosis

Vasomotor Symptoms

A term used to describe the constellation of symptoms commonly referred to as hot flashes or night sweats. VMS are commonly experienced during perimenopause and the menopausal transition as recurrent, transient episodes of flushing accompanied by a sensation of warmth to the upper body and/or face.

History

- Hot flashes, flushing of the face with severe sweating
- Night sweats, sleep disturbances
- May have associated heart palpitations

Physical Examination

- Nonspecific, unless VMS occur during the physical exam

Considerations

- Triggered by caffeine, alcohol, smoking, clothing that is too warm, environmental temperature, stress, eating spicy foods, medications, and co-occurring health conditions
- VMS have been associated with diminished quality of life for some women

PHYSICAL EXAMINATION DOCUMENTATION

EXAMPLE OF NORMAL FINDINGS FOR BREAST ASSESSMENT

Breasts symmetric. No retractions, nipple discharge, skin changes, or lesions. No palpable masses, tenderness, or axillary lymphadenopathy.

EXAMPLE OF NORMAL FINDINGS FOR FEMALE GENITALIA EXAM

External genitalia has no lesions or discharge. No inguinal lymphadenopathy. Vulva without lesions, erythema, or discharge. No tenderness to Bartholin or Skene's glands. Vagina pink, rugae present, no lesions or discharge. Cervix pink, no lesions or discharge. Nulliparous os. Bimanual exam without pain, no cervical motion tenderness. Uterus: Normal size, shape, position, and contour. No adnexal tenderness or palpable masses. Anus: No hemorrhoids, fissures, or lesions. Rectal wall intact, no masses or tenderness.

REFERENCES

References for this chapter draw from Chapter 17, "Evidence-Based Assessment of the Breasts and Axillae," and Chapter 20, "Evidence-Based Assessment of the Female Genitourinary System," of the textbook *Evidence-Based Physical Examination: Best Practices for Health and Well-Being Assessment*. The references may be accessed in the digital version of the handbook at https://connect.springerpub.com/content/book/97808-8261-6466-7/chapter /ch14

15

Evidence-Based Obstetric Assessment

CLINICAL CONSIDERATIONS

- Women should be considered active participants in their care during pregnancy and encouraged to share decision-making with their clinician.
- Recognize that the childbearing year is a time of great growth, stress, and excitement for the entire family unit.
- The clinician should ask about fetal movement, contractions/cramping, vaginal bleeding, and loss of fluid at each visit.
- Collaboration with generalist obstetric providers or perinatologists is key for women with more complicated health histories.
- Many concerns in pregnancy are considered normal. The clinician's job is to determine when these concerns may actually be abnormal and to know how to assess for concerns.
- The initial prenatal visit is an opportunity to provide a wealth of information to patients about their health and pregnancy, as well as an opportunity for the clinician to screen for problems that may arise in later pregnancy.
- The vast majority of women will have a healthy pregnancy.

SUBJECTIVE HISTORY

REASON FOR SEEKING CARE

Pregnancy, pregnancy-related concerns

HISTORY OF PRESENT ILLNESS

- Last menstrual period date, unknown, approximate, definite
- Last normal menstrual period date (if different than LMP)
- Age at menarche
- Age at estimated due date
- Typical cycle length (28–30 days most reliable in terms of dating)

- Is this a planned pregnancy? Was any contraception used at the time of conception?
- Is this a desired pregnancy? If not, discussion of pregnancy options—continuing pregnancy and keeping child, continuing pregnancy and adoption, pregnancy termination.
- See **Box 15.1** for methods of determining EDD.

HEALTH HISTORY

Past Medical History

- History of HTN or diabetes mellitus (also relevant: PCOS or insulin resistance)
- History of asthma or allergic rhinitis

BOX 15.1

METHODS OF DETERMINING ESTIMATED DUE DATE

- The first day of the LMP may be used if the LMP is certain, cycles are regular (ideally every 28–30 days), and the LMP was normal for that woman. The accuracy of this can be compromised by several factors: Some women may not know their LMP, some may ovulate later in their cycle than others, and some may have some early pregnancy bleeding that they mistake for a period. Naegele's rule is based on an LMP from a 28-day menstrual cycle. The formula for Naegele's rule is the first day of LMP +7 days–3 months = EDD. This is the basis for the calculations performed by most pregnancy wheels and apps. The variation in EDDs obtained by these methods is 1 to 7 days (King et al., 2019).
- If the pregnancy is conceived using ART, such as IUI or IVF, the date of insemination or embryo transfer may be used as the LMP.
- Ultrasound may also be used to confirm an EDD. First trimester ultrasound (performed before 14 weeks and 0 days) is most accurate (within 5–7 days). Second trimester ultrasound is less accurate in terms of dating the pregnancy, with a variance of 7–14 days.

ART, artificial reproductive technologies; EDD, estimated due date; IUI, intrauterine insemination; IVF, in vitro fertilization; LMP, last menstrual period.

- History of autoimmune disorders including thyroid disorders
- History of anxiety/depression/postpartum depression or other mental health disorders
- History of varicella (disease or vaccination? If vaccination, how many doses?)
- History of CMV
- History of clotting disorders

Obstetric History (If Relevant)

- GTPAL: **G**ravida (number of pregnancies), **T**erm (number of full-term births), **P**reterm (number of preterm births, after 20 weeks' gestation), **A**bortions (number of elective terminations and/or miscarriages, including births prior to 20 weeks' gestation), **L**iving (number of living children)
- Method of prior births (if vaginal—spontaneous, vacuum, or forceps? If cesarean section—what kind of incision and what was the reason for cesarean?)
- Length of labor
- Complications during previous pregnancies and/or births: Gestational diabetes mellitus (diet-controlled, controlled with oral medication, controlled with insulin), essential hypertension, gestational hypertension, preeclampsia, eclampsia, HELLP, postpartum hemorrhage, shoulder dystocia, retained placenta, 3rd or 4th degree perineal laceration, issues with child's health
- If history of elective termination or miscarriage—any complications? Required D&C?
- If history of miscarriage(s), age of fetus at time of miscarriage?
- History of preterm labor or birth (20 weeks' 0 days–36 weeks' 6 days)?
- History of fetal/neonatal demise?
- History of ectopic pregnancy?
- A poor outcome in previous pregnancy increases the risk for a poor outcome in the next pregnancy.

Gynecologic History

- Last Pap test?
- History of abnormal Pap(s)?
- History of LEEP or cone biopsy? If yes, there is an increased risk for cervical incompetence/preterm labor/preterm birth.
- History of gynecologic surgery?
- History of endometriosis?

Medications

- Prescribed and OTC medications or supplements, including dose and frequency (specifically pregnancy category C, D, and X medications)
- Prenatal vitamins

Allergies

- Allergies to medications or seasonal, environmental, and/or food allergies? If "yes," clarify reaction.

FAMILY HISTORY

- Genetic disorders: Known or suspected genetic disease, multiple malformations, multiple miscarriages, recurrence of the same or similar disorders, intellectual disability, autism spectrum disorders, and consanguinity
- Type 2 DM
- Preeclampsia

SOCIAL HISTORY

- Married/single/divorced/widowed/partnered?
- Is partner involved? If not, who is support?
- Does partner have any other children?
- Who does she live with?
- Housing situation?
- Feels safe at home?
- Tobacco use? If yes, assess readiness to quit.
- Alcohol use?
- Illicit drug use (marijuana may or may not be legal depending on state, but still need to counsel on unknown effects during pregnancy)?
- History of alcohol/drug use or addiction?
- Occupation: Exposure to workplace hazards (e.g., chemicals/fumes, radiation, chemotherapeutic agents, patients with CMV)
- Screen for intimate partner violence?
- Any history of reproductive or sexual coercion?
- What kind of diet is followed? Is there a concern of malnutrition (undernutrition or overnutrition)?

REVIEW OF SYSTEMS

- **Constitutional**: Fatigue, weight gain, weight loss, change in appetite

- **HEENT**: Visual changes (blurred vision, spots, or floaters), epistaxis, nasal drainage/congestion, bleeding gums, tooth pain
- **CV**: Heart palpitations, leg swelling
- **Respiratory**: Shortness of breath, wheezing, snoring
- **GI**: Nausea, vomiting, food aversions, abdominal pain, constipation, diarrhea
- **GU**: Pelvic pain, vaginal bleeding, vaginal discharge, frequent urination, hematuria, dysuria, urinary urgency, urinary incontinence, STI exposure
- **MSK**: Muscle cramping, muscle pain, joint pain
- **Skin**: Itching, breast tenderness, breast lumps, nipple discharge
- **Neurologic**: Headache, seizure, dizziness, lightheadedness, syncope
- **Mental health**: Anxiety, depression, irritability, suicidality
- **Endocrine**: Heat or cold intolerance
- **Hematologic**: Easy bruising, excess bleeding
- **Allergic**: Hives, seasonal allergies

RED FLAGS IN SUBJECTIVE HISTORY

- Nausea or vomiting that prohibits intake or causes weight loss
- Dysuria
- Reported decreased or absent fetal movement
- Severe headache
- Use of Category D or X medications
- Excessive alcohol use
- Recreational drug use or addiction
- Worsening anxiety or depression
- History of domestic or interpersonal violence

PREVENTIVE CARE CONSIDERATIONS

- Up to date on cervical cancer screening?
- Up to date on mammography screening (if applicable)?
- Up to date on flu vaccine (seasonal, recommended during pregnancy regardless of gestational age), tetanus diphtheria, and pertussis vaccine (recommended between 27 and 36 weeks' gestation during each pregnancy)?
- Depression screening
- Intimate partner violence screening
- Tobacco use counseling if patient uses tobacco (advise them to stop smoking and provide behavioral interventions for cessation)
- Screening for unhealthy alcohol use (provide brief behavioral counseling interventions to reduce unhealthy alcohol use)

- Pets at home? In particular, patients with cats must be counseled on the risk of toxoplasmosis and precautions; patients who own reptiles must be counseled on the risk of listeriosis and precautions
- Recent travel for patient or partner to areas with Zika virus and timing of that travel? If so, any mosquito bites or symptoms?
- Current medications/vitamins/supplements (consider safety profile in pregnancy)?
- Prepregnancy weight?
- Preferred pronouns (he/him, she/her, they/their)?

UNIQUE POPULATION CONSIDERATIONS

Advanced Maternal Age

- Women who will be age 35 or older at their estimated due date are considered to be AMA. There are increased risks with AMA pregnancies, including an increased risk of chromosomal abnormalities, fetal growth restriction, gestational diabetes, gestational hypertension, preeclampsia, placental insufficiency, preterm birth, and stillbirth.

Trauma-Informed Care

- A gynecologic or obstetric exam, labor, or delivery may trigger PTSD symptoms from a history of child maltreatment or sexual violence. Even without a history of abuse or maltreatment, some women are finding themselves traumatized by their care prenatally, or in labor and delivery.
- Clinicians must educate themselves on trauma-informed care, as well as how best to care for these women during pregnancy without re-traumatizing them. Trauma-informed care such as universal screening, clinician comfort with adjusting routine exams and responding to possible reactions of those affected by prior trauma, and the availability of PTSD resources and referrals all play a role in helping to establish a good clinician-patient relationship and contribute to improved perinatal outcomes. For more information on trauma informed care, refer to Chapter 16, "Evidence-Based Assessment of Mental Health and Substance Abuse."

PHYSICAL EXAMINATION

GENERAL SURVEY

- Initial assessment for physiologic stability
- **Vital signs:** Temperature, pulse rate, respiratory rate, blood pressure

- Note whether the patient appears visibly pregnant (fundus above the symphysis pubis)
- Height and weight, weight should be recorded at each visit

INSPECTION

- Inspect the breasts and nipples for symmetry. Note any changes to the skin of the breasts, including dimpling, peau d'orange appearance, erythema, or edema. (For more information on breast examinations, please refer to Chapter 14, "Evidence-Based Assessment of Breasts, Female Genitalia, and Reproductive System.")
- A complete visual inspection of the external genitals should be performed, noting any lesions, erythema, edema, or discharge.
- In early pregnancy, Chadwick's sign may be observed during a speculum exam; the cervix appears bluish-purplish in color or cyanotic. Note the presence of any lesions, erythema, edema, discharge, or bleeding inside the vaginal vault or at the cervix.
- The cervical os has a different appearance and feel in nulliparous women vs multiparous women. In the nulliparous woman, the cervical os is pinpoint in size and rounded. In the multiparous woman, the os has the appearance of a slit.

PALPATION

- If >12 weeks' gestation or if dates are unknown, an abdominal exam to assess if the fundus is palpable in the abdomen is useful. See **Figure 15.1** for changes in fundal height.
  - At 12 weeks' gestation, the fundus should be palpable just caudally to the symphysis pubis.
  - At 16 weeks' gestation, the fundus should be palpable midway between the symphysis pubis and the umbilicus.
  - At 20 weeks' gestation, the fundus should be palpable at the umbilicus.
  - As pregnancy progresses past 20 weeks' gestation, the clinician will measure the fundal height at each visit. This is the measurement in centimeters from the top of the symphysis pubis to the fundus (**Figure 15.2**). The measurement approximately correlates with the current number of weeks of gestation.
  - Clinicians will also assess the fetal presentation by utilizing Leopold's maneuvers after approximately 28 weeks' gestation (**Figure 15.3**).
- Gestational age may be estimated by the size of the uterus, both abdominally and with a bimanual exam. In early pregnancy, the clinician may note Hegar's sign, in which the lower segment of

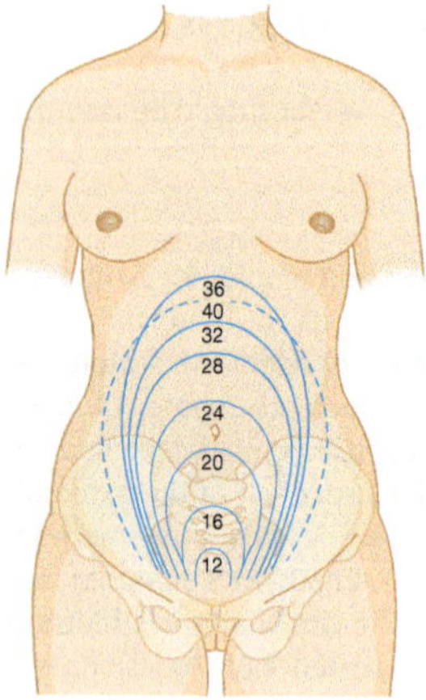

FIGURE 15.1 Changes in fundal height during pregnancy. At 12 weeks' gestation, the fundus of the uterus is palpable just superior to the symphysis pubis. At 16 weeks' gestation, the fundus is palpable midway between the symphysis pubis and the umbilicus. At 20 weeks' gestation, the fundus is in line with the umbilicus. At approximately 28 weeks' gestation, the fundus is palpable midway between the umbilicus and the xyphoid process; the clinician should be able to determine fetal presentation. At 34 weeks' gestation, the fundus is palpable just below the xyphoid process. Sometimes fundal height will decrease at term, as the fetal head engages in the maternal pelvis.

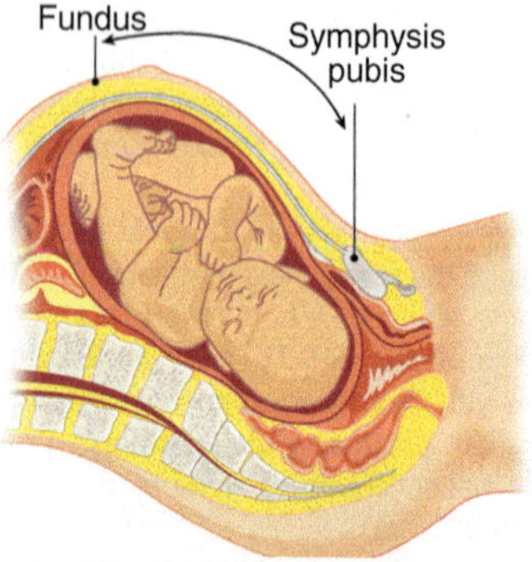

FIGURE 15.2 Measurement of fundal height. Measurement in centimeters from the top of the symphysis pubis to the fundus.

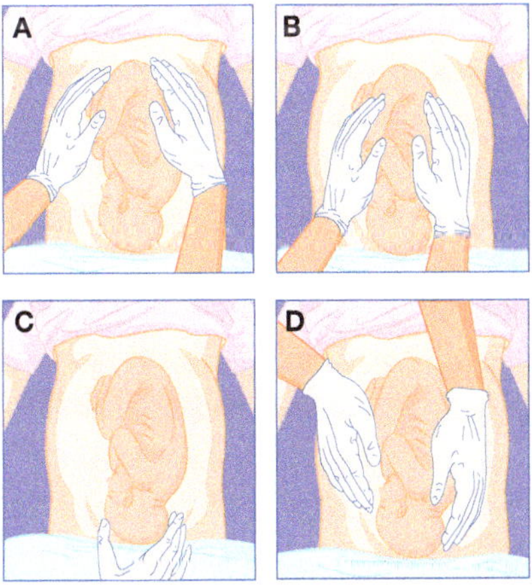

FIGURE 15.3 Performing Leopold's maneuvers. (**A**) Identify fetal part in uterine fundus. (**B**) Using the palmar surface of both hands, identify which side of the uterus contains the fetal back and which contains "small parts" such as hands and feet. (**C**) Use the thumb and third finger to identify fetal presenting part. (**D**) Use both hands to outline fetal presenting part.

the uterus becomes very soft and compressible in early pregnancy. The clinician may also note Goodell's sign, which is softening of the cervix in the first trimester.

- Clinical pelvimetry, or a measurement of the diameters of the pelvis, may be assessed by an experienced obstetric clinician, if indicated or desired. There is mixed evidence for the utility of measurements derived from pelvimetry, although this skill may be more useful during a labor in which cephalo-pelvic disproportion is suspected, or in low-resource countries, where a contracted pelvis may be more common.
- When performing a speculum or bimanual pelvic exam, patient comfort, both physical and emotional, should be considered of the utmost importance. Many exams can be done without the need for stirrups; instead, ask the patient to bend at the knee and come down toward the clinician on the exam table. Appropriate draping is important, as well as eye contact with the patient. It is helpful to ask the patient if they are ready to be touched before the clinician begins a pelvic exam and to initially touch on the inside of the thigh prior to touching the genitals.

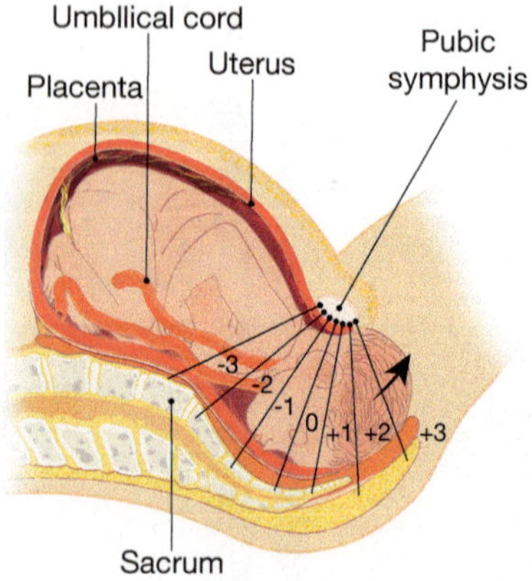

FIGURE 15.4 Fetal station. This is a measurement of the relationship of the presenting part to the ischial spines in the maternal pelvis and signifies the descent of the fetus in the pelvis. Negative numbers (e.g., −2, −1) indicate that the presenting part (typically, the bony aspect of the fetal vertex) is above the ischial spines by that many centimeters. Zero station indicates that the presenting part is in line with the ischial spines. Positive numbers (e.g., +1, +2) indicate that the presenting part is below the ischial spines by that many centimeters. The fetus descends as labor progresses. Most women will feel a spontaneous urge to push around 0 to +2 cm, particularly without an epidural.

- In full-term pregnancy or for concerns prior to term, the clinician may need to perform a cervical exam to evaluate for labor/preterm labor. Five main findings from a cervical exam are dilation, effacement, fetal station (**Figure 15.4**), position of the cervix, and consistency of the cervix.

AUSCULTATION

Fetal heart tones are auscultated at each visit, typically with a Doppler. Fetal heart tones can be heard with a Doppler after 10 to 12 weeks' gestation, depending on the strength of the Doppler. A fetoscope may also be used to auscultate fetal heart tones; however, this requires an experienced clinician and the patient must typically be at least 24 weeks' gestation.

RED FLAGS IN OBJECTIVE EXAM

- Vaginal bleeding
- Loss of fluid

- Contractions prior to 37 weeks
- Upper right abdominal pain
- Changes in vision
- High BP
- Decreased urine output
- Thrombocytopenia
- Impaired liver function
- Proteinuria
- Seizures
- Symptoms of an ectopic pregnancy (severe, unilateral pelvic pain, dizziness, fainting, or rectal pressure in the first trimester)

CONSIDERATIONS

- If maternal BP is elevated at the initial prenatal visit, the clinician should attempt to find pre-pregnancy records to determine if chronic hypertension exists.
- Maternal BMI should be calculated at the initial prenatal visit using the pre-pregnancy weight to guide weight gain recommendations during pregnancy as well as to assess for risk for co-morbid conditions (**Table 15.1**).

TABLE 15.1 Institute of Medicine Weight Gain Recommendations for Pregnancy

Prepregnancy Weight Category	Body Mass Index*	Recommended Range of Total Weight (lbs)	Recommended Rates of Weight Gain 2nd and 3rd Trimesters (lbs; Mean Range [lbs/week])**
Underweight	<18.5	28–40	1 (1.0–1.3)
Normal weight	18.5–24.9	25–35	1 (0.8–1.0)
Overweight	25–29.9	15–25	0.6 (0.5–0.7)
Obese (includes all classes)	>30	11–20	0.5 (0.4–0.6)

*Body mass index is calculated by using the following formula: Weight in pounds / Height in inches x height in inches x 703.
**Calculations assume a 1.1- to 4.4-lb weight gain in the first trimester.

Source: Modified from Institute of Medicine. (2009). *Weight gain during pregnancy: Reexamining the guidelines*. National Academies Press. © 2009 National Academy of Sciences.

EVIDENCE-BASED RESOURCES

American College of Obstetricians and Gynecologists. (2013). ACOG Committee Opinion. No. 548: Weight gain during pregnancy. *Obstetrics & Gynecology, 121*, 210–212. https://doi.org/10.1097/01.aog.0000425668.87506.4c

American College of Obstetricians and Gynecologists. (2015). ACOG Practice Bulletin. No. 156: Obesity in pregnancy. *Obstetrics & Gynecology, 126*(3), e112–e126. https://doi.org/10.1097/AOG.0000000000001211

American College of Obstetricians and Gynecologists. (2016). ACOG Practice Bulletin. No. 175: Ultrasound in pregnancy. *Obstetrics & Gynecology, 128*(6), e241–e256. https://doi.org/10.1097/AOG.0000000000001815

American College of Obstetricians and Gynecologists. (2018a). ACOG Practice Bulletin. No: 189: Nausea and vomiting of pregnancy. *Obstetrics & Gynecology, 131*(1), e15–e30. https://doi.org/10.1097/AOG.0000000000002456

American College of Obstetricians and Gynecologists. (2018b). ACOG Practice Bulletin. No. 190: Gestational diabetes mellitus. *Obstetrics & Gynecology, 131*(2), e49–e64. https://doi.org/10.1097/AOG.0000000000002501

American College of Obstetricians and Gynecologists. (2018c). ACOG Practice Bulletin. No. 202: Gestation hypertension and preeclampsia. *Obstetrics & Gynecology, 133*(1), e1–e25. https://doi.org/10.1097/AOG.0000000000003018

Lockwood, C. J., & Magriples, U. (2020a). Prenatal care: Initial assessment. In V. Berghella (Ed.), *UpToDate*. https://www.uptodate.com/contents/prenatal-care-initial-assessment on August 28, 2018.

Lockwood, C. J., & Magriples, U. (2020b). Prenatal care: Second and third trimesters. In V. Berghella (Ed.), *UpToDate*. https://www.uptodate.com/contents/prenatal-care-second-and-third-trimesters

U.S. Preventive Services Task Force. (2015). *Final update summary: Tobacco smoking cessation in adults, including pregnant women: Behavioral and pharmacotherapy interventions*. https://www.uspreventiveservicestaskforce.org/uspstf/recommendation/tobacco-use-in-adults-and-pregnant-women-counseling-and-interventions

(*continued*)

EVIDENCE-BASED RESOURCES (*CONTINUED*)

U.S. Preventive Services Task Force. (2016a). *Final recommendation statement: Depression in adults: Screening*. https://www.uspreventiveservicestaskforce.org/Page/Document/RecommendationStatementFinal/depression-in-adults-screening1

U.S. Preventive Services Task Force. (2016b). *Final update summary: Gestational diabetes mellitus, screening*. https://www.uspreventiveservicestaskforce.org/Page/Document/UpdateSummaryFinal/gestational-diabetes-mellitus-screening

U.S. Preventive Services Task Force. (2016c). *Final update summary: Low-dose aspirin use for the prevention of morbidity and mortality from preeclampsia: Preventive medication*. https://www.uspreventiveservicestaskforce.org/Page/Document/UpdateSummaryFinal/low-dose-aspirin-use-for-the-prevention-of-morbidity-and-mortality-from-preeclampsia-preventive-medication

ABNORMAL FINDINGS

ACUTE CYSTITIS (URINARY TRACT INFECTION)

An infection of the lower urinary tract.

History

- Dysuria
- Hematuria
- Increased urinary frequency or urgency; incomplete emptying of bladder
- Flank and/or suprapubic pain
- Uterine contractions/cramping

Physical Examination

- Fever
- Pyuria, positive nitrites, and hematuria on urinalysis

Considerations

- Not uncommon in pregnant women due to effects of progesterone on the motility of the ureters.
- The urinary tract is typically sterile. Urinary tract infections occur when bacteria ascends into the urinary tract. The most common organism causing a UTI is *Escherichia coli*.

ANEMIA IN PREGNANCY

A condition in which the blood does not carry enough oxygen to the rest of the body. Iron-deficiency is the most common cause of anemia in pregnancy due to increased maternal iron needs, fetal iron needs, and expanded maternal blood volume.

History

- Fatigue, weakness, shortness of breath, headaches
- Leg cramps
- Cold intolerance
- Reported iron-deficient diet
- Pagophagia or pica
- GI issues affecting iron absorption
- A history of closely spaced pregnancies

Physical Examination

- Pallor
- Tachycardia
- Decreased hemoglobin and ferritin levels

Considerations

- Physiologic anemia is often seen during the second trimester of pregnancy due to increased blood volume.
- Diagnosis and treatment are important as iron-deficiency anemia may contribute to preterm birth, intrauterine growth restriction, decrease in maternal blood reserves during birth and increase in need for transfusion after birth, and decreased milk production.

ASYMPTOMATIC BACTERIURIA

The presence of a high level of bacteria in the urine with no patient-reported symptoms.

History

- No signs or symptoms consistent with UTI

Physical Examination

- High level bacterial growth on urine culture ($\geq 10^5$ CFU/mL). If bacteriuria is due to group B *Streptococcus*, treatment threshold is $\geq 10^4$ and women should be considered to be GBS positive for intrapartum care.

Considerations

- Common in pregnancy and should be treated as these infections have a higher likelihood of ascending to the kidneys.

- Pregnant women should be universally screened for asymptomatic bacteriuria at their initial prenatal visit.
- Asymptomatic bacteriuria may also cause preterm contractions, so it should be a consideration when preterm contractions or persistent cramping are complaints.

CONSTIPATION IN PREGNANCY

A condition that causes hard stools; infrequent or hard to pass bowel movements.

History

- Reports difficult/painful bowel movements, hard stools, and/or straining with bowel movements
- History of infrequent bowel movements (<3 times week)
- Abdominal pain
- Low-fiber diet
- Decreased fluid intake
- Ignoring the urge to have a bowel movement
- Feeling bloated
- History of laxative or opioid use

Physical Examination

- On abdominal exam, hard, palpable stool in the ascending, descending, and sigmoid segments of the colon
- Hard or impacted stool during a rectal exam

Considerations

- Constipation is a common concern during all trimesters of pregnancy, although it is typically more prevalent during the first trimester. Women may also experience constipation due to more pressure on the GI tract from the uterus as it grows throughout pregnancy.
- Prenatal vitamins with iron or the addition of an iron supplement during pregnancy can also contribute to constipation.

FIRST-TRIMESTER BLEEDING

Vaginal bleeding during the first trimester, occurring in approximately 20% to 40% of women.

Benign First-Trimester Bleeding

This bleeding would include implantation bleeding, vaginitis, mistaken hematuria or rectal bleeding, or bleeding from a cervical polyp.

History

- Light spotting/vaginal bleeding
- History of recent intercourse

Physical Examination

- Presence of fetal heart tones at 12 weeks' gestation or more with Doppler
- Presence of fetal cardiac activity/fetal movement on ultrasound
- Increasing levels of hCG

First-Trimester Bleeding That Is Cause for Increased Surveillance or Indicative of Miscarriage

Include blighted ovum, subchorionic hemorrhage (carries increased likelihood of miscarriage), "disappearing" twin gestation, spontaneous abortion (either complete or incomplete), or missed abortion.

History

- History of ectopic pregnancy or previous miscarriage
- History of uterine anomaly
- History of adnexal surgery
- History of PID or endometriosis
- Presence of an IUD
- Varying amount of vaginal bleeding; passing tissue and/or large clots from vagina
- Abdominal cramping; back pain
- Lightheadedness

Physical Examination

- Absence of fetal heart tones at 12 weeks' gestation or more with Doppler
- Absence of fetal cardiac activity/fetal movement on ultrasound
- EDD by LMP inconsistent with crown-rump length on ultrasound
- EDD by LMP inconsistent with uterine size on bimanual exam
- Decreasing levels of hCG

Considerations

- Fifteen to 20% of pregnancies will end in miscarriage and about 80% of those losses will occur in the first trimester.
- It is critical to exclude the possibility of an ectopic pregnancy in any patient with first trimester bleeding, as this can be a life-threatening complication.

GESTATIONAL DIABETES SCREENING

Diabetes (high blood sugar) that is diagnosed for the first time in pregnancy and usually returns back to normal soon after delivery.

History

- Commonly asymptomatic
- May have increased thirst or urination
- Previous history of gestational diabetes, prediabetes, or polycystic ovarian syndrome
- Family history of diabetes
- Lack of physical activity
- Races other than Caucasian are more susceptible

Physical Examination

- Can be overweight/obese
- Elevated blood sugar during 2 step test

Considerations

- The U.S. Preventive Services Task Force (2016b) recommends screening for GD Min all asymptomatic pregnant women after 24 weeks' gestation. The test is typically performed between 24 and 28 weeks' gestation with an oral glucose challenge.
- Infants born to mothers with GDM have an increased incidence of macrosomia, neonatal hypoglycemia, hyperbilirubinemia, shoulder dystocia, and birth trauma.

HYPERTENSIVE DISORDERS

Chronic or Gestational Hypertension

Chronic hypertension is defined as hypertension diagnosed or present before pregnancy or before 20 weeks of gestation. Additionally, cHTN is hypertension diagnosed for the first time during pregnancy that does not resolve during the postpartum period. *Gestational hypertension* is defined as a systolic BP of ≥140 mmHg or a diastolic BP of ≥90 mmHg on two separate occasions in a woman with previously normal blood pressures. Blood pressure readings return to normal in the postpartum period. These measurements must be at least 4 hours apart and after 20 weeks' gestation.

History

- History of kidney disease or diabetes
- Pregnant with multiples
- African American
- May have no signs or symptoms (other than elevated blood pressure)

Physical Examination

- Elevated BP
- Headache
- Edema

- Nausea/vomiting
- May progress to preeclampsia

Considerations

- Gestational hypertension must be distinguished from preeclampsia by the absence of proteinuria or severe features (see next section for diagnostic criteria for preeclampsia).
- A woman with gestational hypertension with severe range BP (a systolic BP of 160 mmHg or greater or a diastolic BP of 110 mmHg or greater) should be diagnosed instead as having preeclampsia with severe features.

Preeclampsia

Hypertension plus proteinuria during pregnancy, with an onset after 20 weeks' gestation. In women with gestational hypertension in the absence of proteinuria, preeclampsia may also be diagnosed with the new onset of any severe features (see the following text for list).

History and Physical Examination

- Proteinuria
- Elevated blood pressure
- Severe features
  - New-onset headache unresponsive to medication and not accounted for by alternative diagnoses
  - New-onset visual disturbances
  - Severe persistent right upper quadrant or epigastric pain unresponsive to medication and not accounted for by alternative diagnoses
  - Thrombocytopenia (platelet count <100,00 × 109/L)
  - Renal insufficiency (serum creatinine >1.1 mg/dL or a doubling of the serum creatinine)
  - Impaired liver function (doubling of liver transaminases)
  - Pulmonary edema

Eclampsia

When preeclampsia is left untreated, it can progress to the serious condition, eclampsia.

History and Physical Exam

- Seizures
- Coma
- Expiry

Consideration

- Up to 50% of women with gestational hypertension will eventually develop preeclampsia during their pregnancy.

Hyperemesis Gravidarum

Severe symptoms of nausea and vomiting that often require inpatient management in the first and second trimesters.

History

- Personal or family history of hyperemesis gravidarum
- Severe nausea
- Having multiples
- Overweight
- Food aversions
- Dizziness/lightheadedness, headaches
- Persistent vomiting (>3–4 times daily)

Physical Examination

- Large ketonuria
- Dehydration
- Weight loss (typically at least 5% of prepregnancy weight)
- Abnormalities with electrolytes, thyroid function, and liver function.

Considerations

- Nausea and vomiting of pregnancy is modulated by increased hCG and estrogen levels.
- Approximately 50% to 80% of pregnant women will report nausea and 50% will experience both nausea and vomiting.
- "Normal" pregnancy-related nausea and vomiting should be differentiated from hyperemesis gravidarum. Unfortunately, there is no widely accepted clinical distinction between the two.

Pruritic Urticarial Papules and Plaques of Pregnancy

A benign, self-limiting rash that occurs during pregnancy and most often resolves within 7 to 10 days after delivery.

History

- Pruritic rash that typically develops in the third trimester
- History of rapid, excessive weight gain or multiple gestation
- More likely to occur in first pregnancies

Physical Examination

- Scattered erythematous papules, most often found on abdomen with a clear area directly around the umbilicus

- Lesions may spread to the extremities, chest, and back; combine to form plaques; in patients with fair skin, white halos may surround the papules
- Lesions started in striae
- No lesions in periumbilical area
- Typically lesions are not on face, palms, or soles

Considerations

- Pruritic urticarial papules and plaques of pregnancy is typically seen in primiparous women toward the end of pregnancy (mean time of onset is 35 weeks' gestation).
- It is benign, self-limiting, and most often resolves within 7 to 10 days after delivery.
- It occurs in 0.3% to 0.6% of pregnancies and is more common with multiple gestation and male fetuses.

Gestational Thrombocytopenia

A platelet count of less than 150 × 109/L. Thrombocytopenia is often asymptomatic and may only be discovered on a routine CBC in pregnancy.

History

- Onset in the mid-second to third trimester
- Women are asymptomatic
- No history of bleeding
- No history of thrombocytopenia outside of pregnancy

Physical Examination

- A platelet count of <150 × 109/L typically found on routine screening
- Thrombocytopenia resolves after pregnancy (within 1–2 months postpartum)

Considerations

- Gestational thrombocytopenia occurs in 5% to 11% of pregnancies.
- A gradual decrease in platelets is expected as pregnancy progresses, but thrombocytopenia may result from both physiologic and pathologic conditions.
- There is no significant maternal or fetal risk with gestational thrombocytopenia, and the diagnosis is one of exclusion. The clinician will want to assess for a history of any bleeding disorders or symptoms associated with platelet disorders, such as petechiae, ecchymosis, epistaxis, gingival bleeding, or a history of menometrorrhagia.

PHYSICAL EXAMINATION DOCUMENTATION

Documentation should include results of inspection, palpation, and auscultation.

EXAMPLE OF NORMAL FINDINGS FROM FIRST PRENATAL VISIT AT 8 WEEKS' GESTATION

BP 120/80, pulse rate 72/min, weight 122 lbs

Well-appearing and afebrile. Heart rate and rhythm regular. Lungs clear to auscultation bilaterally. Breasts engorged, no distinct masses or lymphadenopathy palpable. Abdomen soft, nontender, and nondistended. Speculum exam completed without discomfort: No vaginal discharge, erythema, or edema noted. Cervix is long, posterior, thick, and closed. Uterine size and shape consistent with 8 weeks' gestation; soft lower uterine segment. No palpable adnexal tenderness. Urinalysis: Protein negative. Glucose negative. Labs pending.

EXAMPLE OF NORMAL FINDINGS FROM ROUTINE PRENATAL VISIT (18 WEEKS' GESTATION)

BP 120/80, pulse rate 72/min, weight 130 lbs

Well-appearing and afebrile. Weight is increased 4 pounds from her visit 4 weeks ago and BP is unchanged. No facial or peripheral edema noted. Fundal height 2 cm below the umbilicus. Fetal heart tones 140 beats/min.

REFERENCES

References for this chapter draw from Chapter 21, "Evidence-Based Obstetric Assessment," of the textbook *Evidence-Based Physical Examination: Best Practices for Health and Well-Being Assessment*. The references may be accessed in the digital version of the handbook at connect.springerpub.com/content/book/97808-0-8261-6466-7/chapter/ch15

King, T. L., Brucker, M. C., Osborne, K., & Jevitt, C. M. (2019). *Varney's midwifery* (6th ed.) Burlington, MA: Jones & Bartlett Learning.

16

Evidence-Based Assessment of Mental Health and Substance Use

CLINICAL CONSIDERATIONS

- Normalize discussion of mental health concerns as part of the assessment of health and well-being. Mental status and mental health assessment should be included as part of every health encounter.
- Ask directly about suicidal thoughts, self-harm, and suicide attempts; provide opportunity for individuals to discuss suicidality and mental health concerns openly.
- Be observant for signs and symptoms that suggest a lack of vitality. Lack of energy and/or interest in activities that used to bring enjoyment are key signs of depression.
- When clinicians assess individuals who are struggling with anxiety, depression, and/or substance use, they should also consider that the patient may have additional physical or mental health disorders.
- Trauma, social isolation, genetic factors, and comorbidities increase the likelihood of brain and nervous system changes that lead to mental health and substance use disorders.
- Substance use can be associated with compromised functioning in virtually every system of the body. Medical conditions may develop as a result of the toxicity of the substance, route of administration, and high-risk behaviors in which the patient engages.
- Assessing and engaging effectively with individuals who are unable to control or reduce their use of substances, and/or whose

use continues despite consequences, requires therapeutic communication, empathy, and motivational interviewing. Using an unbiased, empathetic, patient-centered approach, clinicians can recognize and respond effectively to ambivalence, and support substance use treatment and recovery.

SUBJECTIVE HISTORY

COMMON REASONS FOR SEEKING CARE

- Depressive symptoms: Sadness, insomnia, guilt or unworthiness, energy loss, change in appetite, anhedonia or loss of interest, psychomotor changes, suicidality (mnemonic: SIGECAPS)
- Anxiety symptoms: Excessive worry, nervousness
- Substance use concerns, alcohol misuse, smoking cessation

HISTORY OF PRESENT ILLNESS

- HPI questions used to assess mental health concerns can follow the OLDCARTS format, and adapted to determine whether additional screening for mental health disorders is needed. The four examples included (in the text that follows) are intended to show how the HPI assessment can be adapted based on the presenting symptoms for individuals with mental health concerns. Note that "Are the symptoms currently interfering with functioning at work (school) and home?" is a key question, as interference with functioning is often one important indicator of a mental health diagnosis.

HPI Example Incorporating Assessments for Depression and Anxiety

- **Onset:** When did symptoms start, or at what age did you first have these symptoms? Have they been persistent? When are your symptoms better? Worse?
- **Sadness/depressed mood:** Are you feeling sad, helpless, or hopeless? Having trouble concentrating?
- **Insomnia/sleep disturbance:** Are you having difficulty falling asleep? Staying asleep?
- **Guilt or unworthiness:** Are you having feelings of unworthiness?
- **Energy loss or fatigue:** Are you feeling fatigued? Describe your energy level on most days. Has your energy level significantly changed?
- **Changes in appetite:** Has your appetite been decreased? Increased? Has your weight changed? If so, explain.
- **Anhedonia or loss of interest:** Are you finding it difficult to participate in things that you once found enjoyable?

- **Psychomotor changes:** Are you feeling sluggish? Agitated?
- **Suicidality:** Do you have suicidal thoughts? (OR do you think about death or hurting yourself?) Have you ever been suicidal? Have you attempted suicide before? Do you have a plan? Do you have the means to carry out this plan?
- **Severity:** How difficult have these problems made it for you to do your work or take care of things at home, or get along with other people? Are the symptoms currently interfering with functioning at work (school) and home?

HPI Example for the Individual Who Currently Smokes Cigarettes

- **Onset:** Time of first cigarette in the morning, waking at night to smoke?
- **Location**: Smoking at work, home, in the car, around children
- **Duration:** Age that smoking began, previous attempts to quit
- **Characteristics:** Number of cigarettes smoked each day, most recent cigarette; also note whether any additional types of nicotine or tobacco are used
- **Associated symptoms:** Cough, wheezing, or respiratory problems; chest pain; fatigue; and/or symptoms associated with smoking cessation attempts
- **Relieving symptoms**: Coping skills, pharmacological and/or nonpharmacological methods to quit, previous or current counseling
- **Timing or temporal factors:** Use related to stress or need to relax, concurrent use of substances, personal beliefs about need or desire to quit (i.e., readiness to change)
- **Severity:** How difficult has it been for you to continue smoking? To quit smoking?

HPI Example for Individual Who Is Misusing Alcohol

- **Onset:** Time of first drink, amount of drinks per day
- **Location:** Drinking alone, socially, before or associated with driving a motor vehicle
- **Duration:** Occasions of heavy use and binge drinking, average use days per week
- **Characteristics:** Typical amount of alcohol use, type of alcohol use, history of blackouts, most recent use
- **Associated symptoms:** Emotions and beliefs related to use, abstinence; consequences of alcohol use (i.e., unable to attend school or work; effect on relationships; legal issues; health issues, including type 2 diabetes, pancreatitis, cancers, heart disease,

dementia, hepatitis, and cirrhosis); recent intoxication, disinhibition, or stupor

- **Relieving symptoms:** Coping skills, support system, pharmacological and/or nonpharmacological methods to quit, previous or current counseling or involvement in recovery groups, previous periods of sobriety, and what worked to achieve this
- **Timing or temporal factors:** Use related to stress or need to relax, concurrent use of substances, personal beliefs about need or desire to quit (i.e., readiness to change)
- **Severity:** How difficult has it been for you to continue drinking? To quit drinking? Is your drinking, or problems related to your drinking, interfering with functioning at work (school) and home?

HPI Example Incorporating Screening for Substance Use Disorder

- **Onset:** When did symptoms start? At what age did you start feeling this way, and/or using substances?
- **Location:** Location of any pain or physical symptoms?
- **Duration:** Are symptoms persistent?
- **Characteristics** (*incorporate screening tool; CRAFFT tool used in this example is appropriate for use in teens and young adults*): During the past 12 months on how many days did you:
  1. Drink more than a few sips of beer, wine, or any drink containing alcohol?
  2. Use any marijuana (weed, oil, or hash by smoking, vaping, or in food) or synthetic marijuana (like K2 or spice)?
  3. Use anything else to get high (like illegal drugs, prescription or over-the-counter medications, or things that you sniff, huff, or vape)?
  4. Use any tobacco or nicotine products (e.g., cigarettes, e-cigarettes, hookahs, or smokeless tobacco)?

  If "0" for all questions, ask CAR question only.
  Otherwise, ask all six questions that follow:
  1. Have you ever ridden in a CAR driven by someone (including yourself) who was "high" or had been using alcohol or drugs?
  2. Do you ever use alcohol or drugs to RELAX, feel better about yourself, or fit in?
  3. Do you ever use alcohol or drugs while you are by yourself, or ALONE?
  4. Do you ever FORGET things you did while using alcohol or drugs?
  5. Do your FAMILY or FRIENDS ever tell you that you should cut down on your drinking or drug use?
  6. Have you ever gotten into TROUBLE while you were using alcohol or drugs?

- **Aggravating factors:** What makes your symptoms or use worse?
- **Relieving factors:** When are symptoms better? What treatment have you tried?
- **Timing:** What actions or activities decrease the symptoms?
- **Severity and scale:** How difficult have these problems made it for you to do your work or take care of things at home, or get along with other people? Are the symptoms currently interfering with functioning at work (school) and home?

HEALTH HISTORY

Past Medical History

- Hospitalizations, surgeries, emergency department visits
- Previous diagnosis of anxiety, depression, trauma, or mental health disorders
- Previous diagnosis of substance use disorder, alcoholism, addiction
- Previous or current treatment of mental health or SUDs
- Chronic pain
- Recent or current acute pain
- Constitutional changes
- Physical disabilities or reduced mobility
- Poor health status
- Past history of substance misuse
- Motor vehicle accidents
- Chronic physical illness/comorbidities
- Recent or past infectious disease

Medications

Prescribed or OTC medications or supplements, including dose and frequency

Allergies

- Allergies to medications or seasonal, environmental, and/or food allergies

Preventive Health Behaviors

- Physical activity and exercise
- Typical diet, access to fruits and vegetables
- Adequate sleep and rest
- Tobacco cessation
- Alcohol moderation or abstinence
- Vaccine history

- Family, social, and/or community support, including recovery groups
- Removal of triggers (sources of stress, caffeine, nicotine)
- Deep breathing
- Movement therapies (yoga, tai chi)
- Meditation, progressive muscle relaxation, mindfulness-based stress reduction
- Bibliotherapy—Self-help books, workbooks, and psychoeducation
- Counseling, cognitive behavioral therapy

FAMILY HISTORY

- Anxiety, depression, bipolar disorder, schizophrenia
- Other mental health disorders (e.g., ADHD)
- Neurological disorders; seizure disorders
- Substance use disorder; alcoholism or addiction
- Suicide/suicide attempts (trajectory; impact on family)
- Trauma, physical or sexual abuse, neglect
- Other chronic diseases impacted by smoking, alcohol use, or substances

SOCIAL HISTORY

- Home situation and relationships:
    - Married/single/divorced/widowed/partnered?
    - Who lives in the home? Is partner supportive?
    - Substance use in the home?
    - Is housing/home/neighborhood safe? Involved in community activities?
    - Social support system? Close friends? Pets?
- Substance use:
    - Tobacco use? If yes, assess smoking history, readiness to quit
    - Alcohol use? If yes, screen for binge drinking, problematic use
    - Other substances (e.g., medications not prescribed, illicit drugs)?
- Safety (including work or school environment):
    - Trauma history, including adverse childhood events, bereavement, grief, isolation
    - Risk or current victim of violence?
    - Stress, anxiety, burnout related to workplace culture, school or work expectations
    - Financial or career concerns
    - Legal problems, justice involvement, history of driving under the influence

REVIEW OF SYSTEMS

- **Mental health:** Sadness, helplessness, hopelessness, worry, insomnia, hypersomnia, fatigue, headaches; changes in memory, concentration, or mood, memory loss, mood swings, mania, risk-taking, anxiety, worry, guilt, shame; suicidal or homicidal ideation, hallucinations, delusions
- **Neurologic:** Weakness, numbness, loss of consciousness, black outs, headaches, falls, dizziness, idiopathic seizures, confusion
- **Integumentary:** Dryness, itching, bruising, rashes, lesions, burns, sweating
- **HEENT:** Sensory deficits, congestion, sinus pain, sore throat
- **Lymphatic:** Bruising, bleeding, lymphadenopathy
- **CV:** Chest pain, shortness of breath, rapid pulse
- **Respiratory:** Dyspnea, wheezing, cough, breathlessness
- **MSK:** Injury history, pain, stiffness, or swelling
- **GI/GU:** Weight and/or appetite changes, constipation, diarrhea, abdominal pain, nausea, vomiting, incontinence, poor nutrition

PEDIATRIC CONSIDERATIONS

- With children and adolescents, part of the assessment interview will be with parents or caregivers; if the young person can tolerate being separated from their parents, individual time spent with the child/teen is invaluable. In the individual time spent with the clinician (after confidentiality is made clear), the child/teen is often very forthcoming with their own concerns and experiences. The child/teen also can provide the clinician with best treatment options that fit with their values and preferences. Toys and props in the examination room allow the child/teen to keep their hands busy while talking, which is very helpful for their comfort with the interview
- For adolescents, the HEADSS assessment can be helpful in identifying mental health problems:
  - **H**ome: Where is the teen living? Who lives in the home? How is the teen getting along with people in the home? Has the teen ever run away or been incarcerated?
  - **E**ducation and/or **E**mployment: How is the teen functioning in school in terms of grades, performance in class, and teachers/peers? Any recent changes? Have there been any suspensions or missed school days? Any current or past employment? Any problems with work attendance?
  - **A**ctivities: In which extracurricular and sports activities is the teen involved, if any? What do they do with their friends? What does the teen do for fun?

  - **D**rugs: Which drugs, including alcohol, cigarettes, vaping, caffeine, stimulants, or pills, have been used by the teen, their family, and/or friends?
  - **S**exuality: How does the teen express their gender identity? How does the teen identify their sexual orientation? Has the adolescent been sexually active? Are they currently in a relationship? Does the teen use contraception and/or condoms? How many partners have they had? What is the teen's past history of sexually transmitted infections, pregnancy, abortion, and sexual abuse? Has the adolescent been a victim of trauma?
  - **S**uicide: Is there a history of isolation or being withdrawn, emotional outbursts, or impulsive behavior? Has the teen had depression symptoms, including suicidal ideation or a past history of suicide attempts? If there has been suicidal ideation does the teen have a plan and access to the means to commit suicide?
- How to ask sensitive questions and respond effectively to support positive outcomes is a skill that requires empathy, openness, and authenticity; this is true for connecting with teens who are in distress. Being able to develop and sustain a person-centered relationship is central to effective mental healthcare. At the very least, this requires engagement with the adolescent's conceptualization of distress, strengths, and aspiration for the future.

Risk Assessment

- A particularly sensitive part of the mental health assessment is risk assessment for danger to self, danger to others, and danger from others.
- To determine danger to self, it is imperative to conduct a suicide risk assessment. Screen for suicidal ideation, plan, and means. The majority of people who die by suicide visit a clinician within months before their death. Use a valid suicide risk screening tool such as PHQ-9, or Ask Suicide-Screening Questions. Assess history of self-injurious behavior, past attempts, and hospitalizations for suicidal ideation or suicide attempts. Note that the period just following psychiatric hospital discharge is an extremely high-risk time for patients. Ask directly about current ideation, and clarify the plan, including how the patient plans to kill themselves. Also ask about the means or ability to carry out their plan, including access to guns or drugs.

- Another major consideration is substance misuse; asking about the use and availability of substances are critical questions when assessing suicide risk, danger to self, or danger to others. Many individuals with depression will use substances to regulate their depressive symptoms. If the person endorses past suicidal ideation, ask whether there was an attempt or self-injurious behaviors. Ask whether the individual has ever overdosed, nearly overdosed, or has concerns about or has considered overdose with medications or alcohol.
- Homicidal ideation is risk of danger to others. If the patient acknowledges a desire to harm someone else, it is necessary to ask about their plan, intent, available means, and specific target. If the patient identifies someone specifically and has a plan, the intended victim and law enforcement must be informed.
- Screen for trauma and ACEs. Determine current and/or previous experiences of violence, abuse, and neglect. Note that younger and older populations are particularly vulnerable to being in danger from others.
- Identification of personal strengths and priorities for safety can be documented with the free, online, evidence-based Stanley and Brown Patient Safety Plan template (suicidepreventionlifeline.org/wpcontent/uploads/2016/08/Brown_StanleySafetyPlanTemplate.pdf).

RED FLAGS IN SUBJECTIVE HISTORY

- Those who have mental health and/or substance use disorders are at increased risk for suicide; additional risk factors include male gender; increasing age, being single, widowed, or divorced; family history of suicide; and prior suicide attempt.
- Individuals considering suicide may give verbal and/or nonverbal cues that should always be taken seriously. It is important to note warning signs, and directly assess suicidality. Red flags are listed in Box 16.1.
- Individuals exhibiting these symptoms should not be left alone; remove any dangerous objects or drugs that could be used in a suicide attempt and seek immediate help. The U.S. National Suicide Prevention Lifeline can be reached 24 hours a day at 800-273-TALK (8255). The nonprofit Crisis Text Line offers free text counseling; to reach the text line, text "Listen" to 741-741.

BOX 16.1 Red Flags in Subjective History That Indicate Risk of Suicidality (Suicidal Ideation, Plan, and Attempts)

- Threatening to hurt or kill themselves
- Seeking access to pills, weapons, or other means
- Talking or writing about death, dying, or suicide
- Feelings or statements of hopelessness
- Rage, anger, seeking revenge; feeling trapped
- Increased alcohol or other drug use
- Withdrawal from others
- Anxiety and agitation
- Sleep problems; insomnia or hypersomnia
- Dramatic mood changes
- Sudden and/or drastic change in behavior
- Feelings or statements that reflect not having a reason to live

PHYSICAL EXAMINATION

- Completion of a thorough history leads to the determination of which components of a physical examination are completed and how the findings are interpreted. The likelihood of comorbid mental health and substance disorders is significant and should be considered as the clinician completes the physical examination. Although the specific physical exam components are determined on an individual basis, all patient encounters will include an assessment of an individual's mental status.

MENTAL STATUS ASSESSMENT

- An assessment of an individual's mental status provides the basis for identifying signs and/or symptoms related to their overall mental health. A mental status assessment gives the clinician an understanding of the patient's cognitive, emotional, personality, and psychological functioning. This assessment can be done in the course of an individual's routine history and physical examination. Reviewing the reason for seeking care, history of any recent symptoms or problems, as well as the medical and social history provides the clinician with valuable information about mental status and health. With mental status assessment, there is overlap with subjective and objective assessments and findings.

- Within the mental status assessment, the clinician can identify an individual's strengths and coping and note whether there are concerns that require more in-depth or formal assessment of mental health. A mental status assessment incorporates observational assessments which are components of the general survey and neurological status exams. The mental status assessment is performed within the context of the patient's age, developmental level, and cultural norms. Assessments of a person's affect, mood, attention, judgment, and memory can be remembered using the ABC mnemonic:
- ***A: Appearance***
  - Affect: Appropriate for the situation, labile, pleasant, flat, nontoxic
  - Posture: Lying, sitting, or standing; comfortable; obvious limitations or defects
  - Hygiene and grooming: Appropriately dressed for the weather or situation, disheveled or neatly groomed
  - Body habitus: Height, weight, waist circumference, and BMI
- ***B: Behavior***
  - Verbal or nonverbal expressions of pain, anxiety, illness, anger, fear, frustration, contentment, or sadness
  - Interactions: Cooperative, guarded, aggressive, withdrawn
  - Activity level: Calm, active, flat, restless, previous/recent/current impulsivity
  - Body movements and mobility: Coordinated, limited, assistive devices, abnormal movements or involuntary tics present, slowed or very quick movements
- ***C: Cognition***
  - Oriented to time, person, and place; confused; disoriented; delirious
  - Attention and concentration: Able to express coherent, organized thoughts, or rapidly shifting from one topic to the next; any concerns with success in work, school, or at home
  - Speech pattern and pace: Appropriate, rushed, slow, loud or quiet, pressurized, garbled, or clear and articulate.
  - Judgment: Thought content including irrational fears or overwhelming worry; thought patterns including negative patterns of all-or-nothing thinking, catastrophizing, overgeneralization, blaming, emotional reasoning, or always being right

- Altered sensory perceptions: Hearing voices or hallucinations, able to control impulses, insight into personal strengths
- Memory: Able to repeat three unrelated words and remember and repeat these words again in 5 minutes; concerns about memory loss
- Mood: Feelings of sadness, guilt, worry, fear, helplessness, or hopelessness; recent insomnia, hypersomnia, loss of appetite, increased appetite, or difficulty feeling enjoyment; feelings of elation, grandiosity, or mood instability; previous or current suicidal and/or homicidal thoughts and/or plan

PHYSICAL EXAMINATION CONSIDERATIONS

- Assess for signs of acute and chronic disease when individuals present with mental health concerns. As noted previously, mental health disorders, including substance use/misuse, are likely to result in development of comorbidities. Specific health effects of substances to consider when determining components of the physical exam:
  - Excessive alcohol consumption increases the risk of developing type 2 diabetes, pancreatitis, cancers, cardiomyopathy, dementia, hepatitis, and cirrhosis, in addition to the short-term intoxication, disinhibition, stupor, and potential for coma and death.
  - Tobacco use causes damage to nearly every organ in the body, often leading to lung cancer, heart disease, stroke, emphysema, and chronic bronchitis. Exposure to secondhand smoke also causes adverse health effects.
  - Marijuana has not only immediate effects like distorted perception, difficulty problem-solving, and loss of motor coordination, but also has effects with long-term use, including respiratory infections, impaired memory, and exposure to cancer-causing compounds.
  - Opioids not only reduce the perception of pain, but also produce drowsiness, mental confusion, euphoria, nausea, constipation, and respiratory depression. Most overdose deaths from substance use are attributable to opioids.

RED FLAGS IN OBJECTIVE EXAM

- Individuals may present with symptoms resulting from ingestion, withdrawal, and/or chronic use of substances, in addition to the symptoms of mental health disorders that are incompletely treated or untreated. Substance use can be associated with compromised function in any or every body system related to the substance used, how the substance was ingested, and/or the high-risk behaviors in which an individual engages.

- **Box 16.2** includes a list of physical signs that may indicate substance misuse, substance use disorder, or addiction. Note that these signs may indicate intoxication, withdrawal, or heavy use. Signs may be related to the type of substance used or method of use. Presence or absence of these signs are not the sole assessment of substance use.
- While the clinician completes the history and physical exam, how they communicate with the individual who may be misusing

BOX 16.2 Red Flags in Objective Exam Indicating Possible Substance Misuse, Substance Use Disorder, or Addiction

- ***General survey:*** Thin, altered vital signs; unsteady gait
- ***Appearance:*** Poor personal hygiene; smell of alcohol, tobacco, or drug use
- *Mental status:*
    - Combative, aggressive, or bizarre behavior; may appear fatigued, sedated
    - Impaired cognition, confusion, disorientation
    - Slurred speech
- ***Integumentary:*** Jaundice, diaphoresis, lesions/rashes, burns, scars, abscesses, very dry skin
- ***Head, neck, and lymphatics:*** Bruising, bleeding, lymphadenopathy
- ***Eyes:*** Eye redness or drainage, pupil dilation or constriction
- ***ENT:*** Rhinorrhea, deviations or deformities in nasal septum, including perforation, atrophy of the nasal mucosa, epistaxis, pharyngitis
- ***Respiratory:*** Cough, wheezing, respiratory depression or tachypnea
- ***Cardiovascular:*** Hypertension, hypotension, tachycardia, edema
- ***GI/GU/GYN:*** Hepatomegaly, splenomegaly, abdominal distention, signs of sexually transmitted infection
- ***Neurologic:*** Weakness, numbness, loss of consciousness, jitteriness, seizure activity
- ***Musculoskeletal:*** Pain with movement; neck pain, stiffness, or swelling

substances is a priority. Clinicians should continue to employ the framework of screening, brief intervention, and referral to treatment and avoid implicit bias when completing the assessment of an individual using and/or misusing substances in order to avoid triggering shame, guilt, and resistance to treatment. The use of therapeutic communication strategies, including motivational interviewing, while interacting with the patient is foundational to evidence-based practice and effective patient outcomes. The use of motivational interviewing includes nonjudgmental listening and allows an individual to identify their own motivation for changing behavior.

EVIDENCE-BASED RESOURCES

Mental Health and Substance Use Screening Tools

- These evidence-based screening tools are intended to identify concerning signs and/or symptoms that may indicate or raise red flags for mental health diagnoses. These evidence-based tools allow clinicians to assess individuals effectively and efficiently, including those who do not initially present with mental health concerns. Although these screenings are highly important for helping to identify mental health disorders, diagnoses must be confirmed with careful diagnostic clinical evaluation, which goes beyond screening.

Patient Health Questionnaire (PHQ-9 and PHQ-2) Depression Scales

- The PHQ-9 is a widely used, valid and reliable nine-item tool for screening and monitoring the severity of depression. Question 9 of the tool screens for the presence and duration of SI. This screening tool and an instruction manual are available at no cost (www.phqscreeners.com).
- The brief PHQ-2 consists of the first two questions of the PHQ-9, and screens for core symptoms of major depressive disorder; the two questions:
  - Over the past 2 weeks, how often have you been bothered by the following problems?
    1. Little interest or pleasure in doing things
       - Not at all (0)
       - Several days (+1)
       - More than half the days (+2)
       - Nearly every day (+3)

(*continued*)

EVIDENCE-BASED RESOURCES (CONTINUED)

2. Feeling down, depressed, or hopeless
   - Not at all (0)
   - Several days (+1)
   - More than half the days (+2)
   - Nearly every day (+3)

- The total scoring from the PHQ-2 ranges from 0 to 6. If the score is 3 or greater, depressive disorder is likely. Patients who screen positive should be further evaluated.

Generalized Anxiety Disorder Scale (GAD-7 and GAD-2)

- The seven-item GAD-7 is a validated screening tool for anxiety that includes a severity assessment scale. Free download is also available (www.phqscreeners.com).
- The abbreviated GAD-2 screening consists of the first two questions of the GAD-7:
  - Over the past 2 weeks, how often have you been bothered by the following problems?
    1. Feeling nervous, anxious, or on edge
       - Not at all (0)
       - Several days (+1)
       - More than half the days (+2)
       - Nearly every day (+3)
    2. Not being able to stop worrying
       - Not at all (0)
       - Several days (+1)
       - More than half the days (+2)
- Nearly every day (+3) b
- The scoring for the GAD-2 is similar to the PHQ-2, with a range from 0 to 6. The recommended cutpoint for a positive screening is a score of 3 or greater. The GAD-2 and PHQ-2 can be used together (referred to as the *PHQ-4*) to screen for depression and anxiety.

Single-Question Screenings for Substance Use

- Evidence suggests that single-screening questions can be effective tools to identify substance misuse. Note that screening negatively for the misuse of one substance does not negate the need to screen for misuse of other substances. Responses to these single questions serve as the foundation or basis for further dialogue and assessment. A response of one or more is considered a positive screen.

- Single-question screen to identify illicit substance use: "How many times in the past year have you used an illegal drug or used a prescription medication for nonmedical reasons?" If clarification of "nonmedical reasons" is needed, provide the explanation, "For instance, because of the experience or feeling it caused."
- Single-question screening for alcohol misuse: "How many times in the past year have you had *x* or more drinks in a day?" where *x* is five for men and four for women.

PRACTICE GUIDELINES FOR MENTAL HEALTH AND SUBSTANCE USE ASSESSMENT

- **American Academy of Pediatrics:** https://www.aap.org/en-us/Documents/substance_use_screening_implementation.pdf
- **American Psychiatric Association:** https://dsm.psychiatryonline.org/doi/book/10.1176/appi.books.9780890425596
- **American Psychological Association:** https://www.apa.org/pi/lgbt/resources/guidelines
- **Choosing Wisely Campaign:** http://www.choosingwisely.org/
- **National Institute of Mental Health:** https://www.nimh.nih.gov
- **National Institute on Drug Abuse:** https://www.drugabuse.gov
- **Substance Abuse and Mental Health Services Administration:** https://www.samhsa.gov
- **U.S. Preventive Services Task Force:** https://www.uspreventiveservicestaskforce.org

MENTAL HEALTH DISORDERS

The mental health disorders listed in this section of the chapter are in alphabetical order, not in order of prevalence. The list is not exhaustive.

ANXIETY AND ANXIETY DISORDERS

Chronic conditions characterized by excessive and persistent worry, tension, and apprehension that cause difficulty functioning in home, school, work, or social situations. The *DSM-5* criteria for diagnosis of mild, moderate, or severe anxiety or anxiety disorders are embedded in the GAD-2 and GAD-7 screenings.

History

- Excessive worry, fear, feeling of impending doom
- Inability to concentrate, racing thoughts
- Hypervigilance, restlessness, irritability
- Insomnia
- Fatigue

Physical Examination

- Racing heart rate (with palpitations)
- Sweating, trembling
- Mental status exam may reveal racing thoughts, restlessness

Considerations

- Types of anxiety disorders include GAD, OCD, panic disorder, and social phobia or social anxiety disorder. Although PTSD can be considered an anxiety disorder, the diagnosis is formally classified as a trauma- and stressor-related disorder.
- Comorbidities are common, including depression, ADHD, and substance use disorder
- Some conditions are misdiagnosed as anxiety (e.g., hyperthyroidism, lead intoxication, migraine headaches, substance misuse, and asthma)
- When screening for excessive worry, nervousness, and anxiousness, clinicians should recognize that this is a good time to also ask about the patient's usual coping strategies.

Pediatric Considerations

- Anxiety disorders are the most common mental health disorder in children and teens. Anxiety and fear are normal components of development, but should not be excessive, interfere with functioning, or persist beyond what is appropriate for an individual's developmental stage.
- Children with anxiety disorders often present with somatic symptoms, such as abdominal pain, headaches, or chest pain.

Key History Questions for Children and Adolescents

- Is the anxiety appropriate for the age of the child/teen?
- Do they have symptoms in response to a specific trigger (e.g., social situations)?
- Has the child/teen experienced a traumatic event?
- Is there a history of recent stressful events, including marital transition?
- Does their anxiety or worry interfere with functioning?
- What impact does anxiety have on their sleep, concentration, appetite, energy, and relationships?
- What medications, prescribed or OTC, are they taking? For example, antihistamines, antidepressants, stimulants, decongestants, caffeine, steroids, or asthma medications
- Is the child or teen using substances to regulate anxiety symptoms?

ATTENTION DEFICIT HYPERACTIVITY DISORDER

Diagnosis of ADHD involves assessment for a constellation of symptoms and is best understood as one of a spectrum of neurological, developmental, cognitive, and genetic disorders. ADHD is often comorbid with other mental disorders and can present in adulthood. Individuals with ADHD show a persistent pattern of inattention and/or hyperactivity/impulsivity that interferes with function or development. Symptoms occur often (not always) and include:

- Inattention:
  - Fails to give close attention to details or makes careless mistakes
  - Has trouble holding attention on tasks or playing activities
  - Does not seem to listen when spoken to directly
  - Does not follow through on instructions and fails to finish schoolwork, chores, or duties in the workplace (e.g., loses focus, side-tracked)
  - Has trouble organizing tasks and activities
  - Avoids, dislikes, or is reluctant to do tasks that require mental effort over a long period of time
  - Loses things necessary for tasks and activities (e.g., school materials, pencils, books, tools, wallets, keys, paperwork, glasses, cell phones)
  - Is easily distracted
  - Is forgetful in daily activities
- Hyperactivity and impulsivity:
  - Fidgets with or taps hands or feet, or squirms in seat.
  - Leaves seat in situations when remaining seated is expected
  - Runs about or climbs in situations where it is not appropriate (adolescents or adults may be limited to feeling restless).
  - Unable to play or take part in leisure activities quietly
  - Is "on the go," acting as if "driven by a motor"
  - Talks excessively
  - Blurts out an answer before a question has been completed
  - Has trouble waiting for their turn
  - Interrupts or intrudes on others (e.g., into conversations or games).
- In addition, the following conditions must be met:
  - Several symptoms present before age 12 years
  - Several symptoms present in two or more settings (such as at home, school, or work; with guardians, friends, or relatives; in other activities)
  - Symptoms interfere with, or reduce the quality of, social, school, or work functioning.
  - Symptoms are not better explained by another mental disorder (such as a mood disorder, anxiety disorder, dissociative disorder, or a personality disorder).
- Children, adolescents, and adults can have ADHD that predominantly presents as inattention, or hyperactivity-impulsivity, or

both. Because symptoms can change over time, the presentation may change over time as well. ADHD often lasts into adulthood. Symptoms might look different at older ages. For example, in adults, hyperactivity may appear as restlessness.

DEPRESSION AND MOOD DISORDERS

Mood disorders are mental health conditions characterized by disturbances in mood, including elevated mood (mania or hypomania), depressed mood (unipolar depression or major depressive disorder), or cycling between elevated and depressed moods (bipolar depression). Criteria for the diagnosis of depression (mild, moderate, and severe) are embedded in the evidence-based screenings reviewed. The mnemonic SIGECAPS is helpful to remember the signs and symptoms of depression:

- **S**leep: Increased (hypersomnia) or decreased (insomnia)
- **I**nterest: Decreased, loss of ability to enjoy activities that were once enjoyed
- **G**uilt: Feelings of worthlessness, hopelessness
- **E**nergy: Change in energy level, fatigued or restless
- **C**oncentration: Difficulty making decisions
- **A**ppetite changes, and/or weight increase or decrease
- **P**sychomotor activity: Increased (agitation) or decreased (slowed)
- **S**uicidal ideation: Recurrent thoughts of suicide, plans for committing suicide

If the screening or history is positive for depression, obtain a sense of how long the depressive symptoms have been present. When was the first episode of depression? Persistent depressive disorder, or dysthymia, is a chronic form of depression. Depression can be related to medical illness, induced by substances including medication, and/or may be related to additional internal or external factors, such as premenstrual dysphoric disorder or seasonal affective disorder. The person with depression has a lack of energy, lack of interest, lack of initiative, and fewer interactions with others. Depression is more accurately a lack of vitality, not a disorder of "being sad." Sadness is a normal emotion, often triggered by loss. Depression is a disorder characterized by self-diminishing negative patterns of thought.

Signs and symptoms of mood disorder include periods of mood instability and changes in mood that can be daily or weekly. Screening for mania is key to identifying assessments that may indicate bipolar disorder; these include not needing sleep for days, excessive enthusiasm, and periods of great excitement and obsession. DIGFAST is a mnemonic that can help the clinician to remember symptoms of mania:

- **D**istractibility: Difficulty blocking unimportant distractions
- **I**ndiscretion: Excessive involvement in pleasurable activities
- **G**randiosity: Feelings of invulnerability
- **F**light of ideas: Racing thoughts, rapid shifting of ideas
- **A**ctivity increase: Dramatic periods of excitement, enthusiasm
- **S**leep deficit: Decreased need for sleep
- **T**alkativeness: Pressured speech

Identifying symptoms of mania to differentiate unipolar and bipolar mood disorders significantly informs an individual's treatment plan. Antidepressants prescribed to persons with bipolar disorder can activate mania, often with negative outcomes for that person. Note that bipolar disorder can present first as a depressive disorder. The usual age of onset of serious mental disorders (bipolar disorder, thought disorders, and severe persistent mental health disorders) is generally in late adolescence and young adulthood, but can occur earlier or later.

Pediatric Considerations

Important points to note regarding the assessment of depression in children and teens include:

- Young children less than 7 years of age with depression are often misdiagnosed with ADHD as they frequently present with inattention, impulsivity, and hyperactivity
- Anger is often a presenting symptom in adolescents.
- The mean age of onset for major depressive disorder is 14 years.
- Reoccurrence rate is as high as 60% to 70% and often reoccurs in adulthood; 40% to 70% of affected children/teens have comorbid mental health conditions, so it is critical to assess for other mental health disorders (e.g., anxiety, substance use, ADHD).

Key History Questions for Children and Adolescents

- Mood: Have you been feeling sad, down, blue, or grouchy most days, or more days than not? Do you find yourself crying a lot? Have you been getting into arguments more than usual?
- Anhedonia: Are you able to enjoy things you used to enjoy? Do you feel bored or tired a lot of the time?
- Negative self-concept: How do you feel about yourself on a scale of 0 (not good at all) to 10 (really good)?
- Relationships with friends: Do you have friends? Are you liked by your peers?

- Neurovegetative signs: Do you have trouble falling asleep or staying asleep? Do you have trouble concentrating? How is your appetite?
- Somatic symptoms: Do you have headaches and/or stomachaches?
- SIs: Do you ever wish you were dead? Do you think about death or hurting yourself? Have you ever hurt yourself?
- Current health and medications
- Substance use, including caffeine, nicotine, alcohol, marijuana, OTC drugs

Always assess a depressed teen presenting with depressive symptoms for bipolar disorder, including elevated or irritable mood, inflated self-esteem, decreased sleep, more talkative, flight of ideas, distractibility, and excessive involvement in activities that have adverse consequences (e.g., buying sprees, drug use, and promiscuity).

Note that mood disorder symptoms can be nonspecific. Diagnoses that should be ruled out for children, teens, and adults include hypothyroidism, anemia, mononucleosis, eating disorders, substance use or withdrawal, premenstrual syndrome, diabetes, and lead intoxication.

THOUGHT DISORDERS AND SEVERE, PERSISTENT, MENTAL ILLNESS

If the clinician has a difficult time following the patient's conversation while completing the history and physical exam, additional assessments may be needed for delusions, hallucinations, or disordered thoughts. These assessments help the clinician to identify red flags associated with severe, persistent mental illnesses, which are disorders defined by their level of severity and disability. The SPMI category includes the symptomatology of disordered thought processes that can be associated with severe major depressive disorder, schizoaffective bipolar disorders, schizophrenia, psychoses, and borderline personality disorder. SPMIs are characterized by marked difficulties in self-care, marked restriction of ADL, frequent deficiencies of concentration, and significant difficulties in maintaining social functioning.

Delirium

Key Assessments

- Fluctuating level of consciousness (i.e., decreased awareness and attention)
- Restless, agitated, combative behavior that may wax and wane; may be withdrawn

- Acutely disoriented; may have hallucinations, bizarre delusions, abnormal behavior

Considerations

- Suspect delirium when a new onset or an acute deterioration in behavior, cognition, or function occurs, especially in individuals who are elderly or depressed
- In elderly, delirium is often the presenting symptom of an underlying illness

Delusions

Key Assessments

- Thoughts not based in reality: for example, "I am the king of this country."
- Usually has some level of paranoia associated
- Associated irritability, anger, especially if delusion is challenged

Considerations

- Symptom of severe, persistent mental illness, such as schizophrenia, delusional disorder, schizoaffective disorder, and schizophreniform disorder
- Can be a symptom of acute or chronic medical or neurologic disorder
- False belief is not related to religious, cultural, or educational background
- Strongly held false beliefs; individual is absolutely convinced of its truthfulness

Dementia

Key Assessments

- Memory loss, difficulty concentrating, mood changes
- Increasing difficulty with completing familiar tasks
- Confused about time, place; disrupts daily life
- Confusion worse in unfamiliar environments
- Repeated forgetting of recent events, names, faces
- May progress to language and communication problems, personality changes, lack of awareness, mobility issues, incontinence, dysphagia

Considerations

- Types include Alzheimer's, vascular, Lewy bodies, and mixed dementia
- Signs and symptoms vary depending on type of disease/disorder, usually progressive

Hallucinations

Key Assessments

- Sensory perception in the absence of real stimulus, caused by physical/mental disorders
- May be auditory, visual, or tactile

Considerations

- Associated with schizophrenia, psychotic disorder, or psychosis
- May be associated with substance use
- Also associated with Parkinson's disease, epilepsy, dementia, brain tumor, migraines

TRAUMA- AND STRESSOR-RELATED DISORDERS

Trauma- and stressor-related disorders have many of the same symptoms as anxiety disorders; however, the conditions can be linked to traumatic experiences or significant stress. Diagnostic criteria include:

1. Exposure to actual or threatened death, serious injury, or sexual violation in either:
   - Directly experiencing the traumatic event
   - Witnessing, in person, the event as it occurred to others
   - Learning that the event occurred to a close family member or close friend
   - Experiencing repeated or extreme exposure to aversive details of the traumatic event (e.g., first responders on site experiences, exposure to details of child abuse)
2. Presence of the following symptoms:
   - Intrusive thoughts: Intrusive memories, flashbacks, recurrent nightmares
   - Negative mood: Inability to experience happiness, good emotions
   - Dissociation: Altered sense of reality, inability to remember aspects of the trauma
   - Avoidance symptoms: Efforts to avoid reminders, triggers of the event (isolation); efforts to avoid memories
   - Arousal symptoms: Hypervigilance, sleep disturbance, irritable, angry outbursts, exaggerated startle response, problems with concentration

With trauma- and stressor-related disorders, note that the symptoms are a normal human response to extreme stress and/or trauma. Diagnoses include:

- **Adjustment disorders:** Occur within 3 months of the onset of the stressor. Differential diagnoses include adjustment disorders with depressed mood; anxiety; mixed depressed mood and anxiety; disturbance of conduct, which might apply to children/ teens who have experienced trauma; and disturbance of emotions and conduct.
- **Acute stress disorder:** Symptoms begin at time of event and last 3 days to 1 month.
- **PTSD:** Symptoms or disturbance occur after 1 month. There are specific diagnostic criteria for PTSD for ages 6 to adulthood. In children under 6 years, if it is determined at the time of the assessment that a child has experienced trauma or extreme ACEs, it is best to document the examination/assessment and refer to a pediatric trauma specialist. Interestingly, young children respond very quickly to trauma-focused interventions, with much quicker response to treatment than adults.

SUBSTANCE USE DISORDERS

This section includes definitions of terms related to substance use, substance misuse, substance use disorder, addiction, binge drinking, alcoholism, neonatal abstinence syndrome, and recovery.

MISUSE OF SUBSTANCES

Substance use is defined as the use, even once, of any psychoactive compound or substance. Substance misuse is the use of any substance in a manner, situation, amount, or frequency that can cause harm to users or to those around them

SUBSTANCE USE DISORDER DIAGNOSES

SUD is a medical illness caused by repeated misuse of a substance or substances. SUD is characterized by clinically significant impairments in health, social function, and impaired control over substance use and is diagnosed through assessing cognitive, behavioral, and psychological symptoms. SUDs range from mild to severe and from temporary to chronic. SUD typically develops gradually over time, leading to changes in brain chemistry and function. Multiple factors influence whether and how rapidly a person develops an SUD. These factors include the substance itself and the genetic vulnerability of the user. Diagnostic criteria are listed in **Box 16.3**, and withdrawal symptoms that may be associated are listed in **Box 16.4**.

BOX 16.3
DIAGNOSTIC CRITERIA: SUBSTANCE USE DISORDER

Signs and Symptoms Consistent With Substance Use Disorder

1. Substance used in larger amounts or over longer periods than intended
2. Unsuccessful efforts to cut down or control substance use, despite the desire to do so
3. Considerable time spent in activities necessary to obtain and use substance or to recover from the effects of substance use
4. Craving or a strong desire to use the substance leading to onset of repeated substance use
5. Tolerance resulting in need for increased amounts of the substance to attain the desired effect, or diminished effect with continued use of the same amount of the substance
6. Withdrawal symptoms experienced, or the substance used to relieve or avoid withdrawal symptoms
7. Recurrent substance use resulting in failure to fulfill major role obligations at work, school, or home
8. Continued substance use despite having persistent or recurrent social or interpersonal problems
9. Social, occupational, or recreational activities discontinued or reduced as a result of substance use
10. Recurrent substance use in hazardous situations or environments
11. Continued substance use despite knowledge of having a persistent or recurrent physical or psychological problem that is likely to have been caused or exacerbated by the substance

Mild SUD is defined by two or three signs/symptoms of the 11 listed.
Moderate SUD is defined by four to five signs/symptoms.
Severe SUD manifests as six or more.

Source: Adapted from American Psychiatric Association. (2014). *Diagnostic and statistical manual of mental disorders* (5th ed.). American Psychiatric Publishing. https://dsm.psychiatryonline.org/doi/book/10.1176/appi.books.9780890425596

BOX 16.4
SUBSTANCE-SPECIFIC WITHDRAWAL SYMPTOMS

Alcohol withdrawal

Two or more of these symptoms:

- Autonomic hyperactivity
- Increased hand tremor
- Insomnia
- Nausea or vomiting
- Transient visual, tactile, or auditory hallucinations
- Psychomotor agitation
- Generalized tonic–clonic seizures

Cannabis withdrawal

Three or more of these symptoms:

- Irritability, anger, or depression
- Nervousness or anxiety
- Sleep difficulties (e.g., insomnia or disturbing dreams)
- Decreased appetite or weight loss
- Restlessness
- Depressed mood
- Physical symptom that causes significant discomfort (abdominal pain, shakiness/tremors, sweating, fever, chills, or headache)

Opioid withdrawal

Three or more of these symptoms:

- Moodiness
- Nausea or vomiting
- Muscle aches
- Lacrimation or rhinorrhea
- Yawning
- Pupillary dilation, piloerection, or sweating
- Diarrhea
- Fever
- Insomnia

Stimulant withdrawal

Two or more of these symptoms:

- Fatigue
- Vivid, unpleasant dreams
- Insomnia or hypersomnia
- Increased appetite
- Psychomotor retardation or agitation

(continued)

BOX 16.4
SUBSTANCE-SPECIFIC WITHDRAWAL SYMPTOMS *(CONTINUED)*

Tobacco withdrawal
Four or more of these symptoms:

- Irritability, frustration, or anger
- Anxiety
- Difficulty concentrating
- Increased appetite or weight gain
- Restlessness
- Depressed mood
- Insomnia
- Decreased heart rate

Source: American Psychiatric Association. (2013). *Diagnostic and statistical manual of mental disorders* (5th ed.). https://dsm.psychiatryonline.org/doi/book/10.1176/appi.books.9780890425596

Addiction

The most severe form of SUD, addiction, is a chronic brain disease characterized by compulsive or uncontrolled use of one or more substances. This disorder has the potential for relapse (recurrence after a significant time of abstinence), resistance to treatment, and recovery. Alcoholism is the disease of addiction to alcohol, characterized by heavy drinking, dependence, tolerance, and use despite consequences.

Alcohol Use Disorder

The mild, moderate, or severe repeated misuse of the consumption of alcohol. Additional terms are provided for clarity; note that alcoholism is defined by disease progression and consequences, and not by quantity of alcohol consumed, although alcohol misuse is characteristic.

- **Standard drink:** Based on the 2015 to 2020 Dietary Guidelines for Americans, a standard drink contains 14 g (0.6 ounce) of pure alcohol, which equates to one 12-ounce can of beer, one 5-ounce glass of wine, or one shot of 1.5 ounces of a distilled beverage.
- **Moderate drinking:** Up to 1 standard drink/day for women, and 2 drinks/day for men.

- **Low-risk drinking:** For women, low-risk drinking is defined as no more than 3 drinks on any single day and no more than 7 drinks/week. For men, it is defined as no more than 4 drinks on any single day and no more than 14 drinks/week.
- **Heavy drinking:** Binge drinking on 5 days or more in the past month.
- **Binge drinking:** Consuming an excessive amount of alcohol on a single occasion, or in about 2 hours. For men, this is defined as drinking five or more standard drinks, and for women, four or more standard drinks. By definition, binge-drinking episodes have the potential for producing harm, and yet this type of substance misuse is often overlooked as socially appropriate, or misunderstood as developmentally acceptable, despite increasing an individual's risk of developing addiction.

Opioid Use Disorder

Characterized by the persistent use of opioids despite the adverse consequences of its use.

Tobacco Use Disorder

The most common SUD, characterized by nicotine dependence and withdrawal symptoms with tobacco cessation attempts.

LIFE-SPAN AND FAMILY CONSIDERATIONS

Newborns and Neonatal Abstinence Syndrome

Newborns who are exposed to substances during fetal growth and development can experience short and long-term sequelae. When an infant is exposed to opiates in utero, the constellation of signs, symptoms, and problems that result is known as *neonatal abstinence syndrome*. The characteristic symptoms of NAS are highly variable, serious, and include central nervous system hyperirritability and autonomic nervous system dysfunction. Pregnancy complications associated with opiate use include intrauterine growth restriction, placental abruption, preterm delivery, oligohydramnios, stillbirth, NAS, and maternal death. Opiate use during pregnancy is a major public health crisis, and clinicians are cautioned to carefully assess women of reproductive age, pregnant women, newborns, children, and adolescents regarding use and exposure to substances.

Adolescent Considerations

The American Academy of Pediatrics defines *addiction* as a developmental disorder and recommends screening for SUD as a routine part of adolescent care. This position is based on the understanding of neurobiology and the neuroadaptations that result from substance use, which can be more dramatic and happen more quickly during adolescence. Trauma, social isolation, genetic factors, and comorbid physical and mental health disorders increase the likelihood of changes within the brain and nervous system that lead to SUD.

Considerations for the Older Adult

The prevalence rates of SUD are underestimated for older adults. Aging presents risks for harm; biological changes increase the effect of alcohol, medications, and illicit drugs in older adults, causing an increased vulnerability to their effects and interactions. The diagnosis and treatment of comorbid sleep disorders, cognitive impairment, and chronic illnesses are complicated by concurrent use of alcohol, tobacco, and prescription medications.

Impact on Families

Consequences of substance misuse and SUD are experienced by each member of a family; there are emotional, developmental, social, and/or behavioral effects that can have an impact across time and generations. Clinicians should screen for negative outcomes and provide intervention and support to family members experiencing the effects of substance use. Family environments in which a parent or primary caregiver has an SUD are associated with higher rates of abuse and trauma, poor parenting skills, and poor quality parent–child interactions, all of which are risk factors for the development of addiction. Assessment should include screening for comorbid developmental delays, mental and physical health disorders, abuse, neglect, and safety issues; early intervention in families leads to better outcomes for all family members.

RECOVERY

Although resistance to treatment and relapse are common, individuals with SUD can recover. Recovery is a process of change through which individuals improve their health and wellness, live a self-directed life, and strive to reach their full potential. Being "in recovery" indicates that positive sustained changes have become part of a voluntarily adopted lifestyle. Individuals in recovery have unique and personal stories about their lives before recovery, what happened to motivate their change, and what their lives are like now. Clinicians who want to support continued recovery for individuals with SUD can approach these individuals in a manner similar to any individual with a chronic illness.

- Assess their health in all dimensions of wellness.
- Ask whether they have a safe and secure place to live.
- Support their involvement in ADL that give them purpose.
- Assess their connections to others, their relationships, and their social networks.
- Ask about sponsorship and sobriety.
- Recognize that positive clinician feedback can be a significant part of breaking the cycle of shame, guilt, stigma, and secrecy.

PHYSICAL EXAMINATION DOCUMENTATION

Physical exam components are individualized based on subjective history and patient presentation; minimally includes observation/inspection to assess mental status.

EXAMPLE OF NORMAL PHYSICAL EXAM FINDINGS

Affect pleasant. Dressed appropriately for the weather and situation. Well groomed. No repetitive or unusual postures or movements. Judgment intact. Thoughts coherent; able to articulate health history with clarity. Remote and recent memories intact. PHQ-4 screening for depression and anxiety negative; total score 2. Single-question screenings for substance use negative.

EXAMPLE FOR CHILD WITH ANXIETY

Note that this example includes both history and physical exam findings. Zachary, a healthy-appearing, 9-year-old, fourth grader, presents with significant anxiety symptoms that are interfering with his functioning at school. History per mother who accompanies him: In the past 4 to 6 months, Zachary has had increased periods of difficulty concentrating, frequent stomachaches that require visits to the school nurse, frequent expressed fears that something bad may happen to his family, and increased anxiety when his dad is working out of town. Anxiety symptoms increased when his dad was promoted to the role of regional manager, which requires him to be out of town two to three times a week. Zachary has friends; many strengths, including building abilities; and a close supportive family. A GI disorder has been ruled out by a pediatric practitioner/GI service.

No evidence of thought disorder, no depressive/mood disorder, no suicidal ideation, no history of trauma. Appetite and sleep OK. Has occasional bad dreams, worries that keep him awake. Grades are still B's and A's (previously all A's). Mood anxious, affect congruent with content of conversation. Good eye contact. Related warmly with his mom and conversed easily with interviewer. Speech normal rate/rhythm. Friendly and looking forward to summer building projects with his dad.

REFERENCES

References for this chapter draw from Chapter 22, "Evidence-Based Assessment of Mental Health," Chapter 23, "Evidence-Based Assessment of Substance Use Disorder," Chapter 24, "Evidence-Based Assessment and Screening for Traumatic Experiences: Abuse, Neglect, and Intimate Partner Violence," and Chapter 25, "Evidence-Based Therapeutic Communication and Motivational Interviewing in Health Assessment," in *Evidence-Based Physical Examination: Best Practices for Health and Well-Being Assessment*. The references may be accessed in the digital version of the handbook at https://connect.springerpub.com/content/book/97808-0-8261-6466-7/chapter/ch16

Index

abdomen and gastrointestinal and urological systems, 287–317
abdominal aortic aneurysm, 310
abdominal pain, 304–306
abdominal palpation, 296
abdominal percussion technique, 293
abnormal findings, 303–304
acute pancreatitis, 305
allergies, 289
appendicitis, 307
auscultation, 292
of abdominal aorta, 293
of renal arteries, 293
Blumberg's sign, 299–300
celiac disease, 315
cholecystitis/cholelithiasis, 305–306
clinical considerations, 287
constipation, 303
Cullen's sign, 292–293
deep palpation, 296
diarrhea, 303–304
differential diagnoses according to localization of abdominal pain, 304
digital rectal examination, 301
documentation, physical examination, 316–317
family history, 290
general survey, 291–292
GERD/dyspepsia, 311
Hackett's grading system for palpable spleen, 298
health history, 288–290
heel drop test (Markle test or heel jar test), 300–301
hepatitis, 306
history, 303
of present illness, 288
immunizations, 289
inspection, 292
irritable bowel syndrome, 311–312
left lower quadrant pain, 309–310
left upper quadrant pain, 308–309
light palpation, 296
liver palpation, 296
lower urinary tract infection, 313–314
McBurney's point, 299
medications, 289
Murphy's sign, 301
older adults, 301
palpation, 295–299
past medical history, 288–289
pediatric considerations, 289–290, 301
peptic ulcer disease, 312

percussion, 292–295
peritonitis, 313
periumbilical/epigastric pain, 310–313
physical examination, 291, 302–303
psoas test, 300
pyelonephritis, 314
reasons for seeking care, 287
regional ileitis/Crohn's disease, 307
renal colic (urolithiasis, ureterolithiasis), 315
review of systems, 290–291
right lower quadrant pain, 306–307
right upper quadrant pain, 304–306
Rovsing sign, 300
scratch test, 297
sigmoid diverticulosis/diverticulitis, 309
small bowel obstruction, 313
social history, 290
special tests for the abdomen, 299–301
subjective history, 287–288
Traube's space, 294
ulcerative colitis, 309–310
urinary incontinence, 315–316
urinary system, abnormal findings, 313–314
abdominal aortic aneurysm, 64
abdominal reflex, 231
Achilles reflex, 233
acne, 118
acute bronchitis, 93–94
acute coronary syndrome, 64–65
acute mild traumatic brain injury (concussion), 158
acute respiratory distress, red flags, 92
adnexal masses, 375
adults. *See also* older adults
BMI classification, 27
documentation of general survey, example, 42
hypertension, 38
overweight/obesity, 40
anal fissures, 338
anaphylactic shock, 39
ankle/foot anatomy, 274
anorectal agenesis/imperforate anus, 331
anterior drawer test, 271
aorta, coarctation, 68–69
ASCVD risk calculator, 66
asthma, 94
atherosclerosis, 65–67
atrialseptal defect, 67
attention deficit hyperactivity disorder, 419–421
axillae, 137–139

balanitis and balanoposthitis, 334
Barlow–Ortolani maneuvers, 281
Bartholin gland cyst, 373
basal cell carcinoma, 119–120
bed bug bites, 120
Bell's palsy, 238–239
benign prostatic hyperplasia, 339
blood pressure, 50–51
body habitus
BMI calculation, 27
body fat, 28–30
height, 26
waist and other circumferences, 28
weight, 26–27
body mass index
body fat percentage, 28–30

calculation, 27
waist and other circumferences, 28
breasts
abnormal findings of the breast and axillae, 359–360
accessory breast tissue, 359–360
allergies, 347
benign breast mass or lump, 360–361
breast cyst, 360–361
clinical considerations, 343–344
clinical exam, 349–356
family history, 347
fibroadenoma, 361
health history, 345
history of present illness, 344
inflammatory breast cancer, 361–362
inspection, 350
invasive ductal carcinomas, 362
invasive lobular carcinomas, 362–363
mastalgia or mastodynia, 363–364
mastitis, 364
medications, 347
nipple discharge, galactorrhea, 364–365
Paget's disease of the breast, 363
palpation methods, 351
past health history, 347
quadrants, 350
reasons for seeking care, 344
review of systems, 348
sexual history, 346–347
social history, 348
subjective history, 344
bronchial breath sounds, 90
bronchiolitis, 94–95
bronchophony, 90–91
bronchovesicular breath sounds, 90
Brudzinski sign, 237

cachexia, 41
cardiogenic shock, 39
carpal tunnel syndrome, 277–278
cat scratch disease, 141–142
cellulitis, 120–121
cervical intraepithelial neoplasia and cervical malignancies, 374
cervical spine, 255–257
chlamydia, 365–366
chest inspection, 51
children
BMI classification, 27
developmental assessment, 32–36
documentation of general survey,example, 42–43
growth measurement, 30–32
overweight/obesity, 40
rashes, 111–115
vital signs, 24–26
with development delay, 36
chronic venous insufficiency, 68
congestive heart failure, 69–70
contact dermatitis, 121–122
COPD, 95
coronary artery disease, 65–67
COVID-19, 95–96
crackles, 90

De Quervain's syndrome, 278
deep vein thrombosis, 70–71

drug- and toxin-induced
 shock, 39
Dupuytren contracture, 278

ears, nose, and throat, 202–215
 adult ear exam technique, 194
 air and bone conduction, 195–197
 allergic rhinitis, 208
 allergies, 192
 aphthous ulcer, 212–213
 audiometry, 197
 auditory acuity, 195
 cholesteatoma, 203–204
 clinical considerations, 189
 conductive and sensorineural hearing loss, 207
 documentation of physical examination, 215–216
 epistaxis, 210
 eustachian tube dysfunction, 204–208
 evidence-based assessment, 189, 209
 family history, 192
 finger rub test, 195
 health history, 190–192
 hearing loss, 205–206
 herpangina, 213
 history, 202, 203, 204
  of present illness, 190
 immunizations, 192
 inspection, 193–194
 inspection and palpation of the tongue, 200
 leukoplakia, 213–214
 lips, 198
 malignant otitis externa, 207–208
 medications, 192
 mouth, 198–199
 nasal/oral cancers, 215
 nasal polyp, 210–211
 nonallergic rhinitis, 208–209, 209
 nose, 208–211
 nose and sinuses, 197–198
 oral candidiasis, 214–215
 oral cavity and posterior pharynx, 199
 oral examination, 199
 otitis media with effusion, 203
 otoscope, use of, 198
 palpation, 194–195
  of mouth and jaw, 199–200
 paranasal sinuses, 209
 pediatric considerations, 192, 197, 200
 physical examination, 193–197, 202–204, 207
 pneumaticotoscopy, 194
 posterior pharynx, 199
 reasons for seeking care, 189
 review of systems, 193
 Rinne test, 196
 septal perforation, 211
 sinusitis, 209
 social history, 192–193
 subjective history, 189
  red flags, 193
 temporal mandibular joint, 200
 tinnitus, 207
 tongue, 198–199
 Weber screening test, 195–196
ectopic pregnancy, 376
eczema (atopic dermatitis), 122
edema, 61
egophony, 91
elbow, 263, 265

empty can test, 262
endocrine shock, 39
environmental exposure
nervous system, 220
respiratory diseases, 82
epidermoid cyst (a sebaceous cyst), 122–123
epididymitis, orchitis, and scrotal cellulitis, 335
epidural hematoma, 156–157
epilepsy, 239–240
epispadias and hypospadias, 332
erythema migrans, 123
external rotation resistance test, 263
eye
accommodation reflex, 169
acute angle closure glaucoma, 167, 179
allergic conjunctivitis, 176–177
allergies, 165
bacterial conjunctivitis, 177
cataracts, 175–176
clinical considerations, 163
conjunctivitis, 176–178
corneal abrasion, 178
corneal light reflex, 167–168
dacryostenosis, 178–179
diplopia, 179
direct ophthalmoscopy, 171–172
documentation of physical examination, 188
episcleritis, 185
evidence-based considerations, 175
extraocular muscles, 170–171
family history, 165
glaucoma, 179–180
Hirschberg test, 167
history of present illness, 164
inspection, 167
macular degeneration, 180–182
medications, 165
older adult, 174
open-angle glaucoma, 180
optic neuritis and retrobulbar neuritis, 180–181
orbital and periorbital cellulitis, 181–182
past medical history, 164–165
pediatric binocular assessment, 168
pediatric considerations, 173–174
physical examination, 167
pingueculum, 182
pregnancy considerations, 174
preventive care considerations, 165
pterygium, 182
pupillary light reflex, 168–169
reasons for seeking care, 164
red flags
in objective exam, 174–175
in subjective history, 166–167
red reflex, 172
retinal abnormalities, 182–183
retinopathy, 183–184
review of systems, 166
scleritis, 185
Snellen visual acuity chart, 173

eye (*continued*)
- social history, 166
- strabismus, 185–186
- sty (hordeolum), 186–187
- subconjunctival hemorrhage, 187
- uveitis, 187–188
- viral conjunctivitis, 177–178
- visual acuity, 172–173
- visual field testing, 169–170

FABER test, 269
facial fractures, 157
fallot, tetralogy, 76
fever,37
female genitalia, and reproductive system, 343–379. *See also* vaginitis/vaginosis
- abnormal findings of the female genitalia, 365–378
- Bartholin gland cyst, 373
- chlamydia, 365–366
- genital herpes, 368
- genital warts, 367
- gonorrhea, 365
- health history, 345–346
- history, 367
- physical examination, 349, 351–356
- red flags in subjective history, 348–349
- sexually transmitted infections, 365–369
- syphilis, 366–367
- trichomonas, 366
- urethral caruncle, 373

finger-to-nose test,228
Finkelstein test, 267
flexion, abduction, and external rotation test, 269
folliculitis, 123–124

general survey and developmental assessment
- abnormal findings, 37
- body habitus, 26–30
- cachexia, 41
- clinical assessment, 13
- documentation of physical exam, 42–43
- evidence-based considerations, 36
- family history, 16
- history of present illness, 14–15
- hypertension, 37–38
- malnutrition, 39
- mental status assessment, 19
- nutritional assessment, 17–18
- overweight/obesity, 40
- pain assessment, 18–19
- past medical history, 15–16
- pediatric growth and development, 30–135
- physical examination, 19
- physiologic stability, 14
- prescribed and OTC medications, 16
- reasons for seeking care, 13–14
- red flags in emergent distress, 15
- review of systems, 17
- sarcopenia, 41–42
- shock, 38–39
- social history, 16–17
- undernutrition, 39
- vital signs, 19–25
- weight gain, 40
- weight loss, 40–41

genital herpes, 368
genital warts, 367
genetic counseling, 4
gonorrhea, 365
gout, 279
Gower's sign, 281

hand and wrist bones, 266
Hawkins–Kennedy test, 261
headache, 155–156
head and neck
  acute, mild traumatic brain injury (concussion), 158
  allergies, 149
  auscultation and percussion, 152
  clinical considerations, 147
  cluster headaches, 156
  documentation, physical examination, 161–162
  epidural hematoma, 156–157
  evidence-based considerations, 154–155
  facial fractures, 157
  family history, 149
  headache, 155–156
  head injury or trauma, 156–158
  history of present illness, 148
  hyperparathyroidism, 159
  hyperthyroidism, 160
  hypoparathyroidism, 158–159
  hypothyroidism, 159–160
  immunizations, 149
  inspection, 150
  medications, 148–149
  migraine headache, 155
  palpation, 151–152
  parathyroid disorders, 158–159
  past medical history, 148
  pediatric considerations, 153–154
  pediatric craniofacial disorders, 161
  reasons for seeking care, 147
  red flags
    in objective exam, 154–155
    in subjective history, 150
  review of systems, 149–150
  secondary headache, risk indicators, 150
  skull fractures, 157–158
  social history, 149
  TBI red flags, 154
  tension-type headache, 155–156
  thyroid cancer, 160–161
  thyroid disorders, 159–161
head injury or trauma, 156–158
heart and circulatory system
  abdomen, 59
  abdominal aortic aneurysm, 64
  abnormal findings, 64
  acute coronary syndrome, 64–65
  allergies, 47
  aorta, coarctation, 68–69
  ASCVD risk calculator, 66
  atherosclerosis, 65–67
  atrialseptal defect, 67
  auscultation, 51–52, 54, 58
  blood pressure and vital sign assessment, 50–51
  chest inspection, 51
  chronic venous insufficiency, 68
  clinical consideration, 45
  congestive heart failure, 69–70
  coronary artery disease, 65–67
  deep vein thrombosis, 70–71
  documentation, physical examination, 77–78
  edema, 61
  evidence-based consideration, 63

heart and circulatory system (*continued*)
- extremities, 59–60
- family history, 48
- general survey, 50
- history of present illness, 45–46
- hypertension, 71–72
- jugular venous pressure, 56–58
- medications, 47
- mitral valve prolapse, 72–73
- older adults, 63
- palpation, 51, 54–56, 58
- past medical history, 46–47
- pediatric considerations, 47–48
- pericarditis, 73
- peripheral artery disease, 74
- peripheral vascular examination, 56–58
- physical examination, 49
- pulses, grading scale, 61
- reasons for seeking care, 45
- red flags in subjective history, 49, 63
- Raynaud's phenomenon, 75
- review of systems, 48–49
- rheumatic heart disease, 75–76
- seated position examination, 50–53
- social history, 48
- supine position, 54–56
- tetralogy of Fallot, 76
- ventricular septal defect, 76–77
- Well's clinical protection tool, 71

heel-to-shin test, 228
hernia, 326
herpes zoster (shingles), 124–125
hip, 268–269
history taking
- adult chronic patients, 9–10
- chronic care management, 8–9
- episodic visit, 1–2
- family history, 3–4
- history of present illness, 2–3
- key consideration, 7–8
- past medical history, 3
- preventive care considerations, 6
- process, 1–2
- reasons for seeking care, 2
- review of systems, 6–7
- social determinants of health, 5–6
- social history, 5
- therapeutic communication, 10–11
- wellness exam, 7–8

HIV/AIDS, 142
hydrocele, 332
hyperparathyroidism, 159
hypertension, 71–72
hyperthermia, 37
hypoparathyroidism, 158–159
hypothermia, 37
hypothyroidism, 159–160
hypovolemic shock:, 39

immunizations, 81, 103, 134, 149, 192, 219,289
infants
- growth measurement, 30–32
- skin, hair, and nails, 106, 117

inguinal, 140
Inguinal hernias, 327

jugular venous pressure, 56–58

knee, 269–270

Lachman test, 272
lag test, 263
lateral epicondylitis (tennis elbow), 279
Legg–Calve–Perthes diseases, 279–280
lifestyle behaviors
- respiratory disease, 82
- nervous system, 220

lumbar spine, 259
lung cancer, 97
lungs and respiratory system
- acute bronchitis, 93–94
- allergies, 81
- asthma, 94
- auscultation, 89–91
- breathing patterns, 93
- bronchiolitis, 94–95
- clinical consideration, 79
- COPD, 95
- COVID-19, 95–96
- cystic fibrosis, 96
- documentation, physical examination, 99
- evidence-based consideration, 92–93
- family history, 82
- history of present illness, 79–80
- immunizations, 81
- influenza, 96
- lung cancer, 97
- medications, 81
- obstructive sleep apnea, 97
- older adult, 91
- palpation, 86–87
- past medical history, 80–81
- pediatric considerations, 81–82, 91
- percussion, 87–88
- peripheral assessment, 85
- pertussis, 97–98
- physical examination, 84
- pneumonia, 98
- pulmonary embolus, risk indicators, 84
- reasons for seeking care, 79
- red flags
  - in acute respiratory distress, 92
  - in objective exam, 92
  - in subjective history, 84
- review of systems, 83
- social history, 82
- thoracic cage and chest movement, 85–86
- tuberculosis, 98

lymphadenitis, 142–143
lymphangitis, 143
lymphatic filariasis, 143–144
lymphatic system
- axillae, 137–139
- cat scratch disease, 141–142
- clinical consideration, 133
- documentation, physical examination, 146
- family history, 135
- head and neck, 137
- history of present illness, 133–134
- HIV/AIDS, 142
- immunizations, 134
- inguinal, 140
- inspection, 136
- lymphadenitis, 142–143
- lymphangitis, 143
- lymphatic filariasis, 143–144
- lymphedema, 144
- lymphoma, 145
- medications, 134
- mononucleosis (or mono), 145
- older adult, 141
- palpation, 137
- past medical history, 134

lymphatic system (*continued*)
pediatric considerations, 141
physical examination, 136
reasons for seeking care, 133
red flags
in objective exam, 141
in subjective history, 135–136
review of systems, 135
social history, 135
lymphedema, 144

male genital candidiasis, 335
male genitalia, prostate, rectum, and anus, 319–341
abnormal findings, 331–340
abnormalities, 337
additional assessments for specific conditions, 326–328
anal fissures, 338
anorectal agenesis/imperforate anus, 331
assessment for hernia, 326
balanitis and balanoposthitis, 334
benign prostatic hyperplasia, 339
clinical considerations, 319–320
condyloma, 336
congenital or developmental abnormalities, 331–334
cremasteric reflex, 326
digital rectal examination, 328
documentation, physical examination, 340–341
epididymitis, orchitis, and scrotal cellulitis, 335
epispadias and hypospadias, 332
external and internal hemorrhoids, 338–339
health history, 320–324
history of present illness, 320
hydrocele, 332
infection or inflammatory disorders, 334–336
inguinal hernias, 327
inspection, 325
male genital candidiasis, 335
manifestations of systemic conditions, 337
nonspecific urethritis, 336
older adults, 330
other abnormalities, 337–338
palpation test, 325–326
pediatric considerations, 328–330
digital rectal examination, 329
Peyronie's disease, 337
phimosis/paraphimosis, 332–333
physical examination, 325
prostate cancer, 339
reasons for seeking care, 320
rectal polyps and rectal cancer, 340
red flags
in objective exam, 330–331
in subjective history, 324–325, 325
review of systems, 324
sexually transmitted infections, 336
skin cancer, 337
subjective history, 320–324

technique for assessing inguinal hernias, 327
testicular torsion, 333
testicular tumor/ malignancy, 338
transillumination, 326
undescended testes, 333
varicocele, 334
malnutrition, 39
McMurray's test, 272
melanoma, 125
mental health and substance use, 403–433
addiction, 429
adolescent considerations, 431
alcohol use disorder, 429–430
allergies, 407
anxiety and anxiety disorders, 418–419
attention deficit hyperactivity disorder, 419–421
clinical considerations, 403–404
considerations for the older adult, 431
depression and anxiety, 404–405
depression and mood disorders, 421–423
documentation, physical examination, 432–433
evidence-based considerations, 416–417
example for child with anxiety, 432–433
example of normal physical exam findings, 432
family history, 408
health history, 407–408
history of present illness, 404–407
impact on families, 431
life-span and family considerations, 430–431
medications, 407
mental health disorders, 418–426
mental status assessment, 412–414
ABC mnemonic, 19
newborns and neonatal abstinence syndrome, 430
past medical history, 407
pediatric considerations, 409–410
physical examination considerations, 414
practice guidelines for mental health, 418
preventive health behaviors, 407–408
reasons for seeking care, 404
recovery, 431–432
red flags
in objective exam, 415–416
review of systems, 409
risk assessment, 410–411
single-question screenings for substance use, 417–418
social history, 408
subjective history, 404–407, 410–412
substance use screening, 416–417
tobacco use disorder, 430
trauma and stressor-related disorders, 425–426
migraine headache, 155
mitral valve prolapse, 72–73
mononucleosis (or mono), 145
muscle strength scale, 254
muscular dystrophy, 280

musculoskeletal system, 249–285
- abnormal findings, 277
- ankle/foot anatomy, 274
- anterior drawer test, 271
- apprehension test, 273
- area of snuffbox tenderness, 267
- carpal tunnel syndrome, 277–278
- cervical spine, 255–257
- clinical considerations, 249
- De Quervain's syndrome, 278
- dermatomes/myotomes of the lower and upper extremity, 256, 259
- documentation physical examination, 285
- hand and wrist bones, 266
- Hawkins–Kennedy test, 261
- head, 255
- health history, 250–251
- hip, 268–269
- history, 281
- history of present illness, 250
- knee, 269
- Neer test, 261
- Osgood–Schlatter disease, 280–281
- osteoarthritis, 281–282
- painful arc test, 262
- palpation, 253
  - of spinal processes, 258
- pediatric considerations, 276
- Phalen's test, 267
- physical examination, 252–253, 281
- radial head subluxation, 282–283
- range of motion and special tests, 253
- reasons for seeking care, 249
- red flags in history and physical exam, 275–276
- review of systems, 252
- rheumatoid arthritis, 283
- rotator cuff tear, 283–284
- scoliosis, 276
- shoulder bones, 260
- slipped capital femoral epiphysis, 284
- social history, 252
- spinal column, 258
- Spurling test, 257
- squeeze test, 275
- Stinchfield test, 269
- straight leg raise, 259
- subjective history, 249
- Thomas test, 269
- thoracic/lumbar spine, 257–259
- Tinel's sign, 265
- Trendelenburg test, 269
- types of movement, 254
- valgus stress test, 265, 271
- wrist/hand, 265

nervous system, 217–218, 217–247
- Achilles reflex, 233
- allergies, 219
- Bell's palsy, 238–239
- biceps and brachioradialis, 230
- biceps reflex, 232
- brachioradialis reflex, 232
- Brudzinski sign, 237
- cerebral palsy, 239
- clinical considerations, 217

comorbidities or risk factors related to neurological diseases, 219
cortical sensory function, 236–237
corticospinal, basal ganglia, and cerebellar motor pathways, 229
cranial nerve documentation, 247
deep tendon reflexes, 231–233
documentation of physical examination, 246–247
epilepsy, 239–240
evidence-based considerations, 238
family history, 220
finger abduction, 230
foot/ankle, 231
graphesthesia, 237
grip strength, 230
health history, 218–220
hemorrhagic stroke, 240–241
hip, 231
history and physical exam, 237–238
history of present illness, 217–218
immunizations, 219
intracranial tumor, 241
ischemic stroke, 241–242
joint position sense, 236
Kernig's sign, 237
knee, 231
medications, 219
meningitis, 242–243
mental status examination, 222–227
multiple sclerosis, 243–244
muscle strength, 230–231
myasthenia gravis, 244
neurological disorders, 220
Parkinson's disease, 244–245
past medical history, 218–219
patellar reflex test, 233
pediatric considerations, 220
peripheral neuropathy, 245–246
physical examination, 221–227
primary sensory functions, 235
primitive reflex testing in infancy, 233–234
pronator drift testing, 230
proprioception and cerebellar function, 227–231
reasons for seeking care, 217
reflexes, 231–234
review of systems, 221
sensory function, 234–236
social history, 220–221
special tests, 236–237
subjective history, 217–218
thumb opposition, 230
trauma, 218–219
triceps reflex, 233
trigeminal neuralgia, 246
tuning fork, vibration testing, 235
two-point discrimination test, 236
wrist, 230
neurogenic shock, 39
neuropathic pain, 18
nociceptive pain, 18
nutritional status, 17–18

obstetric assessment, 381–401
  advanced maternal age, 386
  allergies, 384
  clinical considerations, 381
  family history, 384
  gynecologic history, 383
  health history, 382
  history of present illness, 381–382
  medications, 384
  obstetric history (if relevant), 383
  past medical history, 382–383
  preventive care considerations, 385–386
  reasons for seeking care, 381
  review of systems, 384–385
  social history, 384
  subjective history, 381–382
   red flags, 385
  trauma-informed care, 386
  unique population considerations, 386
  obstructive sleep apnea, 97
older adults
  chronic conditions, 9–10
  heart and circulatory system, 63
  lungs and respiratory system, 91
  lymphatic system, 141
  mental health and substance, use, 403–433
  prostate cancer, 339
  skin, hair, and nails, 103–104, 117
onychomycosis, 125–126
ovarian cancer, 376
ovarian cysts, 375
overweight/obesity, 40
pain
  assessment, 18
  evidence-based tool, 18–19
  types, 18
parathyroid disorders, 158–159
Parkinson's disease, 244–245
pediatric considerations
  anogenital examination, 328–330
  anxiety disorders, 418–419
  depression, 421–423
  ear, nose, throat, 192, 197
  gastrointestinal and urological systems, 301
  head and neck, 153–154
  hearing problem, 200
  heart and circulatory system, 47–48
  lungs and respiratory system, 81–82
  lymphatic system, 141
  male genitalia, prostate, rectum, and anus, 328–330
  mental health problems, 409–410
  musculoskeletal system, 251, 276
  nervous system, 220
  respiratory disease, 91
  skin, hair, and nails, 103, 106
  vision assessment, 173–174
peripheral artery disease, 74
peripheral assessment, lungs and respiratory system, 85
pertussis, 97–98
pityriasis rosea, 126–127
plantar reflex, 231
pleural rub, 90
pneumonia, 98
posterior drawer test, 271
pregnancy, 386–390
  abnormal findings, 393

- acute cystitis (urinary tract infection), 393
- anemia in pregnancy, 394
- asymptomatic bacteriuria, 394–395
- auscultation, 390
- changes in fundal height, 388
- chronic or gestational hypertension, 397–398
- constipation, 395
- eclampsia, 398
- fetal station, 390
- first-trimester bleeding, 396
  - benign, 395–396
- general survey, 386–387
- gestational diabetes screening, 396–397
- gestational thrombocytopenia, 400
- hyperemesis gravidarum, 399
- hypertensive disorders, 397–400
- inspection, 387
- Leopold's maneuvers, 389
- measurement of fundal height, 388
- miscarriage, 396
- objective exam, 390–391
- palpation, 387
- physical examination documentation, 401
- population considerations, 386
- preeclampsia, 398
- pruritic urticarial papules and plaques of pregnancy, 399–400
- weight gain, 391

preterm infants,
- skin, hair, and nails, 106

prostate cancer, 339
psoriasis, 127
pulmonary embolus, risk indicators, 84
pulses, grading scale, 61

Raynaud's phenomenon, heart and circulatory system, 75
rheumatic heart disease, 75–76
rheumatoid arthritis, 283
rhonchi, 90
Rinne test, 196–197
rosacea (acne rosacea), 127–128

sarcopenia, 41–42
scabies, 128
scoliosis, 276
sensory function, 234–236
- monofilament test, 234–235
- primary sensory functions, 235–236
- testing superficial pain with Wartenberg wheel, 235
- testing vibration with a low-pitched tuning fork, 235

septic shock, 38
shock
- definition, 38
- septic, 38
- types, 38–39

shoulder, 259–261
skin, hair, and nails
- abnormal findings, 118–131
- acne, 118
- allergies, 103
- basal cell carcinoma, 119–120
- bed bug bites, 120
- cellulitis, 120–121
- childhood rashes, 111–115s
- clinical consideration, 101
- contact dermatitis, 121–122

skin, hair, and nails (*continued*)
  documentation of physical examination, 131–132
    eczema (atopic dermatitis), 122
    epidermoid cyst (a sebaceous cyst), 122–123
    erythema migrans, 123
    evidence-based practice, 117–118
    family history, 104
    folliculitis, 123–124
    herpes zoster (shingles), 124–125
    history of present illness, 101–102
    immunizations, 103
    infants, children, and adolescents, 106, 117
    inspection, 106
    medications, 103
    melanoma, 125
    older adults, 103–104, 117
    onychomycosis, 125–126
    palpation, 106
    past medical history, 102
    pediatric considerations, 103
    physical examination, 106
    pityriasis rosea, 126–127
    preterm infants, 106
    primary and secondary skin lesions, 107–110
    psoriasis, 127
    race and ethnic considerations, 117
    reasons for seeking care, 101
    red flags
      in objective history, 117
      in subjective history, 105
    review of systems, 104–105
    rosacea (acne rosacea), 127–128
    scabies, 128
    social history, 104
    squamous cell carcinoma, 129
    Tanner stages (female and male development), 116
    tinea corporis, 129–130
    tinea versicolor, 130
    urticaria (hives), 130–131
    verruca vulgaris (warts), 131
skull fractures, 157–158
slipped capital femoral epiphysis, 284
spinal column, 255
Spurling test, 257
squamous cell carcinoma, 129
squeeze test, 275
Stinchfield test, 269
straight leg raise, 259
stridor, 90
substance use disorders, 426–430
    diagnostic criteria, 427
    misuse of substances, 426
    substance-specific withdrawal symptoms, 428–429
superficial reflexes, 231
systemic inflammatory response syndrome, 38

Tanner stages (female and male development), 116
testicular torsion, 333
testicular tumor/malignancy, 338
Thomas test, 269
thoracic/lumbar spine, 257–259
thought disorders and severe mental illness, 423–425
    delirium, 423–424
    delusions, 424
    dementia, 424
    hallucinations, 425

thyroid cancer, 160–161
throat, 211–215
acute pharyngitis, 211–212
aphthous ulcer, 212
strep pharyngitis, 212
tinea corporis, 129–130
tinea versicolor, 130
Tinel's sign, 265
tobacco use disorder, 5 A's intervention steps, 83
tracheal breath sounds, 90
transillumination, 326
Traube's space, 294
Trendelenburg test, 269
triceps reflex, 233
tuberculosis, 98

ulcerative colitis, 309–310
undernutrition, 39
urinary incontinence, 315–316
urticaria (hives), 130–131
uterus bimanual exam, 354–356
uterine fibroids, 377

vaginitis/vaginosis, 369–370
bacterial vaginosis, 369–370
menopause, 370
genitourinary syndrome, 371–373
vulvar cancers, 372
valgus stress test, 265, 271
varicocele, 334
varus stress test, 271
ventricular septal defect, 76–77
verruca vulgaris (warts), 131
vesicular breath sounds, 90
vital signs
assessment, 50–51
blood pressure, 22–24
pulse rate, 21–22
respiratory rate, 22
temperature measurement, 19–21

weight gain, 40
weight loss, 40–41
Wells' clinical prediction tool, 71
wheezes, 90
whispered pectoriloquy, 91
wrist/hand, 265